Anaphylactic Reactions in Anesthesia and Intensive Care
Second Edition

Jerrold H. Levy, M.D.
Associate Professor of Anesthesiology
Emory University School of Medicine
Division of Cardiothoracic Anesthesiology and Critical Care
Emory Clinic

Associate Director
Cardiothoracic Intensive Care Unit
Emory University Hospital
Atlanta, Georgia

Butterworth–Heinemann
Boston   London   Oxford   Singapore   Sydney   Toronto   Wellington

Copyright © 1992 by Butterworth-Heinemann, a division of Reed Publishing (USA) Inc.
All rights reserved.

No part of this publication may be reproduced, stored in a retrieval system, or transmitted, in any form or by any means, electronic, mechanical, photocopying, recording, or otherwise, without the prior written permission of the publisher.

Every effort has been made to ensure that the drug dosage schedules within this text are accurate and conform to standards accepted at time of publication. However, as treatment recommendations vary in the light of continuing research and clinical experience, the reader is advised to verify drug dosage schedules herein with information found on product information sheets. This is especially true in cases of new or infrequently used drugs.

∞ Recognizing the importance of preserving what has been written, it is the policy of Butterworth-Heinemann to have the books it publishes printed on acid-free paper, and we exert our best efforts to that end.

Library of Congress Cataloging-in-Publication Data

Levy, Jerrold H.
　　Anaphylactic reactions in anesthesia and intensive care / Jerrold
　H. Levy.—2nd ed.
　　　p.　　cm.
　　Includes bibliographical references and index.
　　ISBN 0-7506-9064-X (case bound : alk. paper)
　　1. Anaphylaxis.　2. Anesthesia—Complications and sequelae.
　3. Critical care medicine—Complications and sequelae.　I. Title.
　　[DNLM: 1. Anaphylaxis—chemically induced.　2. Anesthesia—adverse
　effects.　　QW 900 L668a]
　RD82.7.A48L48　1992
　616.97'5—dc20
　DNLM/DLC
　for Library of Congress　　　　　　　　　　　　　　　　　　　91-47872
　　　　　　　　　　　　　　　　　　　　　　　　　　　　　　　　　　　　　CIP

British Library Cataloguing in Publication Data

Levy, Jerrold H.
　Anaphylactic reactions in anesthesia and intensive care—2nd ed
　I. Title
　616.975

ISBN 0-7506-9064-X

Butterworth-Heinemann
80 Montvale Avenue
Stoneham, MA 02180

10　9　8　7　6　5　4　3　2　1

Printed in the United States of America

Contents

Preface v

PART I
Mechanisms of Anaphylaxis 1

1 Anaphylaxis, Allergy, and Immunology 3

2 Initiation and Clinical Manifestations of Anaphylaxis 13

3 Mediators of Anaphylactic Reactions 31

4 Complement and Contact Activation 51

5 Nonimmunologic (Pharmacologic) Histamine Release 63

PART II
Management of Anaphylaxis 81

6 Common Anaphylactic and Anaphylactoid Reactions Seen by the Anesthesiologist 83

7 Preoperative Considerations of the Allergic Patient 121

8 General Approach to Anaphylactic Reactions 135

9 Pharmacologic Therapy for Anaphylaxis 143

10 Management of Anaphylaxis 161

11 Managing Sequelae in the Recovery Room and Intensive Care Unit 175

12 Human Physiologic Responses During Anaphylactic or Anaphylactoid Reactions   185

Summary: Preventing Anaphylactic Reactions   205

References   207

Index   240

Preface

Anaphylaxis, which is often unpredictable and sudden in onset, represents one of the most serious, potentially lethal emergencies in medical practice. Anesthesiologists routinely administer foreign substances, including anesthetic agents, antibiotics, blood products, and other drugs, and monitor patients during injections of contrast media during diagnostic studies. Because all of these substances can produce anaphylaxis, anesthesiologists and other clinicians must be prepared to deal with the acute cardiovascular and pulmonary dysfunction that might occur.

This book provides anesthesiologists, intensivists, and other interested physicians and health care professionals with a practical approach to the recognition, understanding, and management of these life-threatening reactions. Lessons learned from the treatment of acute cardiopulmonary dysfunction during cardiovascular surgery and in the intensive care unit, including the importance of vasoactive drug administration (i.e., epinephrine), have proven invaluable in dealing with anaphylaxis that occurs perioperatively.

The second edition of *Anaphylactic Reactions in Anesthesia and Intensive Care* has been revised and updated. The extensive bibliography serves as a comprehensive guide to the literature on anaphylaxis. The second edition includes new information on the mechanisms of action of histamine and other mediators that produce cardiopulmonary dysfunction, as well as more extensive data on peptide and lipid mediators. Chapter 4 reviews the importance of complement activation and its interaction with contact activation, and the plasma proteins of the coagulation, fibrinolytic and kinin-generating pathways. Chapter 5 discusses nonimmunologic histamine release by drugs and peptides and the direct effects of drugs on vascular responses. This edition elaborates on management of the allergic patient and reviews drug allergy and diagnostic tests. The list of agents implicated in anaphylaxis has been updated to include latex, newer anesthetic drugs, antibiotics, and peptides (i.e., insulin, streptokinase). It includes more comprehensive data regarding muscle relaxants, protamine, and new drugs on the horizon. Chapters 9 and 10 update pharmacologic approaches to and therapeutic plans for anaphylaxis, including experimental therapeutic approaches to inhibiting complement activation and reversing pulmonary vasoconstriction and plans for treating bronchospasm and right ventricular failure.

I would like to acknowledge the contributions made by other investigators to the elucidations of, and therapeutic approaches to, anaphylactic reactions in anesthesia and intensive care around the world, including Drs. Carol Hirshman and N. Franklin Adkinson, Jr. at Johns Hopkins; Dr. Michael Weiss at the University of Washington; Dr. Roberto Levi at Cornell; Dr. Jonathan Moss at the University of Chicago; Drs. Marie-Claire Laxenaire, Denise Moneret-Vautrin, and Daniel Vervloet in France; Drs. Wilfred Lorenz and Alfred Doenicke in Germany; Drs. Malcolm Fisher, Brian Baldo, and David Harle in Australia; Dr. David Sage in New Zealand; and Drs. John Watkins and Richard Clark in the United Kingdom. I especially thank Dr. Roberto Levi for reviewing Chapters 2 and 3; Drs. Michael Weiss, N. Franklin Adkinson, Jr., Roberto Levi, and Lawrence Schwartz for their help in developing new ways to investigate perioperative anaphylaxis; and Kathleen Mainland for her assistance and editorial guidance for the first and second editions. Finally, I would like to thank Gilbert and Vivian Levy for all of their support through the years.

JHL

PART I

Mechanisms of Anaphylaxis

1

Anaphylaxis, Allergy, and Immunology

Anaphylaxis was first reported by Charles Richet and Paul Portier in 1902 to describe a profound hypersensitivity response—shock and death—in dogs after a second sublethal injection of a sea anemone toxin (*Actinia sulcata*) (Portier and Richet, 1902). The term *anaphylaxis* was proposed from the Greek terms *ana*, meaning against, and *phylaxis*, meaning protection, to indicate the reverse of prophylaxis. Previous administration of toxin at sublethal dosages did not confer protection to subsequent injections as Richet intended but sensitized the animals to the foreign protein. For anaphylaxis to occur, previous exposure to an antigen or substance of similar structure is necessary to achieve a sensitization state.

Anaphylaxis, defined 90 years after the first report, is a life-threatening *immediate hypersensitivity reaction* characterized by the presence of an immediate generalized response, including symptoms of upper airway obstruction, dyspnea with or without wheezing, syncope, or hypotension (Austen, 1974; Bochner and Lichtenstein, 1991; Kelly and Patterson, 1974; Sheffer, 1985). The complex of sudden physiologic changes involving the cardiovascular, respiratory, and cutaneous systems is produced by an allergic reaction. A reaction is considered allergic when it is produced by immunologic mechanisms; therefore, pharmacologic idiosyncracy, direct toxicity, drug overdosage, drug interactions, or reactions that mimic allergy are not considered allergic reactions (Patterson, 1984; Parker, 1975). Immunologic reactions have two major characteristics: 1) they involve the interaction of both antigens with antibodies, specific effector cells, or both; and 2) they are reproducible when rechallenged with specific antigens (the anamnestic response) (DeSwarte, 1986; Watkins et al., 1982). Anaphylactic reactions represent only some of many different immunologic reactions in humans. The terms *anaphylaxis* and *immediate hypersensitivity reaction* used in the text describe a specific clinical syndrome; however, not all immediate hypersensitivity reactions are anaphylactic. Therefore, a review of antigens, antibodies, and concepts of immunologic reactions provides a framework for understanding anaphylaxis.

PROPERTIES OF AN ANTIGEN

Molecules capable of stimulating an immune response when injected (i.e., immunospecific antibody production or lymphocyte activation) are called *antigens*. Antibodies are large protein molecules capable of binding to antigens. The specificity of the immunologic response to produce unique antibodies directed against a chemical structure represents an important characteristic. A molecule's ability to act as an antigen to stimulate an immune response is called its *immunogenicity*. Specificity and immunogenicity characteristics include molecular size and degree of foreignness to the recipient (Butler and Beiser, 1973). Antigens can also be low-molecular-weight substances that bind to host proteins in a hapten mechanism (e.g., drugs), or larger molecules that stimulate an immune response by themselves (e.g., proteins). Only a few large-molecular-weight drugs (e.g., streptokinase, chymopapain, and insulin) are complete antigens (Table 1.1). Smaller-molecular-weight polypeptides, such as protamine (molecular weight 4500 to 5000), are probably also complete antigens; however, most commonly used drugs are small organic compounds with a low molecular weight of around 1000 daltons. For a small molecule to become immunogenic, it must form a stable bond with a circulating or tissue macromolecule. When drugs bind to larger molecules to become antigenic, they are called *haptens*. Fortunately most drugs are not sufficiently reactive in the human body to form a stable complex with larger molecules. Based on the extensive work on penicillin allergy, it is probable that reactive drug metabolites bind with a carrier protein to become complete antigens. For most other allergic drug reactions, the formation of reactive metabolites and their conjugations with macromolecules can only be inferred.

The foreignness of a molecule is important in determining its ability to stimulate an immune response. Normally people do not show an immune response to their own proteins, but proteins of phylogenetically different species are immunogenic and produce lymphocyte activation and perhaps antibody formation. Although healthcare workers administer blood products that contain

Table 1.1 Different Molecules That Function as Antigens to Induce Sensitization and IgE Production

Complete Antigens	*Haptens*	*Mirror Molecules*
Protamine	Penicillin	Succinylcholine
Streptokinase	Thiobarbiturates	Atracurium
Insulin	Sulfa drugs	Symmetric biquaternary ammonium compounds
Antisera		

a variety of foreign cellular and protein antigens, the incidence of acute allergic reactions after additional transfusions is low. This response may reflect structural similarities of proteins. Previous administration of horse sera for tetanus or antithymocyte globulin often produces profound acute allergic reactions if a second dose is required, however. This immediate hypersensitivity response may reflect a human immunosurveillance system requiring immediate rejection of foreign antigens that are present on bacteria or parasites.

ANTIBODIES

Antibodies are protein macromolecules with the unique ability to combine with the antigen that stimulated their production. Immunoglobulins represent proteins of a specific structure that function as antibodies. Although all antibodies are immunoglobulins, not all immunoglobulins have antibody function. The structure of the basic antibody unit is Y shaped, as shown in Figure 1.1. The base of the antibody molecule provides the biologic diversity responsible for different physiologic functions, such as cellular binding or complement activation. Proteolytic enzymes cleave the antibody molecule to produce two antibody fragments known as Fab (antibody binding) and Fc (cell membrane binding) regions. The two combining sites on the molecules can cross-link two antigen groups on cells or bacteria to produce clumping, complement activation, or recruitment of other immunosurveillance systems.

Synthesis

After antigenic exposure and transformation of specific B cell-derived lymphocytes in a complex process, antibodies are synthesized in plasma cells and lymphocytes are activated in the lymph nodes, Peyer's patches of the intestine, and other reticuloendothelial organs involving regulatory thymus-derived (T cell) lymphocytes. After synthesis, immunoglobulins are released into the blood,

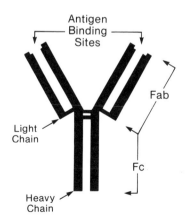

Figure 1.1 Simplified basic structural configuration of antibody molecule representing human immunoglobulin G. Immunoglobulins are composed of two heavy chains and two light chains bound by disulfide linkages (represented by cross bars). Papain cleaves the molecule into two Fab fragments and one Fc fragment. Antigen binding occurs on the Fab segments whereas the Fc segment is responsible for membrane or complement activation.

saliva, and other secretory systems to function as antibodies. Antibodies such as immunoglobulin E remain primarily bound to mast cells or basophils, whereas antibodies such as immunoglobulin A are released in the saliva and other secretions.

Immunoglobulin Classes

Differences in the Fc region (constant region) of immunoglobulins determine the biologic behavior of each molecule. The differences among the classes of immunoglobulins are summarized in Table 1.2. Functioning as serum antibodies, they may 1) recognize and neutralize antigens in the circulation (i.e., immunoglobulin G or M), 2) bind to cells both intravascularly or in tissues to produce immediate hypersensitivity responses after antigen exposure, or 3) act as specific cell receptor molecules interacting with antigens to cause lymphocyte proliferation and differentiation into antibody-secreting cells (i.e., immunoglobulin D [IgD]).

Immunoglobulin G

Immunoglobulin G (IgG) comprises approximately 70% of the serum immunoglobulins. The IgG molecule has a molecular weight of 150,000 and represents the classic antibody structure with two light chains and two heavy chains. After the Fab regions have combined with a bivalent antigen, conformational changes occur in the Fc region of the molecule to activate complement. Different subclasses of IgG molecules exist depending on differences in the gamma chain. IgG_1 and IgG_3 readily activate complement but also are bound by phagocytic cells. IgG_2 is less active in complement binding, whereas IgG_4 does not bind complement but may bind to mast cells.

Immunoglobulin D

IgD appears to function as a receptor, acting as the principal membrane receptor for lymphocytes. It is present at very low levels in the serum.

Immunoglobulin E

Immunoglobulin E (IgE), also called *reaginic antibody*, is the antibody responsible for anaphylaxis and other type I immediate hypersensitivity reactions (see following section). This class of immunoglobulins is present in low serum concentrations, is heat labile, and can be inactivated by heating the serum to 56°C for 2 hours. The epsilon chain has a high carbohydrate content, which characterizes the Fc region of the molecule. Mast cell and basophil surface membranes avidly bind the Fc portion of the IgE molecule.

Immunoglobulin M

Immunoglobulin M (IgM), the largest of the immunoglobulins, has the basic structure of the IgG molecule and appears as a pentamer of IgG. IgM molecules are the first antibodies formed after immunization. Although certain

Table 1.2 Biologic Characteristics of Immunoglobulins

Characteristic	IgE	IgG	IgM	IgA	IgD
Molecular weight	188,000	160,000	900,000	170,000	184,000
Mast cell binding	+	−*	−	−	−
Complement activation	−	+*	+	−	−
Function	Sensitize mast cells/basophils for anaphylaxis	Major antibody involved in host defense; crosses placenta	Antibody to blood groups	Antibody in body secretions	Membrane receptor on lymphocytes
Serum concentration (g/L)	<0.001 × 10³	6–14	0.5–1.5	1–3	<0.1

* IgG$_4$ does not activate complement but binds to mast cells.

IgM molecules fix complement, most do not participate in allergic reactions. Naturally occurring antibodies to the ABO blood groups in humans are IgM molecules, also called *isohemagglutinins*. Antibodies of this class are synthesized against blood groups not occurring on their own red blood cells. Apparently antibody production occurs through antigenic stimulation by carbohydrate allergens in plants. IgM does not cross the placenta.

Immunoglobulin A

Immunoglobulin A (IgA), a secretory antibody found in saliva and gastrointestinal and respiratory secretions, represents an immunologic paint coating the mucosal surface to provide host protection against pathogenic organisms (Tomasi, 1968). The basic unit of IgA resembles IgG but is linked to a small peptide called the J chain. IgA molecules are synthesized in lymphocytes, released into the lamina propria, and transported across the mucosal cells. A secretory component of the mucosal cells is attached to the IgA chain. IgA deficiency occurs in approximately 1 in 850 people even in the absence of apparent immunologic deficiencies (Ammann and Hong, 1971; Kolstinen, 1975).

CLASSIFICATION OF IMMUNOLOGIC REACTIONS

Immunologic reactions can be classified into four types based on the antibody involved, the type of cell modulating the reaction, the nature of the antigen, and the duration of the reaction. Although the different reactions are classified as functionally distinct, the immune system is highly complex and interacts at different levels for autoregulation. For example, one drug, such as penicillin, may produce type I, II, III, or IV immunologic reactions in different patients. The different reactions have also been referred to as *hypersensitivity reactions* because the exaggerated responses lead to destruction or injury of the host's tissues (DeSwarte, 1986; Watkins et al., 1982). Nonetheless, the classification of Gell and Coombs still provides a basic understanding of the pathophysiology and spectrum of immunologic reactions seen clinically (Gell et al., 1975). A summary of type I through IV immunologic reactions in included in Table 1.3.

Type I

Anaphylactic reactions are examples of type I reactions; they are also called *immediate hypersensitivity reactions*. The antibody mediating the response is an IgE type that attaches to the surface of mast cells and basophils. When an antigen binds to the IgE antibody on the surface of these cells, cellular activation and degranulation ensue with the release of a variety of pharmacologically active substances classically producing anaphylaxis (see Chapter 2). Not all type I allergic reactions are anaphylactic, however. Other examples of type I allergy include classic penicillin allergy, bee-sting reactions, extrinsic asthma, and allergic rhinitis. Allergic reactions are considered type I reactions (Roitt et al., 1989).

Table 1.3 Gell and Coombs Classification of Immunologic Reactions

Reaction	Synonyms	Antibody	Chemical Mechanism	Examples
Type I	Immediate hyper-sensitivity	IgE	Antigen binds to IgE on the surface of mast cells and basophils with release of mast cell products	Anaphylaxis Cutaneous wheal and flare Extrinsic asthma
Type II	Cytotoxic	IgG IgM	IgG, IgM binds antigen on cell membranes; complement is activated with liberation of anaphylatoxins and cellular destruction	Transfusion reactions Hemolytic anemia Rh disease
Type III	Immune complex	IgG IgM	IgG, IgM binds antigen in the fluid phase and deposits in small blood vessels; complement is activated with cellular destruction	Serum sickness Glomerulonephritis
Type IV	Delayed hyper-sensitivity Cell-mediated immunity	Not involved	Sensitized thymus-derived lymphocytes bind antigen and release effectors known as lymphokines	Contact dermatitis Tuberculin immunity

Modified from Gell PGH, Coombs RRA, Lachmann PJ, eds. Clinical Aspects of Immunology, 3rd ed. Oxford: Blackwell Scientific Publications, 1975. Reprinted with permission from Levy JH, Roizen MT, Morris JM. Anaphylactic and anaphylactoid reactions. Spine 1986b; 11:282–91.

Type II

Type II reactions are known as *cytotoxic reactions*. Antibodies involved are IgG or IgM types, which are called *cytotoxic antibodies*. The reaction occurs when antibodies bind to immunospecific antigens. The antigens may be integral components of cell membranes (blood group antigens) or haptens, which adhere to the red cell surface (e.g., penicillin). Antigen–antibody interaction activates the complement system, which in turn lyses the cells. Peptide fragments known as anaphylatoxins are released during the activation of complement, producing systemic manifestations. Examples of type II reactions include ABO-incompatible transfusion reactions, Rh disease of the newborn, drug-induced or autoimmune hemolytic anemia, and Goodpasture syndrome.

Type III

Type III reactions are known as *immune complex reactions*. Antibodies and circulating soluble antigens form insoluble complexes that are too small to be filtered by the liver and spleen macrophages of the reticuloendothelial system. Instead the complexes deposit in the microcirculation. The antibodies involved are of the IgG or IgM class. Complement is activated by the interaction of antigen and antibodies, producing inflammation at the deposition site. The anaphylatoxins liberated also cause the migration of other inflammatory cells, producing vasculitis. The complement-mediated attraction and tissue localization of polymorphonuclear leukocytes at the site of immune complex deposition represents the mechanism of tissue damage. A classic example of a type III allergic reaction is so-called serum sickness observed after a second administration of foreign antisera for snake bites, botulism, or as antilymphocyte globulin. Vasculitis after penicillin or drug-induced systemic lupus erythematosus are also examples of type III reactions.

Type IV

Type IV reactions are known as *cell-mediated immune* or *delayed hypersensitivity reactions*. These reactions are independent of antibodies. Instead, lymphoid cells known as *thymus-derived lymphocytes* are activated by cellular antigens or circulatory proteins. The activated T cells can directly kill foreign cells or produce substances known as *lymphokines*, which orchestrate the immune response. Lymphokines mediate inflammation at the site of a foreign antigen. Lymphokines regulate macrophages, polymorphonuclear leukocytes, lymphocytes, and other cell functions directing the killing of foreign cells and organisms. The time course of these reactions is slow to develop, first appearing at 18 to 24 hours, reaching a maximum at 48 hours, and disappearing by 72 to 96 hours. Examples of cell-mediated immune reactions are tuberculin skin testing, graft rejection, and poison ivy allergy.

Abnormalities in cell-mediated immune function produce failures of normal immune surveillance; patients are then at risk for opportunistic infections. Acquired immunodeficiency syndrome (AIDS) is a manifestation of abnormalities in cell-mediated immunity. Subpopulations of T cell lymphocytes known as cytotoxic-suppressor cells are altered by infections with human immunodeficiency virus (HIV), producing defects in immunity. Opportunistic infections such as *Pneumocystis carinii* and lymphoproliferative syndromes such as Kaposi's sarcoma can result.

THE EFFECTS OF ANESTHESIA ON THE IMMUNE RESPONSE

Multiple in vivo and in vitro reports exist in the literature regarding the effects of anesthetic agents on the immune system. Sophisticated studies have evaluated both humoral and cell-mediated immunologic changes associated with anesthesia. A major problem with most studies, however, is separating the effects of intraoperative factors and the associated stress response from the direct effects of anesthetic agents themselves (Stevenson et al., 1990). The contribution of anesthetic agents to alterations in immune responsiveness is poorly understood because there are few studies of prolonged anesthetic exposure without surgery. Many investigators suggest that the changes in immune competence seen in vivo and in vitro in surgical patients are the result of surgical trauma and alterations in the stress response produced by circulating adrenocorticotropic hormone, catecholamines, and corticosteroids and by nonanesthetic drugs rather than the direct result of anesthetic exposure (Slade et al., 1975; Stevenson et al., 1990). Finally, there are no outcome studies that demonstrate any improvements in immunocompetence using one anesthetic regimen rather than another. Most investigators conclude that the trauma of surgery is the main cause of the observed postoperative immunodepression of otherwise normal people (Stevenson et al., 1990).

Determining the effects of anesthetic agents on many important aspects of immune function has been difficult in the past because of the primitive nature of the investigative studies. Recently the elucidation of a host of biologic response modifiers, including interleukins, granulocyte–monocyte colony-stimulating factor, gamma interferon, lymphotoxin, natural killer cell factor, alpha interferon, tumor necrosis factor, and granulocyte colony-stimulating factors, for example, has allowed investigators to identify specific abnormalities and specific immune responses more accurately. Furthermore, the ability of anesthesia to block the increase in sympathoadrenergic responses associated with anaphylactic shock may also have a significant impact on outcome considerations for the patient in acute shock. There are too few data to suggest an advantage in using one agent or anesthetic technique over another in terms of outcome and effects on immunocompetence, however.

2

Initiation and Clinical Manifestations of Anaphylaxis

Anaphylaxis is an immediate-onset allergic reaction produced by the immunologically mediated release of physiologically active substances from mast cells and basophils. These substances produce a clinical syndrome of specific responses in the respiratory, cardiovascular, and cutaneous systems (Figure 2.1). The reaction occurs after exposure to an antigen or molecule similar in antigenic structure to one to which the patient has had previous exposure. Anaphylactic reactions, classically considered to be type I allergic reactions, are due to the immunoglobulin (IgE)-mediated release of mast cell and basophil products. The original reports of anaphylaxis by Richet and Portier used a dog model, which is an immunoglobulin G (IgG)-mediated reaction (Halpern, 1983). IgG antibodies can also produce anaphylaxis in humans by complement activation, which causes the generation of anaphylatoxins (see Chapter 4).

INITIAL CELLULAR ACTIVATION

For anaphylaxis to occur, the antigen must be *polyvalent,* capable of binding two or more adjacent IgE molecules (Geha, 1984; Metzger et al., 1986). After antigen administration in a previously sensitized person, two IgE antibodies on mast cell and basophil surface membranes are bridged by an immunospecific antigen, causing the receptors to undergo conformational changes (Geha, 1984; Ishizaka, 1981). These stereochemical changes stimulate membrane phospholipid metabolism, followed by influx of extracellular and mobilization of intracellular calcium (Rafferty and Holgate, 1989). This intracellular signal produces cellular activation to release primary and secondary mediators (Kazimierczak and Diamant, 1978; Winslow and Austen, 1982). Histamine, heparin, and different chemotactic factors of anaphylaxis are released immediately from the storage granules by fusion of the perigranular and mast-cell membranes (Gomez et al., 1986; Wasserman, 1983). Specific increases in calcium permeability across cellular membranes are essential for histamine release and intracellular activation. In addition to degranulation, a rapid, sequential, oxidative metabolism of arachidonic acid occurs, synthesizing other phospholipid and chemical mediators, including products of cyclooxygenase and lipoxygenase metabolism, as well as platelet-activating factor, which is discussed in more detail in Chapter 3 (Piper, 1976; Wasserman, 1983).

MAST CELLS AND BASOPHILS

Mast cells and basophils are heterogeneous effector cells of anaphylaxis. After activation, both participate in the immediate release and sequential synthesis of physiologically active mediators (Orange et al., 1971). Both possess over 100,000 high-affinity membrane receptors for IgE but they differ in their morphology, location, and biosynthetic products (Conroy et al., 1977a; Winslow and Austen, 1982).

Mast cells are tissue fixed, residing in the perivascular connective tissue and mucosa of the respiratory, gastrointestinal, and cutaneous tissues (Pearce, 1982; Zweiman, 1983). Normal human skin contains approximately 7000 mast cells per square millimeter and duodenal mucosa contains 20,000 mast cells per square millimeter (Mikhail and Miller-Milinska, 1964; Zweiman, 1983), whereas lung tissue contains 2,000,000 mast cells per gram (Metcalf, 1982). Histamine is stored in the electron-dense granules of mast cells complexed ionically to the proteoglycan heparin and protein enzymes (Figure 2.2). The granule size is 0.1 to 0.4 microns, whereas the entire mast cell is 10 to 30 microns (Metcalf, 1982). The half-life of normal human mast cells is unknown but may be from weeks to months (Metcalf, 1982). Connective tissue and mucosal mast cells are subgroups of human mast cells distinguished by differences in granule density and cytochemical staining (Metcalf, 1982). Furthermore, there may be differences in functional characteristics within mast cell populations as well as heterogeneity between mast cells of a given organ (i.e., the gastrointestinal tract is composed of both connective-tissue and mucosal mast cells) (Metcalf, 1982).

Basophils are polymorphonuclear granulocytes comprising 0.5% to 1% of the circulating leukocytes and 0.3% of nucleated cells in the bone marrow (Metcalf, 1982; Schleimer et al., 1983a). Human basophils have a granule size of 1.2 microns and an overall size of 5 to 7 microns (Metcalf, 1982). Basophils can be recruited during a variety of immunologic and inflammatory responses.

The role of mast cells and basophils in the pathogenesis of immediate hypersensitivity reactions is well established; however, the normal physiologic roles are unclear. Mast cells appear to modulate gastric acid secretion and may be involved in vascular permeability control (Schleimer et al., 1983a). Both cell types, including IgE and eosinophils, are involved in the immune system's defense against parasitic infections (Schleimer et al., 1983a). Because mast cells reside in the perivascular spaces of the skin, lung, and intestine, organ systems that interface with the external environment, they appear to play a role in initial host defense against microbiologic intruders.

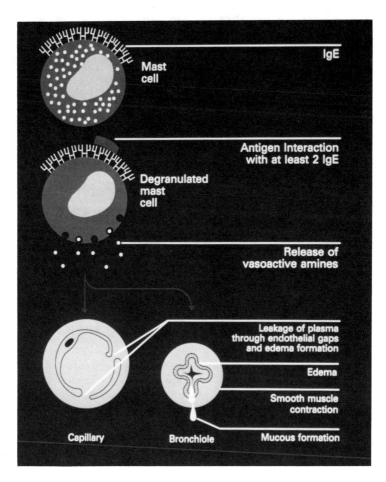

Figure 2.1 IgE anaphylaxis (type I immediate hypersensitivity reaction). When an antigen enters through a parenteral route in a previously sensitized person, either intravenously or intramuscularly, it bridges two IgE antibodies on the surface of mast cells and basophils. In a calcium- and energy-dependent process, the cells release physiologically active substances, producing the severe and life-threatening effects in the respiratory (bronchospasm, airway obstruction, and mucus secretion) and cardiovascular (vasodilation and increased capillary permeability) systems. *Modified with permission from Immunology: A Scope publication. The Upjohn Company, Kalamazoo, MI, 1981.*

Factors Influencing Mast Cell/Basophil Activation

Factors that influence the immunologic response to antigens are complex. At the level of the mast cell and basophil, variations in the clinical manifestation of anaphylaxis may be due to the amount of cell-bound IgE, the concentration of the antigen, the primary site of the reaction, the presence of inhibiting factors, and the physiologic state of the organs (Terr, 1985). There appears to be a graded

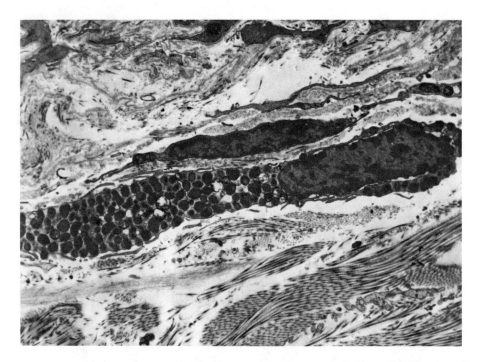

Figure 2.2 Electron micrograph of a human cutaneous mast cell. The cell outline is well defined and the electron-dense cytoplasmic granules that store histamine, tryptase, and chemotactic factors are well delineated. Note the collagen bundles in the lower portion of the micrograph (magnification × 50,000). *Reprinted with permission from Levy JH, Brister NW, Shearin A, et al. Wheal and flare responses to opioids in humans. Anesthesiology 1989;70:756–60.*

response among different people to antibody-dependent and antibody-independent release of histamine. Conroy and others have coined the term *releasibility*, to describe a person's ability to activate mast cells when stimulated (Conroy et al., 1977b).

Role of Calcium

Calcium is considered to be a major component of the cellular system's regulatory effect on mast cell and basophil secretory activity. If these cells are stimulated with antigen without the presence of extracellular calcium, mediator release does not occur (Patkar and Diamant, 1982; Tharp et al., 1982). Experimental data suggest that activation is related to a specific increase in the membrane permeability to calcium (Patkar and Diamant, 1982; Tharp et al., 1982). That is, the concentration of calcium outside the cell is higher than inside (10^{-3} molar compared with 10^{-5} to 10^{-7} molar) (Kazimierczak and Diamant, 1978).

When the divalent antigen binds IgE, phospholipids within the cell membrane are reoriented to allow an increase in calcium (Ca^{2+}) flux through specific channels into the cell (Ishizaka, 1981). After calcium influx, degranulation occurs and arachidonic acid release is triggered by activation of a calcium-dependent phospholipase A_2 (Borgeat et al., 1983). The formation of cyclooxygenase and lipoxygenase products is controlled by mast-cell and basophil phospholipases, which make arachidonic acid available for metabolizing enzymes (see Chapter 3) (Borgeat et al., 1983). This also has important considerations for potential therapeutic approaches to inhibiting mast cell activation (see Chapter 9).

ONSET OF REACTION

In a sensitized person, the onset of the signs and symptoms of anaphylaxis is usually immediate but may be delayed 2 to 20 minutes after parenteral injection of antigen (Figure 2.3) (Delage and Irey, 1972). Retrospective reporting during a postmarketing survey of 164 cases of anaphylaxis after chymopapain injection (Chymodiactin, Smith Laboratories, Chicago) revealed that 54% of manifestations occurred within 5 minutes, 30% within 10 minutes, and 10% within 20 minutes. Anaphylaxis may also occur with oral or respiratory exposure to allergens; however, manifestations may occur at unpredictable times (Delage and Irey, 1972). The severity of the reaction is suggested to be directly proportional to the rapidity of onset (Terr, 1985).

A previous history of allergy or exposure to the responsible allergen may be unknown to the patient (Delage and Irey, 1972). Furthermore, the reaction is unpredictable, and the clinical manifestations vary from mild hypotension to life-threatening cardiopulmonary dysfunction. Familiarity with and alertness to the signs and symptoms are necessary for early recognition of an impending anaphylactic reaction.

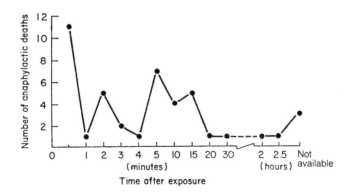

Figure 2.3 Onset of anaphylaxis (in minutes) after exposure to agent in 43 cases of fatal anaphylaxis. *Data from Delage C, Irey NS. Anaphylactic deaths: a clinicopathologic study of 43 cases. J Forensic Sci 1972;17:525–40.*

Table 2.1 Recognition of Anaphylaxis During Regional and General Anesthesia

System	Symptoms	Signs
Respiratory	Dyspnea Chest discomfort	Coughing Wheezing Sneezing Airway obstruction Laryngeal edema Decreased pulmonary compliance Fulminant pulmonary edema Acute respiratory distress
Cardiovascular	Dizziness Malaise Retrosternal oppression	Disorientation Diaphoresis Loss of consciousness Hypotension Tachycardia Dysrhythmias Decreased systemic vascular resistance Pulmonary hypertension Cardiac arrest
Cutaneous	Itching Burning Tingling	Urticaria (hives) Flushing Perioral edema Periorbital edema

SIGNS AND SYMPTOMS

The effects of mediators on different receptors in the lungs, heart, and vasculature produce the physiologic manifestations of anaphylaxis. Patients who have these reactions may manifest some or all of the following signs and symptoms (Table 2.1) (Kelly and Patterson, 1974; Pavek et al., 1982).

Respiratory System

Patients may complain of nasal stuffiness or itching, chest tightness, difficulty in breathing, a sense of retrosternal oppression, hoarseness, an oral tingling sensation, or the sensation of a lump in the throat (from laryngeal edema). Examination may reveal coughing, wheezing, tachypnea, stridor, intercostal and suprasternal retraction, cyanosis, or acute pulmonary edema. The patient may be in acute respiratory distress and laryngoscopy may reveal upper airway edema. Acute decreases in pulmonary compliance manifested by increased airway pressures may occur during positive pressure ventilation.

Cardiovascular System

Patients may complain of dizziness and there may be changes in consciousness. Varying levels of hypotension, including complete loss of detectable blood pressure, may occur. Electrocardiographic changes can vary from tachydysrhythmias and nonspecific ST segment and T wave changes to ventricular dysrhythmias, atrioventricular conduction defects, and ventricular fibrillation. Patients with invasive hemodynamic monitoring may demonstrate profound reductions in systemic vascular resistance. Furthermore, acute pulmonary hypertension may occur as a result of transfusion or protamine reactions.

Integumentary System

Complaints may include generalized itching, warmth, perioral/orbital or extremity edema, or ocular itching. Patients may have the characteristic wheal and flare of a histamine reaction with the appearance of small wheals that enlarge and coalesce together. Angioedema, defined as mucosal swelling, often localizes to the face, tongue, pharynx, and larynx.

Gastrointestinal System

Nausea, vomiting, diarrhea, or abdominal pain may occur as isolated symptoms, caused by smooth muscle contraction in the visceral organs or in association with other organ dysfunction.

INTRAOPERATIVE ANAPHYLAXIS

Hypotension, cyanosis, and respiratory distress manifest themselves most often during severe, fatal intraoperative anaphylactic reactions (Laxenaire et al., 1982). Urticaria and other cutaneous manifestations are not readily visible in patients who are under general anesthesia and are usually covered with surgical drapes. Furthermore, after hymenoptera (bee sting) challenges in patients with a specific anaphylactic history, the highest observed histamine levels were associated with hypotension but not cutaneous manifestations (Smith et al., 1980).

Anaphylactic reactions in intubated patients may involve any combination of cardiovascular, pulmonary, or cutaneous signs, as shown in Table 2.2. The sine qua non of intraoperative anaphylaxis is severe cardiovascular collapse. In a study of 100 reported cases of anaphylaxis during anesthesia, Laxenaire and coworkers found that circulatory collapse accounted for 68% of all cases, and cardiac arrest accounted for an additional 11% (Laxenaire et al., 1982). Bronchospasm and widespread flushing were less reliable manifestations, occurring in 23% and 55% of patients, respectively (Laxenaire et al., 1982).

The cardiovascular changes associated with eight anaphylactic/anaphylactoid reactions in patients with hemodynamic monitoring who underwent cardiac surgery are shown in Table 2.3. Systolic, diastolic, and mean arterial pressures decreased in all the patients whereas ventricular rate did not change. Systemic

Table 2.2 Recognition of Anaphylaxis in Intubated Patients

System	Signs
Respiratory	Cyanosis
	Wheezing
	Increased peak airway pressure
	Acute pulmonary edema
Cardiovascular	Tachycardia
	Dysrhythmias
	Hypotension
	Pulmonary hypertension
	Decreased systemic vascular resistance
	Cardiovascular collapse
Cutaneous	Urticaria
	Flushing
	Perioral edema
	Periorbital edema

Table 2.3 Hemodynamic Parameters During Anaphylactic/Anaphylactoid Reactions

Parameter*	Baseline	Reaction	Recovery
Heart rate (beats/min)	79 ± 11	80 ± 13	85 ± 11
SAP (mmHg)	119 ± 7	72 ± 8†	119 ± 13
DAP (mmHg)	62 ± 7	39 ± 8†	62 ± 4
MAP (mmHg)	81 ± 9	50 ± 7†	80 ± 6
Cardiac output (L/min)	4.6 ± 0.6	6.5 ± 1.2‡	5.0 ± 1.3
Stroke volume (mL/beat)	49 ± 11	83 ± 22§	62 ± 19
SVR (dyne/sec/cm^{-5})	1294 ± 137	563 ± 127†	1196 ± 310
MPAP (mmHg)	16 ± 5	16 ± 10	17 ± 6
CVP (mmHg)	7 ± 3	5 ± 3	7 ± 2

All values expressed as mean ± standard deviation (SD). The P values refer to a comparison between baseline and anaphylactoid reactions.

* SAP = systolic arterial pressure; DAP = diastolic aortic pressure; MAP = mean arterial pressure; SVR = systemic vascular resistance; MPAP = mean pulmonary arterial pressure; CVP = central venous pressure.

† $P < 0.001$.

‡ $P < 0.005$.

§ $P < 0.02$.

From Levy JH. Anaphylactic/anaphylactoid reactions during cardiac surgery. J Clin Anesth 1989a;1:426–30.

vascular resistance decreased and cardiac output and stroke volume increased in all patients. Although mean pulmonary artery and central venous pressures showed no significant changes, isolated pulmonary hypertension occurred after blood and protamine administration in 2 patients (Figure 2.4). There were cutaneous manifestations consisting of a wheal or flare in 2 patients, and bronchospasm was noted in only 1 patient.

Fisher and Moore reported epidemiologic studies and clinical observations of perioperative anaphylaxis. In their series of anaphylactic episodes in 116 Australian patients flushing was the most common manifestation, occurring in 44 patients (38%; Table 2.4) (Fisher and Moore, 1981). Bronchospasm was found in 25 patients, 19 of whom were asthmatic. Bronchospasm represented the most difficult feature to treat and was associated with the highest mortality (3 of 4 deaths). Fisher later reported on 227 patients who developed perioperative anaphylaxis (Fisher, 1986). Cardiovascular collapse, defined as a blood pressure below 40 mmHg, occurred in 205 patients. It was the most severe feature in 155 patients and was described as unrecordable at some point in 83 patients. Supraventricular tachycardia occurred in 153 patients and 4 patients subsequently developed ventricular fibrillation.

PATHOPHYSIOLOGY
Cardiovascular Collapse

Clinical observations, pathologic studies, and epidemiologic findings of anaphylaxis indicate that the cardiovascular system is a primary target (Assem, 1989; Levi, 1988). Cardiovascular collapse during anaphylaxis results from the

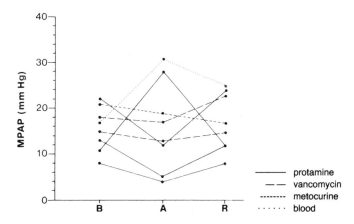

Figure 2.4 Cardiovascular changes during anaphylaxis. Changes in individual values of mean pulmonary artery pressure (MPAP) during baseline (B), anaphylactic reaction (A), and recovery (R) in eight patients during anaphylaxis.

Table 2.4 Manifestations of Anaphylaxis in 116 Patients

Manifestation	No.
Flushing	44
Bronchospasm	25
Pulse not palpable	15
Coughing	7
Subjective complaint	6
Urticarial rash	7
Edema	5
Cyanosis	4
Wound not bleeding	1
Loss of consciousness	2

Data from Fisher MM, More DG. The epidemiology and clinical features of anaphylactic reactions in anaesthesia. Anaesth Intensive Care 1981;9:226–34.

effects of multiple mediators on both the heart and peripheral vasculature. Fisher suggests that intraoperative cardiovascular collapse is primarily caused by vasodilation and fluid loss due to increased capillary permeability (Fisher, 1986). Vasodilation can result from a spectrum of different mediators, as shown in Table 2.5. The interaction of different mediators with the endothelium to produce endothelium-derived relaxing factor, or their direct effects on vascular smooth muscle, are the mechanisms responsible for vasodilation. Individual mediators and their effects are discussed in Chapter 3.

Biventricular dysfunction, producing a decreased cardiac output, has also been suggested as the factor most often responsible for both hypotension and fatalities during anaphylactic shock (Delage and Irey, 1972). Multiple factors are potentially responsible for a decreased cardiac output, including decreased venous return, dysrhythmias, hemoconcentration with increased blood viscosity, increased pulmonary vascular resistance, right heart failure, and decreased coronary blood flow from hypotension and coronary vasoconstriction (Revenäs, 1979; Sheffer, 1985; Smedegärd et al., 1979; 1981). Thromboxane A_2 can produce both coronary and pulmonary vasoconstriction (Levi, 1988). When pulmonary vascular resistance increases acutely, the right ventricle, which is normally accustomed to ejecting against a low resistance, fails. The right ventricle dilates and shifts the shared intraventricular septum into the left ventricle, altering both compliance and loading, thus preventing systemic flow. Because of the important interactions between the heart and lungs, bronchospasm and overdistention of the lung can also increase pulmonary vascular resistance. Persistent hypotension during anaphylaxis can also produce myocardial ischemia and resultant left ventricular dysfunction (Nicolas et al., 1984).

Table 2.5 Mediators That Produce Vasodilation

Prostaglandins: PGI_2 (prostacyclin), PGE_1, PGE_2, PGD_2, PGA_2

Histamine (H_1 and H_2 effects)

Kinins: bradykinin, kallikrein

Leukotrienes

Platelet-activating factor (PAF)

Substance P

Over the past 15 years, the widespread use of hemodynamic monitoring in patients has allowed measurements of cardiovascular function during anaphylactic reactions. In a patient developing anaphylaxis to nafcillin, a decrease in pulmonary capillary wedge pressure and decreased cardiac output caused hypotension (Silverman et al., 1984). This patient had a previous myocardial infarction and numerous subsequent hospitalizations for acute pulmonary edema, indicating severely compromised ventricular function. Most reports of decreased cardiac output after anaphylaxis were measured long after the initial onset of hypotension. Arterial pressure, pulmonary capillary wedge pressure, pulmonary vascular resistance, systemic vascular resistance, and left ventricular end diastolic volume decreased in a vascular surgical patient who developed anaphylaxis to cefazolin, whereas stroke volume, cardiac output, and ejection fraction increased, as shown by 2-dimensional transesophageal echocardiography (Figure 2.5) (Beaupre et al., 1984). Despite a history of anteroseptal and inferior myocardial infarctions, this patient exhibited enhanced myocardial function during anaphylaxis. Levy and coworkers have also reported increased cardiac output during anaphylactic reactions due to different drugs (Levy, 1989a; Levy et al., 1986a; 1989d). The increased cardiac output and stroke volume observed initially in anaphylactic reactions may be due to both an acute reduction in afterload and the inotropic effect of histamine on the heart, as well as an increase in sympathoadrenergic output that follows histamine release and hypotension (Schellenberg et al., 1991; Vigorito et al., 1983). Hypotension observed initially during anaphylactic shock may be associated with varying cardiac outputs depending on the preload, afterload, contractility, heart rate, and rhythm.

Dysrhythmias and abnormalities in automaticity and atrioventricular conduction may contribute to the alterations in cardiac output during anaphylaxis (Levi, 1988; Levi et al., 1991). Booth proposed the following mechanisms as possible explanations for the observed electrocardiographic changes: 1) a direct antigen–antibody myocardial reaction, 2) a pharmacologic effect of mediators released during anaphylaxis, 3) the effect of catecholamines used for treatment, 4) anoxia, 5) underlying heart disease, and 6) a combination of several of these factors (Booth and Patterson, 1970). Direct histamine infusions in humans have been reported to produce atrioventricular dissociation (Vigorito et al., 1983).

Acute cardiac dysfunction probably results from combinations of the pre-

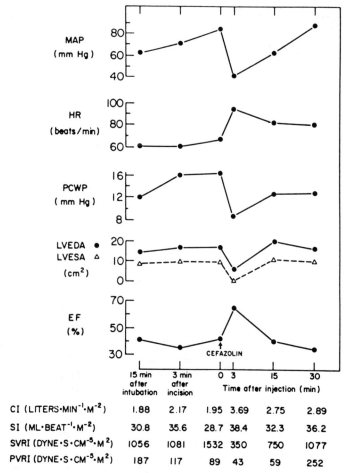

Figure 2.5 Hemodynamic and echocardiographic changes before, during, and after an anaphylactic reaction to cefazolin. EF has increased despite the decrease in PCWP and end-diastolic volumes. MAP = mean arterial blood pressure; HR = heart rate; PCWP = pulmonary capillary wedge pressure; LVEDA and LVESA = left ventricular end-diastolic and end-systolic cross-sectional areas; EF = ejection fraction (LVEDA − LVESA)/LVEDA; CI = cardiac index; SI = stroke index; SVRI = systemic vascular resistance index; and PVRI = pulmonary vascular resistance index. *Reprinted with permission from Beaupre PN, Roizen MF, Cahalan MK, Alpert RA, Cassorla L, Schiller NB. Hemodynamic and two-dimensional transesophageal echocardiographic analysis of an anaphylactic reaction in man. Anesthesiology 1984;60:483.*

viously mentioned factors. Histamine and other mediators can produce coronary vasoconstriction if vascular endothelium is impaired, as in patients with coronary artery disease (see Chapter 3). Hypotension caused by any shock state produces decreased coronary artery perfusion, resulting in myocardial ischemia or infarction, and can release additional mediators with negative inotropic and dromotropic effects (Levi, 1988; Wolff and Levi, 1986). Ventricular dysfunction, resulting from myocardial ischemia, may be the underlying problem, producing secondary irreversible shock after anaphylaxis.

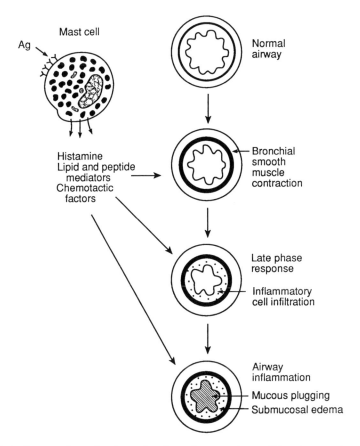

Figure 2.6 Proposed mechanisms for bronchospasm/reversible airway obstruction in patients during anaphylaxis. After mast cell activation and mediator release, patients with normal airways can develop rapid bronchospasm and reversible airway obstruction. The release of chemotactic factors causes the recruitment and migration of inflammatory cells to the airways and can produce persistent airway obstruction, characteristic of late-phase responses. In patients with a history of asthma and airway inflammation, the additional release of histamine, leukotrienes, and prostaglandins can produce further life-threatening airway obstruction.

Airway Obstruction/Bronchospasm

Rapid development and persistence of reversible airway obstruction occurring during anaphylaxis is due to the effects of mediators on both large and small airways, which produce smooth muscle constriction, mucosal airway edema, and hypersecretion of mucus (Figure 2.6) (Goetzl, 1984; Revenäs et al., 1979). Multiple mediators are responsible for these pathophysiologic changes, as shown in Table 2.6. Traditionally, the word *bronchospasm* has been used almost synonymously with *asthma,* and the reversibility of airway obstruction with bronchodilators has been a major criterion for the physiologic diagnosis of asthma (Busse and Reid, 1988). Asthma is much more than bronchoconstriction, however, and considerable emphasis has been placed on the inflammatory component of the airway obstruction and the interaction of eosinophils, other inflammatory cells, and lipid mediators in generating this pathophysiologic response (Barnes, 1989a; Busse, 1989; Gleich et al., 1988; Kay, 1991). Mediator release after anaphylaxis can produce bronchospasm but can also recruit additional inflammatory cells to produce additional injury to the airway, as shown in Figure 2.6.

Asthma, as defined by the American Thoracic Society, is "a clinical syndrome characterized by increased responsiveness of the tracheal bronchial tree to a variety of stimuli" (American Thoracic Society, 1987). Asthmatic responses may be provoked by specific or nonspecific stimuli, including allergens and other irritants. Cardinal features of asthma are the bronchial hyperresponsiveness (an exaggerated bronchoconstrictor response that correlates with the severity of

Table 2.6 Pathologic Features of Respiratory Involvement During Anaphylaxis and Proposed Mediators

Pathologic Feature	Mediators Responsible
Bronchospasm	Histamine (H_1 effect)
	Leukotrienes C_4, D_4, E_4
	Prostaglandin $F2\alpha$
	Thromboxane A_z
	Bradykinin
	Platelet-activating factor
Mucosal edema	Histamine (H_1 effect)
	Leukotrienes C_4, D_4, E_4
	Prostaglandin E_z
	Bradykinin
	Platelet-activating factor
Airway inflammation	Chemotactic factors
	Leukotriene B_4
	Platelet-activating factor

Modified from White MV. The role of histamine in allergic disease. J Allergy Clin Immunol 1990;86:599–605.

disease), frequency of symptoms, and need for treatment (Barnes, 1989a). Asthma is a complex, interactive inflammatory process involving many cell types and inflammatory mediators. Multiple mediators and factors may lead to the pathologic features of asthma, including bronchoconstriction, bronchial hyperresponsiveness, airway secretion, and microvascular leakage.

Patients with preexisting asthma who develop anaphylaxis can be the most difficult to treat (Fisher and Moore, 1981). One explanation for this finding may be that patients with asthma, airway inflammation, and reactive airway disease are more sensitive to the bronchoconstrictor effects of mediator release. Those patients who develop severe airway obstruction after anaphylaxis may have minimal ventilatory exchange. The increased functional residual capacity that results from air trapping and hyperinflated lungs produces increased pulmonary vascular resistance and acute cor pulmonale, thus exacerbating hemodynamic instability.

Urticaria and Angioedema

Urticaria, or hives, is a wheal-and-flare reaction produced by mediator release from mast cells within the superficial dermis. Circumscribed, raised, erythematous, often pruritic, and evanescent areas of edema that involve the superficial portions of dermis are known as *urticaria* (Mathews, 1983). The lesions vary in size from 1 to 2 mm to many centimeters in diameter. When the edematous process extends into the deep dermis or subcutaneous and submucosal layers, it is known as *angioedema* (Mathews, 1983). Angioedema results from increased permeability of subcutaneous blood vessels, producing pharyngeal, perioral, and periorbital edema that can be asymmetrically distributed (Mathews, 1983; Terr, 1985). Angioedema may account for a substantial loss of intravascular volume during anaphylaxis and has a predilection for the face, although it can also occur in the gastrointestinal tract.

The vasoactive effects of histamine and its local interactions with nerve endings are initially responsible for the cutaneous effects. Histamine dilates superficial venules and contracts endothelial cells to form a functional pore, thus increasing vascular permeability (Antohe et al., 1986; Kilzer et al., 1985; Movat, 1987). The wheal corresponds to an area of tissue edema produced by increased capillary permeability and the flare corresponds to local cutaneous vasodilation and detectable redness (Olsson et al., 1988). Histamine can also stimulate cutaneous sensory neurons, which synapse with afferent neurons within the spinal cord to carry the impulses detected as pruritus (Bienenstock et al., 1987; Mathews, 1983). The sensory neurons involved are type C, unmyelinated fibers that originate in proximity to cutaneous mast cells and blood vessels (Bevan and Brayden, 1987; Church et al., 1989a; 1989b). Antidromic conduction is caused by a histamine-induced impulse in one afferent nerve-ending that reaches a branch point and conducts the impulse in the opposite direction along one of the other branches (back toward the skin); this causes the local release of substance P and perhaps other neuropeptides that contribute to the flare reaction (Bienenstock et al., 1987; Church et al., 1989a; 1989b; Payan, 1989). The reflex vasodilation associated with this flare yields an area of redness that is considerably wider than the area within which histamine can diffuse. The combination of vasodilation, increased vascular permeability, and this axon reflex, known as the *triple response of Lewis,* is seen when histamine is injected intradermally or after degranulation of cutaneous mast cells.

The cutaneous mast cells are used as an immunologic window to evaluate antigen–IgE interactions through measurement of the local cutaneous effects after intradermal antigen administration. If the patient is allergic to a drug, he or she will have immunospecific IgE antibodies directed against the drug bound to cutaneous mast cells. Intradermal injection activates the mast cells, releasing histamine and other vasoactive mediators and producing a wheal-and-flare response.

PATHOLOGIC FINDINGS

Autopsy findings after fatal anaphylactic and anaphylactoid reactions have been reported in two separate retrospective studies (Delage and Irey, 1972; James and Austen, 1964). Penicillin was the cause of anaphylaxis in 32 of 43 cases and 3 of 6 cases, respectively. Major pathologic changes, noted primarily in the respiratory tract, are described in the following sections. Clinicopathologic correlations from the two studies suggest that the immediate cause of death can be attributed to asphyxiation from upper airway edema and congestion, acute bronchospasm with hyperinflation of the lung, irreversible shock, or a combination of these factors.

Respiratory System

Delage and Irey noted mild to severe pulmonary congestion in 36 of 40 patients, pulmonary edema in 20 of 40 patients, and intraalveolar hemorrhage in 18 of 40 patients. Severe hypersecretion was noted in only 4 of 40 patients (Delage and Irey, 1972).

Upper respiratory tract edema that included the hypopharynx, epiglottis, and larynx was noted in 15 of 40 and 5 of 6 patients in the two studies, respectively. Delage and Irey noted that 5 of 18 patients demonstrated only microscopic evidence of edematous fluid in the lamina propria of the mucosa without distortion of the laryngeal structures. Six of 18 patients demonstrated gross evidence of laryngeal swelling with ventricular fold obliteration or narrowing but without air passage obstruction, and 4 of 18 patients developed extensive laryngeal structure swelling and distortion, producing complete upper respiratory airway obstruction. James and Austen suggested that upper airway edema contributed to the cause of death in four of six patients.

Hyperinflation (acute pulmonary emphysema) of the lungs was noted in 11 of 40 and 5 of 6 patients in the two studies, respectively. James and Austen noted slight focal thickening of the bronchial basement membrane in 2 of 6 patients, one of whom had a history of asthma. Although none of the 6 patients demonstrated the full morphologic changes associated with asthma, acute bronchospasm produces the same pathologic features of hyperinflation noted in these studies (Terr, 1985).

Autopsy records from 27 cases of fatal dextran-induced anaphylactic reactions suggested the most frequent macroscopic findings were dilation of the right ventricle and acute pulmonary stasis (Ljungstroem et al., 1988). Pulmonary microemboli were noted in 15 of 17 lung specimens. The microemboli had the appearance of hyaline eosinophilic globules and the lung vasculature also contained leukocytes, platelets, and disintegrated erythrocytes. Pulmonary changes consistent with alveolar edema were described as severe in 6 cases and slight in 7 cases. Acute emphysema was present in 4 cases; in 2 cases laryngeal edema was found (Ljungstroem et al., 1988). The dextran antibodies that produced anaphylaxis in these patients were of an IgG class, which mediates its reaction by complement activation (see Chapter 4) (Ljungstroem et al., 1988).

Cardiovascular System

Myocardial ischemia has been noted in a high percentage of cases of anaphylaxis. Acute right ventricular dilation was noted by James and Austen in 2 of 6 patients, suggesting right ventricular failure, perhaps secondary to acute elevations in pulmonary vascular resistance. The increased pulmonary vascular resistance may be due to both 1) acute air trapping that increases total lung capacity and passive increases in pulmonary artery pressure, and 2) thromboxane-mediated vasoconstriction, as discussed in Chapter 3.

Delage and coworkers reported direct histochemical evidence of varying degrees of early myocardial damage in 24 of 30 patients who died from drug-induced anaphylactic shock (Delage et al., 1973). The exact pathophysiologic cause of the histochemical changes is unknown; however, there was no anatomic evidence of preexisting heart disease in any of the 30 patients studied. Although 20 patients received catecholamines for resuscitation, no myocardial changes, such as focal myocytolysis, which has been described in association with vasopressors, were noted in the sections. Delage and coworkers suggested the myocardial lesions could have been caused by either an immunologic reaction on the myofibers or an effect of the inflammatory mediators.

Gastrointestinal Changes

Additional organ dysfunction has been noted in anaphylaxis, including gross congestion; hyperemia; and edema of the liver, spleen, and other visceral organs (James and Austen, 1964). Eosinophils can be found microscopically in the sinusoids of the spleen, liver, and pulmonary blood vessels.

Hemostatic Changes

In a study of experimentally induced hymenoptera anaphylaxis (bee sting), Smith and coworkers noted that titers of fibrinogen, Factor V, Factor VIII, and, to a lesser extent, high-molecular-weight kininogen, were reduced, whereas titers of plasma prekallikrein and Factor XII were unaltered (Smith et al., 1980). Additional hemostatic defects have been demonstrated in other patients, showing elevated prothrombin times (26.5 seconds with a control of 11.5 seconds) and activated partial thromboplastin times (greater than 120 seconds with a control of 26 seconds) 3 hours after wasp-sting anaphylaxis and persisting 14 hours after the initial sting (Ratnoff and Nossel, 1983). One patient's plasma contained an unknown anticoagulant that interfered with the action of thrombin, impeding the release of fibrinopeptide A from fibrinogen (Ratnoff and Nossel, 1983). This thrombin inhibitor could not be equated with heparin or other known thrombin inhibitors. Ratnoff and Nossel also noted profound reductions in Factor V titers and high-molecular-weight kininogen titers with normal Factor XII titers (Ratnoff and Nossel, 1983). Activation of the coagulation system during anaphylaxis has also been demonstrated in the monkey (Smedegård et al., 1980).

# 3

Mediators of Anaphylactic Reactions

The life-threatening responses during anaphylactic reactions result from cardiovascular and pulmonary dysfunction produced as end-organ responses to the preformed mast cell and basophil granular constituents (stored mediators) and the newly synthesized lipid and protein products (unstored mediators), as shown in Table 3.1. As discussed in Chapter 2, a variety of different mediators can collectively produce the clinical manifestations by mechanisms that include 1) direct stimulation of receptors in the vasculature, heart, or lungs to produce organ dysfunction; 2) orchestration of the activation and migration of other inflammatory cells; and 3) potentiation of the effects or release of secondary mediators. This chapter reviews the effects of the individual mediators.

Multiple clinical observations, clinicopathologic findings, and epidemiologic studies indicate that the cardiovascular system is a primary target organ in anaphylaxis (Levi, 1988). The clinical manifestations of cardiovascular collapse are due to mediator-induced systemic vasodilation, alterations in coronary and pulmonary blood flow, and increases in capillary permeability. The net effect of any mediator on a given vascular bed is the result of multiple actions on both the smooth muscle and underlying endothelium. Therefore, the pathophysiology of the vascular effects will be emphasized. Although most information evaluating the physiologic effects of the mediators is from animal studies, human data will be emphasized. Because histamine is the most extensively studied mediator that can be released both immunologically and by different drugs administered in anesthesia and in the intensive care unit, its effects on human tissues and cardiovascular responses will be considered in depth.

STORED MEDIATORS
Histamine
Biochemistry

Histamine is an imidazolylethylamine with a molecular weight of 111 daltons. It is stored predominantly in tissue mast cells and circulating basophils (Beaven et al., 1982). Histamine comprises 5% to 10% of the human mast cell

Table 3.1 Biologic Actions and Clinical Manifestations of Mast Cell/Basophil Mediators

Mediators	Biologic Actions	Manifestations
Histamine	Smooth muscle relaxation	Vasodilation, hypotension
	Smooth muscle contraction	Bronchospasm, coronary spasm, increased GI motility
	Increases capillary permeability	Angioedema, urticaria, efflux of inflammatory cells
	Positive inotropic	Increased myocardial contractility
	Positive chronotropic	Tachycardia
ECF-A	Eosinophil chemotaxis	Inflammation
NCA	Neutrophil chemotaxis	Inflammation
Neutral proteases	Proteolysis	Inflammation
Heparin	Anticoagulant	Coagulopathy
Newly synthesized		
Prostaglandin D_2	Smooth muscle relaxation	Vasodilation, hypotension
	Smooth muscle contraction	Bronchospasm, coronary spasm, increased GI motility
	Stimulates mucus secretion	Broncho/rhinorrhea
	Enhances basophil mediator release	Potentiates reactions
	Inhibits platelet aggregation	Not known
Leukotrienes (C_4, D_4, E_4)	Smooth muscle relaxation	Vasodilation, hypotension
	Smooth muscle contraction	Bronchospasm, coronary spasm, increased GI motility
	Increases capillary permeability	Angioedema, urticaria, efflux of inflammatory cells
	Stimulates mucus secretion	Broncho/rhinorrhea
	Negative inotropic	Myocardial depression, hypotension
PAF	Smooth muscle relaxation	Vasodilation, hypotension
	Smooth muscle contraction	Bronchospasm, coronary spasm, increased GI motility
	Increases capillary permeability	Angioedema, urticaria, efflux of inflammatory cells
	Negative inotropic	Myocardial depression, hypotension
	Neutrophil aggregation	Neutrophil activation
	Platelet aggregation	Platelet activation

ECF-A = eosinophilic chemotactic factor of anaphylaxis; GI = gastrointestinal; NCA = neutrophilic chemotactic factor; PAF = platelet-activating factor.

granule by weight and is ionically bound in mast cell granules by the proteoglycan heparin (Wasserman, 1983). Human lung, intestine, and skin contain high concentrations of histamine stored in tissue-fixed mast cells (Metcalf, 1982; Schleimer et al., 1983a; 1984). The average histamine content of human lung mast cells is about 4 picograms per cell but varies between 1 and 15 pg per cell (Schleimer et al., 1984). Circulating basophils also contain high concentrations of histamine stored in the cytoplasmic granules, averaging 1 pg of histamine per cell (Metcalf, 1982).

The heart itself also contains large quantities of histamine; human right atrial tissue contains 0.9 to 2.8 µg/g (Rydzynski et al., 1988; Wolff and Levi, 1986). Histamine and mast cells are distributed with a craniocaudal, right-to-left gradient; the right atrium has the highest concentration of histamine and the greatest number of mast cells; the left ventricle has the least (Rydzynski et al., 1988; Wolff and Levi, 1986). Wolff and Levi suggest that mast cells are an important repository of cardiac histamine (Wolff and Levi, 1986). The proximity of large quantities of histamine to the sinoatrial and atrioventricular nodes sets the stage for dysrhythmias and ischemia on cardiac mast cell degranulation.

Other tissues have been suggested to contain non–mast-cell histamine or to have the capability for rapid histamine biosynthesis (Beaven, 1976). Vascular endothelium, smooth muscle (Olridge and Hollis, 1982), and endocardial tissue are all potential sites of histamine biosynthesis; however, the exact role or clinical importance of non–mast-cell histamine is presently unknown.

Histamine Receptors

Histamine acts predominantly on two distinct (H_1 and H_2) receptors in different tissues, as shown in Table 3.2. A third H_3 receptor has also been identified. H_1 receptor stimulation produces a variety of adverse effects, including bronchial constriction, increased capillary permeability, coronary vasoconstriction, prostaglandin generation, and enhanced migration of polymorphonuclear leukocytes (Levi et al., 1991; Reinhardt and Borchard, 1982). H_1 receptor-mediated effects on the endothelial cells produce partial disconnection along intercellular junctions of postcapillary venules causing endothelial leaks and increased capillary permeability (Hill, 1990; Majno and Palade, 1961; Majno et al., 1967). This is manifested as either edema formation or wheals. Histamine also causes variable effects on the coronary and pulmonary vasculature depending on the combined effects of H_1 and H_2 stimulation on vascular endothelium and smooth muscle (see following section). H_2 receptor-mediated effects include gastric acid secretion, pulmonary and coronary artery dilation, and positive chronotropic and inotropic effects (Bristow et al., 1982; Reinhardt and Borchard, 1982). H_2 receptor stimulation on mast cells inhibits activation, similar to β_2-adrenergic receptor stimulation (Boyce, 1982; Bristow et al., 1982). H_2 receptor stimulation also inhibits T cell lymphocyte function. Vasodilation of capillaries and venules as well as local cutaneous reactions (wheal and flare) are mediated by both H_1 and H_2 receptor effects (Plaut, 1979; Powell and Brody, 1976). The

Table 3.2 Distribution of H_1 and H_2 Receptors in Different Organ Systems

Organ	Type of Receptor	Histamine-mediated Response
Arteries		
Great	H_1	Vasoconstriction
Small	H_1 and H_2	Vasodilation
Bronchi	H_1 (predominant)	Bronchoconstriction
	H_2 (small fraction)	Bronchoconstriction
Gastric mucosa	H_2	Stimulation of gastric acid production
Heart	H_1	Prolongation of atrioventricular conduction time
	H_1	Coronary vasoconstriction
	H_2	Positive chronotropic effect
	H_2	Positive inotropic effect
	H_2	Adenylate cyclase stimulation of ventricle
	H_1 and H_2	Coronary and pulmonary vasodilation
Mast cells	H_2	Feedback control of histamine release
Venules	H_1	Increased capillary permeability
	H_1 and H_2	Vasodilation

Data from Levi R, Rubin LE, Gross SS. Histamine in cardiovascular function and dysfunction: recent developments. In: Uvnäs B, ed. Handbook of Experimental Pharmacology, Vol 97, Histamine and Histamine Antagonists. Berlin: Springer-Verlag, 1991; Reinhardt D, Borchard V. H_1 receptor antagonists: comparative pharmacology and clinical use. Klin Wochenschr 1982;60: 983–90.

H_3 receptor is thought to be involved in the modulation of neurotransmission and may inhibit mast-cell discharge (Ishikawa and Sperelakis, 1987).

Metabolism

Histamine is rapidly metabolized by tissue enzymatic pathways. Enzymatic destruction of histamine occurs by either ring methylation by histamine N-methyltransferase or oxidative deamination by histaminase (diamine oxidase) (Khandelwal et al., 1982). Rapid tissue uptake and metabolism of histamine produces a short duration of effects. The half-life of histamine in plasma is 102 to 120 seconds (Ind et al., 1982; Lorenz and Doenicke, 1981; Pollock and Murdoch, 1989). The vascular endothelium appears to be the site for histamine metabolism (Gill et al., 1989).

Persistent hypotension and cardiovascular dysfunction during anaphylaxis suggest the effects of other vasoactive mediators, because cardiovascular changes in humans subside within 5 minutes after a histamine infusion is stopped (Vigorito et al., 1983). The body has an amazing capacity for metabolizing histamine to ensure that circulating levels remain relatively low. An elevation of plasma histamine levels implies a significant release from storage sites. To raise plasma histamine levels 1 ng/mL in a 70 kg subject, an infusion rate of 0.1 μg/kg/min was required (Kaliner et al., 1982). Thus, over the course of 30 minutes, 210,000 nanograms were required to sustain this elevation. At an infusion rate of 0.25 μg/kg/min, a dose of 500,000 ng was necessary to increase plasma histamine to 2.5 ng/mL. Sensitive radioenzymatic assays using isolated enzymatic preparations of histamine N-methyltransferase improved the ability to measure histamine release during allergic reactions and during administration of anesthetic drugs (Beaven et al., 1982; Faraj et al., 1983). All muscle relaxants may inhibit histamine N-methyltransferase in vitro and interfere with the radioenzymatic histamine measurement (Futo et al., 1990), but there is no evidence for any in vivo clinical significance (Levy and Adelson, in press). The development of a new radioimmunoassay provides a new, more sensitive method of assaying histamine in plasma (McBride et al., 1988).

Cardiovascular Effects

Hemodynamic Effects in Humans   In volunteers, the intravenous administration of histamine caused vasodilation in systemic arterial and vascular capacitance beds that led to a decrease in intraventricular and systemic blood pressure without effects on pulmonary artery pressure (Marshall, 1984; Vigorito et al., 1983). Increases in histamine levels correlate with hemodynamic manifestations and symptoms (Table 3.3). Although histamine levels of 40 to 140 ng/mL have been reported during human anaphylaxis, small increases in plasma histamine may be associated with hemodynamic changes (see Table 3.3) (Moss et al., 1981; Smith et al., 1980).

Table 3.3   Correlations of Human Plasma Histamine Levels and Symptoms

Condition	Level (ng/mL)
Baseline levels	0.6 ± 0.2
30% increase in heart rate	1.6 ± 0.3
Significant flush, headache	2.39 ± 0.5
30% increase in pulse pressure	2.45 ± 0.3
Increased LV dP/dt, hypotension	4.6 ± 2
Severe hypotension	> 12

Data from Kaliner M, Sigler R, Summers R, Shelhamer JH. Effects of infused histamine: analysis of the effects of H-1 and H-2 histamine receptor antagonists on cardiovascular and pulmonary responses. J Allergy Clin Immunol 1981;68:365–71; Kaliner M, Shelhamer JH, Ottesen EA. Effects of infused histamine: correlation of plasma histamine levels and symptoms. J Allergy Clin Immunol 1982;69:283–9; Lörenz W, Doenicke A, Schoning B, Neugebauer E. The role of histamine in adverse reactions to intravenous agents. In: Thornton JA, ed. Adverse Reactions of Anaesthetic Drugs. Amsterdam: Elsevier/North Holland Biomedical Press, 1981;169–238; Vigorito C, Russo P, Picotti GB, Chiariello M, Poto S, Marone G. Cardiovascular effects of histamine infusion in man. J Cardiovasc Pharmacol 1983;5:531–7.

The most extensive hemodynamic data was reported by Vigorito and co-workers, who administered histamine in four patients undergoing diagnostic cardiac catheterization with normal left ventricular function. Histamine was infused intravenously for 3.5 to 7 minutes at the rate of 0.4 μg/kg/min, producing histamine levels of 4.6 ± 2 ng/mL (mean ± standard deviation). They noted a significant decrease in systolic, diastolic, and mean aortic pressure, systemic vascular resistance, left ventricular end-diastolic pressure, and stroke index and a significant increase in heart rate, cardiac output, and left ventricular dP/dT max (Table 3.4). There were no significant changes in mean pulmonary artery pressure or pulmonary vascular resistance. Plasma norepinephrine but not epinephrine increased significantly. All of the hemodynamic changes started 1 to 2 minutes after the onset of the histamine infusion and returned to baseline within 5 minutes after discontinuation. One patient progressed from first- to third-degree atrioventricular block during the infusion but recovered after it was stopped. The authors concluded that the cardiovascular changes noted were attributable to both a direct effect of histamine and an increase in sympathoadrenergic activity (Vigorito et al., 1983).

Effect on Conduction in the Heart Histamine has a positive chronotropic effect on the sinoatrial node (Wolff and Levi, 1986). This positive chronotropic

Table 3.4 Human Cardiovascular Effects of 0.4 μg/kg/min Histamine Infusion

Parameter	Resting	Histamine Infusion
Heart rate (beats/min)	68 ± 10	97 ± 10
Systolic arterial pressure	137 ± 23	96 ± 21
Diastolic arterial pressure	73 ± 14	47 ± 13
Mean arterial pressure	97 ± 8	61 ± 17
Cardiac index (L/min/m^2)	3.4 ± 0.5	4.2 ± .5
Stroke index (mL/m^2)	50 ± 3	44 ± 3
LVEDP (mmHg)	9 ± 2	4 ± 2
LV dP/dt$_{max}$ (mmHg)	1544 ± 244	1846 ± 335
Systemic vascular resistance	1306 ± 201	656 ± 103
Pulmonary vascular resistance	89 ± 32	75 ± 26
Mean pulmonary artery pressure	13 ± 4	11 ± 2
Histamine (ng/mL)	0.4 ± 0.2	4.6 ± 2
Norepinephrine (pg/mL)	333 ± 19	535 ± 34
Epinephrine (pg/mL)	79 ± 16	80 ± 30

Values expressed as mean ± standard deviation. LVEDP = left ventricular end-diastolic pressure; LV dP/dT$_{max}$ = maximum rate of rise of left ventricular pressure.

Modified with permission from Vigorito C, Russo P, Picotti GB, Chiariello M, Poto S, Marone G. Cardiovascular effects of histamine infusion in man. J Cardiovasc Pharmacol 1983;5:531–7.

effect is produced by H_2-receptor stimulation. Histamine's actions on atrioventricular nodal conduction comprise both direct and indirect effects (Borchard et al., 1986; Wolff and Levi, 1986). The net in vivo effect is that histamine slows atrioventricular nodal conduction, which is independent of its effect to increase sinus rate (Levi et al., 1991). The decrease in atrioventricular nodal conduction can produce complete heart block during histamine infusions in volunteers (Vigorito et al., 1983). Sakuma and coworkers suggest that at least part of the negative dromotropic effect of histamine is mediated by adenosine release (Sakuma et al., 1988). Histamine enhances normal automaticity in sinoatrial and atrioventricular node cells and Purkinje fibers whereas it induces normal automaticity in atrial and ventricular cells (Wolff and Levi, 1986). The enhancement of automaticity by histamine has been attributed to an increase in slow inward current associated with an increase in cyclic adenosine monophosphate (cAMP) (Wolff and Levi, 1986).

Effect on Contractility Histamine increases contractility both in vivo and in vitro in human ventricular muscle. The positive inotropic effect of histamine is principally due to an H_2-mediated increase in cAMP, a mechanism analogous to β_1-adrenergic stimulation (Bristow et al., 1982; Levi et al., 1991). Investigators have used the H_2-receptor agonists impromidine and dimaprit to increase contractility in patients with ventricular dysfunction.

Effect on Regional Vascular Beds The effects of histamine on specific regional vascular beds are variable. Levi and coworkers emphasized that histamine can elicit either vasoconstriction, vasodilation, or a combination of both depending on the dose, route of administration, anatomic location, caliber, and tone of the vessel (Levi et al., 1991). Histamine's net effect on a given regional vascular bed is the result of multiple actions on the smooth muscle and underlying endothelium (Figure 3.1). H_1 receptors on vascular smooth muscle mediate constriction whereas (H_2 receptors) mediate relaxation. Endothelial H_1 receptors promote vasorelaxation through the release of endothelium-derived relaxing factors or prostacyclin (Figures 3.1 and 3.2). Transmembrane signaling mechanisms thought to be involved in the actions of histamine on vascular smooth muscle include phosphoinositide hydrolysis (H_1-mediated vasoconstriction), an increase in cyclic guanosine monophosphate (endothelium-derived relaxing factor-dependent, H_1-mediated vasorelaxation by cyclic guanosine monophosphate [cGMP] production), and an increase in cAMP (H_2-mediated vasorelaxation by cAMP production) (Levi et al., 1991).

When endothelium is removed, the vasculature reacts to histamine with a contractile or a dilatatory response depending on which of the two histamine receptor subtypes predominates in the smooth muscle. Even when the endothelium is intact, however, the release of endothelium-derived relaxing factors may be insufficient to offset the H_1-mediated vasoconstriction (Levi et al., 1991). Vasodilation may also result from the inhibition of sympathetic tone by an action of histamine H_3 receptors on perivascular nerve terminals (Ishikawa and Spere-

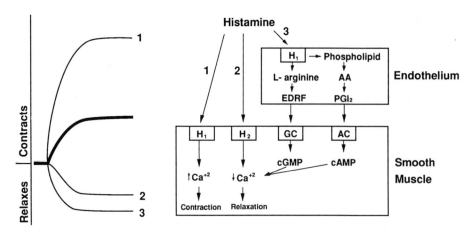

Figure 3.1 Schematic representation of the potential effects of histamine on vascular beds. Histamine produces vascular responses that are the result of multiple actions on the smooth muscle and endothelium (right), which are manifested as vascular relaxation or contraction (left). H_1 receptor stimulation of vascular smooth muscle produces vascular contraction, whereas H_2 receptor stimulation produces relaxation. Stimulation of endothelial H_1 receptors releases endothelium-derived relaxing factor (EDRF) (which derives from L-arginine by the action of nitric oxide synthetase) or prostacyclin (PGI_2). EDRF (nitric oxide) activates guanylate cyclase (GC), which generates cGMP, whereas PGI_2 activates adenylate cyclase (AC), which generates cAMP. The heavy line represents the observed response to histamine predominantly in human coronary arteries, especially those affected by atherosclerotic vascular disease with impaired H_1 receptor-mediated endothelial responses, as shown in reaction 3. The net effect of histamine on different vascular beds in humans with normal vascular endothelium is shown in reactions 2 and 3, which produce predominantly vascular relaxation and vasodilation. *Modified from Levi R, Rubin LE, Gross SS. Histamine in cardiovascular function and dysfunction: recent developments. In: Uvnäs B, ed. Handbook of Experimental Pharmacology, Vol 97, Histamine and Histamine Antagonists. Berlin: Springer-Verlag, 1991; Toda N. Mechanism of histamine actions in human coronary arteries. Circ Res 1987;61:280–6.*

lakis, 1987). Levi and coworkers have suggested that the reported variability of histamine's effects on specific vascular beds and in vessels of different tissues may simply reflect the predominance of one component over another and the loss of relaxing factors due to endothelial destruction from vascular disease (Levi et al., 1991). The specific vascular effects of histamine in different tissues will be considered. Only human data will be reported.

Effects on Coronary Arteries Histamine produces a dose-dependent contraction of isolated human coronary arteries (Ginsburg et al., 1980; 1981; Kalsner and Richards, 1984; Toda, 1983; 1987). Coronary vasoconstriction is diminished or even reversed by H_1 receptor blockade and potentiated by H_2

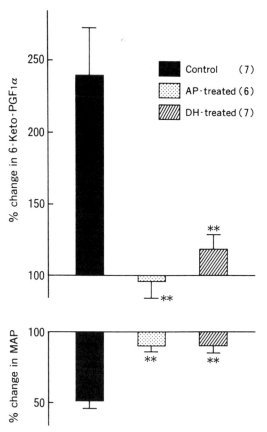

Figure 3.2 Changes (%) in plasma 6-keto-PGF$_{1\alpha}$ concentration (the metabolite of prostacyclin) and in mean arterial pressure (MAP) 2 minutes after bolus administration of 0.6 mg/kg of d-tubocurarine (dTc) in control (left), aspirin-treated (AP) (25 mg/kg) (middle), and diphenhydramine-treated (DH) (1 mg/kg) (right) patients. The values just before dTc administration were taken as 100%. Figures in parentheses indicate the number of patients studied. **$P <$ 0.01, significantly different from control. Pretreatment with aspirin or diphenhydramine attenuated the hypotensive responses to histamine release by dTc by inhibiting either prostacyclin synthesis or decreasing endothelial H$_1$ receptor stimulation. *Reprinted with permission from Hatano Y, Arai T, Noda J, et al. Contribution of prostacyclin to d–tubocurarine-induced hypotension in humans. Anesthesiology 1990;72: 28–32.*

receptor antagonists or endothelium removal (Toda, 1983; 1987; 1988; Keitolu et al., 1988). H$_1$-mediated coronary vasoconstriction is the predominant effect of histamine in humans, however, vasodilating receptors on the smooth muscle (H$_2$) and the endothelium (H$_1$) modulate this effect (see Figure 3.1).

The contribution of endothelium-derived relaxing factor to the coronary vasomotor action of histamine also depends on vascular caliber (Levi et al., 1991). Potassium-constricted human proximal and distal epicardial coronary artery rings that have an intimal thickness less than 200 μm respond to histamine with an endothelium-dependent relaxation, whereas thicker segments respond with a contraction (Keitolu et al., 1988). The magnitude of histamine-induced relaxation is inversely correlated with intimal thickness; the thicker the intima, the smaller the relaxant effect. Levi and coworkers suggest that intimal thickening serves as a diffusional barrier to the short-lived endothelium-derived relaxing factor (Levi et al., 1991). It may also explain why histamine constricts the proximal human coronary artery more than the distal one (Ginsburg et al., 1981).

Coronary vessels obtained from people who died from coronary artery disease contain much more histamine than vessels from people who died from other causes (Kalsner and Richards, 1984). The availability of histamine from cardiac stores and in the perivascular spaces in cardiac patients and the loss of endothelium-dependent vasodilation increases the likelihood that coronary spasm may ensue with its sudden release; this could precipitate angina and potentially fatal dysrhythmias. In a patient with a history of coronary spasm who succumbed to sudden cardiac death, coronary artery adventitial mast cells were found to be greatly increased in number, particularly in the region of narrowing (Forman et al., 1985). Moreover, mast cell degranulation has been confirmed in myocardial biopsies from patients with angina (Dvorak, 1986).

Effects on Coronary Blood Flow Differences between the effects of histamine on proximal and distal coronary arteries are even more pronounced in vivo. Histamine injected into patients with *normal* coronary arteries during cardiac catheterization at a dose of 4 µg produces significant increases in coronary blood flow (65% ± 6%) and a decrease in coronary vascular resistance (-40% ± 3%) with minor changes in the RR interval and mean arterial pressure (Vigorito et al., 1987). H_2 receptor blockade with cimetidine did not affect these changes, whereas H_1 receptor blockade with diphenhydramine significantly reduced the histamine-induced increase in coronary blood flow and decrease in coronary vascular resistance. Histamine-induced coronary vascular changes persisted after H_2 receptor blockade. In patients with normal coronary arteries, Vigorito and coworkers demonstrated that histamine induces a direct dilation of the small resistance coronary arteries that is predominantly, but not completely, mediated by H_1 receptor responses (Vigorito et al., 1987).

The same investigators also evaluated selective H_1 receptor activation on coronary hemodynamics in patients with normal coronary arteries and those with spontaneous angina with coronary artery disease (Vigorito et al., 1986). Selective H_1 receptor stimulation was achieved by infusing 0.5 µg/kg/min of histamine intravenously for 5 minutes after pretreatment with the H_2 receptor antagonist cimetidine at a massive dose of 25 mg/kg. Heart rate was maintained constant by coronary sinus pacing. In patients with normal coronary arteries, mean arterial pressure fell from 99 ± 5 to 77 ± 4 mmHg. Coronary vascular resistance decreased from 1.07 ± 0.17 to 0.82 ± 0.14 mmHg/mL/min. Coronary blood flow and myocardial oxygen consumption remained unchanged. None of the patients with normal coronary arteries developed angina during histamine infusion. In the five patients with spontaneous angina, however, four of whom had significant ($> 70\%$) coronary artery stenosis and one of whom had normal coronary arteries, two (40%) developed angina during histamine infusion accompanied by ST-T elevation, a decrease in coronary blood flow, and a decrease in coronary vascular resistance without significant average changes in hemodynamics. In one of the two patients, circumflex coronary artery spasm was demonstrated angiographically during histamine-induced angina.

Vigorito and coworkers suggest that H_1 receptor stimulation induces a reduction in coronary vascular resistance, probably resulting from vasodilation of small coronary resistance vessels (Vigorito et al., 1986). H_1 receptor-induced vasoconstriction of large capacitance coronary arteries may prevail over peripheral vasodilation in patients with vasospastic angina, however. The pathophysiologic effects of histamine on coronary blood flow may have practical relevance, especially in patients undergoing treatment with H_2 receptor-blocking drugs (Vigorito et al., 1986). The response is most likely due to stimulating vasoconstricting H_1 receptors of large epicardial coronary arteries; however, in some patients there may also be a change of geometry or stenosis secondary to hypotension, peripheral coronary vasodilation, or the loss of endothelium-derived relaxing factors due to atherosclerotic disease. The data also support the concept that histamine may precipitate coronary artery spasm in patients with vasospastic angina with or without coronary artery disease who are undergoing treatment with H_2 receptor-blocking drugs.

Effects on Pulmonary Vessels Histamine can produce dual effects on the pulmonary vasculature. In vitro, histamine is a more potent constrictor than prostaglandin F2α (PGF2α), serotonin, or angiotensin II (Boe, 1983). Potassium-depolarized ring preparations from human intralobar pulmonary arteries and veins, presumably with intact endothelium, have also been reported to relax in response to low histamine concentrations and contract when exposed to higher ones; pretreatment with histamine H_1 receptor antagonists inhibits both phases (Mikkelsen et al., 1984). Removal of the endothelium or treatment with indomethacin abolishes the histamine-induced relaxation and potentiates the vasoconstriction of human pulmonary artery, suggesting that prostacyclin mediates the vasodilating effect of histamine (Schellenberg et al., 1986). Histamine releases prostacyclin from human endothelial cells in culture (Baenziger et al., 1980; 1981). When infused to levels of 4.6 ± 2 ng/mL in volunteers, histamine did not increase pulmonary artery pressures or pulmonary vascular resistance (Vigorito et al., 1986).

Effects on Vascular Permeability Histamine H_1 receptor stimulation produces increased capillary permeability and leakage of plasma proteins from various vascular beds. This change in vascular permeability occurs in postcapillary venules and is produced by endothelial cell contraction and the formation of junctional gaps of up to 1 μm between adjacent endothelial cells (Hill, 1990). This represents a pharmacologic effect of histamine on the contractile state of the endothelium rather than pathologic damage. Endothelial cells possess the necessary contractile proteins, actin and myosin, for such a mechanism, and H_1 receptors have been detected in endothelial cells.

Effects on Veins H_1-mediated contraction and H_2-mediated relaxation of de-endothelialized segments of human saphenous vein have been reported (Schoeffter and Godfraine, 1989).

Pulmonary Effects

Histamine stimulates airway smooth muscle contraction through H_1 receptor activation and increases pulmonary epithelial permeability when infused intravascularly or inhaled (Rafferty and Holgate, 1989). Histamine can also modulate prostaglandin production from lung mast cells by an H_1 receptor-mediated effect. Many additional mediators, including prostaglandins and leukotrienes, contract airway smooth muscle directly, increase microvascular leakage, increase airway mucous secretion, and attract and activate other inflammatory cells, however (see Table 2.6). Barnes suggests that although a single mediator may have widespread effects, it is unlikely that it could account for all of the pulmonary dysfunction in asthma or even anaphylaxis (Barnes, 1989a). Even though potent antihistamines may attenuate the immediate bronchoconstrictor response to an allergen, they do not have a beneficial effect in clinical asthma. Therefore, as Barnes suggests, it is possible that interaction between histamine and other inflammatory mediators might account for the bronchoconstriction, increased airway secretion, microvascular leakage, and chemotaxis of other inflammatory cells.

Chemotactic Factors

Because mast cell degranulation results in the influx of eosinophils, neutrophils, and lymphocytes, mast cells can recruit these secondary cells to the sites of immediate hypersensitivity reactions by releasing chemotactic factors (Serafin and Austen, 1987). A chemotactic factor stimulates the directed migration of cells from a region of low mediator concentration to one of high concentration. Both neutrophilic and eosinophilic factors have been described. Eosinophilic chemotactic factor of anaphylaxis is an acidic peptide with a molecular weight of 500 to 600 daltons; stored in the mast cell granules, it is chemotactic for eosinophils (Wasserman et al., 1974; Wasserman, 1983a). The exact role of the eosinophil in the allergic response is not clear; however, during phagocytosis, eosinophils release histaminase and arylsulfatase (Schatz et al., 1978). These enzymes can inactivate histamine and leukotrienes and may function to limit the inflammatory response.

Different factors released after mast cell activation have been demonstrated to possess both chemotactic and chemokinetic activity for neutrophilic polymorphonuclear leukocytes in humans (Atkins and Wasserman, 1983; Wasserman, 1983a). Although other mast-cell-derived factors, including oxidative products of arachidonic acid, platelet-activating factor, or histamine, possess neutrophil-directed activities, a high-molecular-weight neutrophilic chemotactic factor is also liberated after immunoglobulin E (IgE) or mast-cell-mediated reactions (Wasserman, 1983a). This factor is released into the circulation 1 to 5 minutes after mast cell activation; its peak activity occurs within 5 to 15 minutes and persists for up to several hours (Wasserman, 1983a). Although the exact role of chemotactic factors in anaphylaxis is unclear, they may help modulate the appearance and functions of released mediators, interact to promote further tissue destruction to prolong the local inflammatory response, or help terminate the local effects of mediators (Atkins and Wasserman, 1983). They also produce the second wave of inflammation, occurring 3 to 6 hours after antigen challenge to produce the late-phase reactions and ongoing inflammation after anaphylaxis.

Enzyme Mediators

Tryptase, chymase, lung Hageman activator, acid hydrolases, and peroxidase are stored in the secretory granules of mast cells and basophils (Schwartz, 1983; 1990; Wasserman, 1983a). The role of these different enzymes is uncertain, but they may suppress coagulation and fibrin deposition at mast cell sites and recruit other inflammatory mediators to amplify inflammatory pathways (Schwartz, 1983). Tryptase and chymase are found in human mast cells only, except for minute quantities in basophils (0.04 pg/cell) (Matsson et al., 1991). Tryptase is present in mucosal mast cells of the small bowel and lung and skin mast cells at concentrations of 10 to 35 pg/cell (Matsson et al., 1991). Tryptase is a tetrameric protease with a molecular weight of 134,000 (Matsson et al., 1991). Normal tryptase levels in serum or plasma are less than 2.5 ng/mL, although levels greater than 10 ng/mL have been found in all patients with anaphylaxis and may reach as high as 1000 ng/mL (Schwartz et al., 1987; Schwartz, 1990). Schwartz suggests that tryptase levels can first be detected within 15 to 30 minutes after antigenic challenge, peak at 1 to 2 hours, and decline with a half-life of about 2 hours (Schwartz et al., 1989; Schwartz, 1990). This is in marked contrast to histamine, which peaks within minutes and can be released by nonimmunologic stimuli. Tryptase is released from mast cells only and provides a useful diagnostic tool to evaluate suspected anaphylactic reactions (see Chapter 7).

Heparin

Heparin, a proteoglycan ionically bound to histamine in granules, is stored in human lung and cutaneous mast cells. These cells contain approximately 5 μg of heparin (molecular weight 60,000 daltons) per 1,000,000 cells (Metcalf, 1982). Heparin used in clinical practice is derived from both cow and pig lungs because of the high mast cell content. Human basophils do not contain heparin as the proteoglycan; they contain chondroitin 4 and 6 sulfates, which possess a molecular weight of 300,000 (Wasserman, 1983a).

SYNTHESIZED MEDIATORS

Additional lipid-derived and protein-derived mediators are not formed until mast cell or basophil activation. The lipid mediators synthesized de novo include arachidonic acid metabolites and the phospholipid derivative platelet-activating factor. The kinins can be formed from their larger molecular weight precursors. Both lipid-derived and peptide-derived mediators will be reviewed.

Arachidonic Acid Metabolites

After IgE–antigen interactions in mast cells and basophils, arachidonic acid is liberated from membrane lipids by phospholipase A_2 or phospholipase C and diacylglycerol lipase (Mathé et al., 1977; Parker, 1982; Serafin and Austen, 1987). Arachidonic acid is processed into cyclooxygenase products, including prostaglandins, thromboxanes, and prostacyclin, and 5-lipoxygenase products—leukotrienes. Both cyclooxygenase and lipoxygenase are enzymes that catalyze the stereospecific insertion of molecular oxygen into various positions of arachidonic acid (Lewis et al., 1990). The 5-lipoxygenase and cyclooxygenase products will be considered separately.

Leukotrienes

The involvement of mast cells, basophils, and eosinophils, all of which can produce leukotrienes, has implicated their role in allergic disease (Lewis et al., 1990). Leukotrienes are potent mediators, requiring only nanomolar concentrations to produce their effects. Composed of fatty acids with sulfidopeptide linkages, they are synthesized by the oxidative metabolism of arachidonic acid through the 5-lipoxygenase pathway, a calcium-dependent pathway (Lewis et al., 1990). Slow-reacting substance of anaphylaxis (SRS-A), generated during antigenic challenge of sensitized lung, is composed of three leukotrienes (leukotrienes C_4, D_4, and E_4) (Goetzl, 1980). Leukotrienes have been studied both in vitro and in vivo and will be considered separately.

Leukotriene B_4 Experimentally, leukotriene B_4 has only weak direct effects on smooth muscle, but induces prolonged bronchoconstriction by stimulating the cyclooxygenation of endogenous arachidonic acid and thromboxane generation locally in airway tissues, producing neutrophil influx, edema formation, and increased airway mucus secretion (Goetzl, 1980; 1984). In animal models, leukotriene B_4 causes a conspicuous and reversible adhesion of leukocytes to the endothelium in postcapillary venules (Dahlén et al., 1981). Although it has no effect on coronary artery blood flow or myocardial contractility when injected into the circumflex coronary artery of sheep, leukotriene B_4 caused profound neutropenia, reflecting the potent chemotactic and chemokinetic properties of this compound (Michelassi et al., 1983).

Leukotriene C_4 Mast cells and polymorphonuclear leukocytes are thought to synthesize leukotriene C_4 in humans. Leukotriene C_4 is the predominant product of IgE–antigen-activated pulmonary mast cells (Samuelsson et al., 1980). Inhaled, it is a potent bronchoconstrictor, affecting small airways more than large ones, and is 600 to 9500 times more potent than histamine in producing decreases in maximal expiratory flow rate at 30% of vital capacity above residual volume (Weiss et al., 1982). The effects have a slow onset with changes occurring at 10 minutes, peak effects near 15 minutes, and changes persisting for 25 to 30 minutes (Weiss et al., 1982). In animal experiments leukotriene C_4 produced coronary artery vasoconstriction and negative inotropic effects when infused into circumflex coronary arteries (Burke et al., 1982; Ezra et al., 1983; Michelassi et al., 1983). In the hamster cheek pouch model, increased capillary permeability resulted from postcapillary venules after infusion (Dahlén et al., 1981). Injection of leukotriene C_4 into monkeys produced bronchoconstriction and decreased pulmonary dynamic compliance; its cardiovascular effects were transient pulmonary and systemic hypertension followed by a prolonged hypotensive period associated with decreased cardiac output, hemoconcentration, and leukopenia (Smedegard et al., 1982). In human endothelial cells, leukotrienes C_4 and D_4 stimulate platelet-activating factor release, which activates neutrophils and platelets (McIntyre et al., 1986b).

Leukotriene D_4 Leukotriene D_4 produces potent constriction of bronchial smooth muscle, affecting small airways more than large ones. Its peak effect is appreciable within 2 to 7 minutes and returns to baseline by 14 minutes (Weiss et al., 1983). On a molar basis administered by inhalation, it is 5900 times as potent as histamine in producing an identical decrement in maximal expiratory flow rate at 30% of control vital capacity above residual volume, a measure of airway constriction (Weiss et al., 1983). Leukotriene D_4 produces other systemic effects including pulmonary vasoconstriction, decreased lung compliance, and increased microvascular permeability (Casey et al., 1982; Dahlén et al., 1981; Hanna et al., 1981). Michelassi and coworkers, while studying the effects of leukotriene D_4 in animals, demonstrated potent coronary vasoconstriction as well as impaired regional ventricular wall motion (Michelassi et al., 1983).

Cyclooxygenase Products

Prostaglandins, prostacyclin, and thromboxane are unsaturated fatty acids synthesized de novo from arachidonic acid by the enzyme cyclooxygenase during an anaphylactic reaction (Mathé et al., 1977). Prostaglandins are potent mediators of the inflammatory response and can induce bronchospasm, pulmonary artery hypertension, and peripheral vasodilation. Mast cells in human lung parenchyma may be major source of prostaglandin synthesis. Anaphylactic challenge of human lung tissue in vitro primarily liberates prostaglandin D_2, but also liberates thromboxane A_2 and prostaglandin $F_{2\alpha}$ (Adkinson et al., 1980). Human lung contains macrophages and endothelial cells in addition to mast cells, which may account for the thromboxane A_2 release.

Prostaglandin D_2 Mast cells are the major source of prostaglandin D_2 (Wasserman, 1983a). Prostaglandin D_2 increases nondirected migration of polymorphonuclear leukocytes and inhibits enzyme release induced by other agents. Prostaglandin D_4 causes bronchoconstriction in the lungs, producing a significant fall in specific airway conductance when inhaled by normal patients (Hardy et al., 1984). In the vasculature, prostaglandin D_2 produces slight enhancement of microvascular permeability and systemic vasodilation. Intradermal injection produces cutaneous vasodilation and a wheal and flare response (Lewis and Austen, 1984; Stenson and Parker, 1983).

Prostaglandin E_2 Mast cells and neutrophils are the major synthetic source of prostaglandin E_2 (Stenson and Parker, 1983), which inhibits mitogenesis, lymphokine production, cytotoxicity, and antibody production and stimulates differentiation of lymphocytes while stimulating nondirected migration (chemokinesis) of polymorphonuclear leukocytes (Stenson and Parker, 1983). Prostaglandin E_2 induces fever, erythema, and increased vascular permeability (Stenson and Parker, 1983). On mast cells, it inhibits antigen-induced histamine release and activation (Tauber et al., 1973). Prostaglandin E_2 and E_1 are bronchodilators (Rosenthal et al., 1971), blocking antigen-induced histamine release in the vasculature and producing peripheral, coronary, and pulmonary artery vasodilation by direct effects on the vascular smooth muscle (Figure 3.3) (Sczeklik et al., 1978).

Prostaglandin $F_{2\alpha}$ Macrophages and mast cells synthesize prostaglandin $F_{2\alpha}$ (Stenson and Parker, 1983). Its effects on the vasculature include vasoconstriction and slight decrease in microvascular permeability (Mathé et al., 1977; Stenson and Parker, 1983). Prostaglandin $F_{2\alpha}$ is a potent bronchoconstrictor and is presumed to play an important role in asthma (Mathé et al., 1977).

Thromboxane A_2 Neutrophils, platelets, and pulmonary macrophages are the major sources of thromboxane A_2 (Schulman et al., 1981), which produces platelet aggregation, bronchoconstriction, and vasoconstriction. Thromboxane A_2 is a potent pulmonary and coronary artery vasoconstrictor that can initiate coronary spasm, platelet trapping, and additional mediator formation (Levi, 1988). Thromboxane A_2 is also the mediator responsible for pulmonary hypertension after protamine reactions in humans and experimental animals (Conzen et al., 1989; McIntyre et al., 1986a; Morel et al., 1987) (see Figure 3.3).

Prostacyclin (Prostaglandin I_2) Mast cells in human lung and vascular endothelium synthesize prostacyclin during anaphylaxis in vitro, antagonizing many of the effects of thromboxane A_2 (Stenson and Parker, 1983). In addition, stimulation of endothelial H_1 receptors induces prostacyclin synthesis (Figure 3.3) (Baenziger et al., 1980; Hatano et al., 1990). Prostacyclin has direct effects on vascular smooth muscle that increase cAMP and produce vasodilation and increase microvascular permeability (Furchgott and Vanhoutte, 1989; Mathé et al., 1977). Longer-acting analogues of prostacyclin (iloprost) have been used to inhibit platelet aggregation (Kraenzler and Starr, 1988).

Platelet-Activating Factor

Platelet-activating factor (acetyl-glyceryl-ether-phosphoryl-choline), an unstored lipid synthesized in activated neutrophils, monocytes, and platelets by

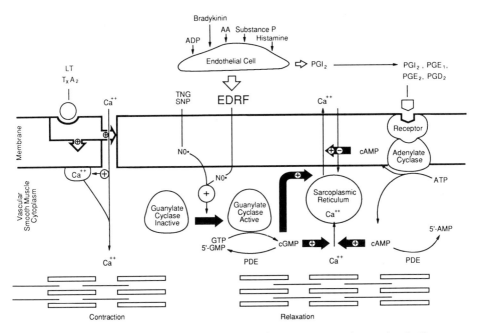

Figure 3.3 The action of any mediator on vascular responses is the result of effects on vascular endothelial cells and direct responses on vascular smooth muscle. Leukotrienes (LT), thromboxane A_2 (TxA_2), and histamine (H_1 receptor effects) produce vascular contraction by increasing calcium release or entry in vascular smooth muscle. Bradykinin, substance P, histamine (H_1 receptor effects), and other mediators stimulate endothelial cells to release both endothelium-derived relaxing factor (EDRF) and prostacyclin (PGI$_2$), which produce vasodilation by vascular relaxation. EDRF, like nitroglycerin (TNG) or sodium nitroprusside (SNP), generates nitric oxide (NO·), which activates guanylate cyclase. Guanylate cyclase generates cGMP, which causes calcium uptake into the sarcoplasmic reticulum and extrusion from the cell to produce vascular relaxation and vasodilation. PGI$_2$, PGE$_1$, and other prostaglandins directly stimulate receptors on vascular smooth muscle that are coupled to adenylate cyclase. Stimulation of these prostaglandin receptors increases cAMP, which also increases calcium uptake into the sarcoplasmic reticulum and extrusion from the cell to produce vascular relaxation and vasodilation. The cyclic nucleotides in vascular smooth muscle cytoplasm are broken down by various phosphodiesterase enzymes (PDE) as shown.

the action of phospholipase A_2 on membrane phospholipids, is an extremely potent biologic material producing physiologic effects at concentrations as low as 10^{-10} M (O'Flaherty and Wykle, 1983; Serafin and Austen, 1987; Wasserman, 1983a). Platelet-activating factor binds, aggregates, and activates human platelets and leukocytes to release inflammatory products (McIntyre et al., 1986b; O'Flaherty and Wykle, 1983). When injected into human skin, as little as 0.2 nmol causes a profound wheal and flare response (Serafin and Austen, 1987; Wasserman, 1983a). In the lung, platelet-activating factor attracts human eosinophils, produces contraction of bronchial smooth muscle, and increases capillary permeability and mucosal edema (Barnes, 1989a). In the heart, platelet-activating factor has a negative inotropic effect in animals and either potentiates or inhibits the effects of other mediators (Levi, 1988). Inhaled platelet-activating factor causes bronchoconstriction and increased bronchial responsiveness (Barnes, 1989a). Leukotrienes C_4 and D_4 release platelet-activating factor from human endothelial cells that bind neutrophils and platelets to create a potentially prothrombotic surface (McIntyre et al., 1986b).

Kinins

Kinins are small-molecular-weight polypeptides that possess many different biologic properties, including contracting or relaxing the smooth muscle, increasing vascular permeability, and producing pain. Bradykinin is a 9 to 11 amino acid peptide with residues that can be liberated from the parent kininogen molecule by different proteases, including kallikrein. Plasma kinins, including prekallikrein and bradykinin, have been identified in anaphylaxis of various species and may be important in the human physiologic response (Brocklehurst and Lahiri, 1952; Eyre and Lewis, 1972). They are low-molecular-weight peptides that dilate certain blood vessels and may constrict small airways. Bradykinin produces endothelium-derived relaxing factor-dependent vasodilation and also contracts endothelial cells, causing the formation of intercellular gaps to enhance capillary permeability. In vitro IgE-mediated release of a prekallikrein activator has been demonstrated from human lung (Meier et al., 1983). Purified human prekallikrein was converted to the active form (kallikrein) by the lung protease. The kallikrein produced was shown to generate bradykinin from purified human high-molecular-weight kininogen. The prekallikrein activator provides a physiologic mechanism by which kallikrein can be formed during anaphylaxis in humans. Several processes independent of IgE can also generate kinins. These are discussed in Chapter 4.

Kinins circulate in plasma as precursors that include a high-molecular-weight kininogen (110,000 d) and a low-molecular-weight kininogen (70,000 daltons). Bradykinin is cleaved from the larger molecule. High-molecular-weight kininogen exists in blood as a complex with prekallikrein or Factor XI (Colman, 1984). Both plasmin and trypsin can liberate kinins from kininogen. Kallikreins are trypsinlike serine proteases that release lys-bradykinin from kininogen and possibly function physiologically in maintaining fluid balance.

Physiologic Effects

Kinins can relax or contract smooth muscle and increase vascular permeability independent of other mediators. Their exact role in the physiology of anaphylaxis and other inflammatory states is unclear, however, perhaps because of the multiplicity of mediators released or the lack of antagonists specific to kinins that would help to define the role that kinins actually play. The mechanisms by which kinins affect cell activity are unclear, but calcium, arachidonic acid, and cyclic nucleotide metabolism all appear to play an important role

(Wiggins and Cochrane, 1984). Kinins appear to act on blood vessels partly through cellular signals such as the release of endothelium-derived relaxing factor and prostaglandins. These messengers alter cyclic nucleotide-dependent protein kinase, which regulates actin–myosin–adenosine triphosphate (ATP) interaction under the influence of different regulatory proteins and mediators.

Kinins alter vascular permeability by endothelial cell contraction of the postcapillary venule, which widens intercellular junctions (Wiggins and Cochrane, 1984). Although the role of the kallikrein–kinin system is poorly understood, bradykinin in the cardiovascular system has direct effects on cardiac muscle, producing dilation of arteries and venoconstriction with an increase in the number of functioning capillaries and increased vascular permeability (Wiggins and Cochrane, 1984).

Metabolism

Different enzymatic systems are responsible for inactivation of the kinins, including a I and II kininase enzyme. Kininase I, or carboxypeptidase N, is a zinc-containing metalloenzyme with a 300,000 molecular weight that is normally present in plasma at a concentration of 30 to 40 μg/mL (Wiggins and Cochrane, 1984). It cleaves the C-terminal amino acid from several biologically active peptides, including bradykinin, lys-bradykinin, fibrinopeptides, and the complement-derived anaphylatoxins C3a, C4a, and C5a (Erdos, 1979). Investigators have demonstrated that protamine inhibits carboxypeptidase-N, implicating this inhibition as one mechanism responsible for protamine reactions (Tan et al., 1989).

Kininase II (angiotensin-converting enzyme) is similar to carboxypeptidase-N. It is a peptidyl dipeptidase with 150,000 molecular weight that cleaves the two C-terminal amino acids (phenylalanine and arginine) from bradykinin to inactivate them (Wiggins and Cochrane, 1984). The active enzyme is present on the surface of endothelial cells, primarily in the lung, the major site of kinin metabolism (Erdos, 1979; Pitt, 1984). The enzyme also cleaves the two C-terminal amino acids to convert angiotensin I to angiotensin II, a potent vasoconstrictor. The angiotensin-converting enzyme (ACE) inhibitors prevent the formation of angiotensin II and also inhibit the breakdown of bradykinin, which may explain the severe angioedema in some patients who receive ACE inhibitors (Orfan et al., 1990).

4

Complement and Contact Activation

The mediators of anaphylaxis can be liberated by other pathways independent of immunoglobulin-E (IgE) antibodies to produce a clinically identical symptom complex. Multiple effector processes can generate biologically active mediators to produce an immediate hypersensitivity reaction that includes 1) activation of the complement cascade by immunoglobulin-G (IgG), immunoglobulin-M (IgM)–antigen interactions, or independent of antibodies; 2) activation of the coagulation and fibrinolytic systems, and the kinin-generating sequence by contact with foreign surfaces; or 3) nonimmunologic (pharmacologic) histamine release by drugs to liberate a similar spectrum of vasoactive substances (Figure 4.1).

Various terms have appeared in the literature to describe immediate hypersensitivity reactions. The most important consideration is whether or not patients have antibodies to the agent in question, because rechallenge in this group of patients produces reactions. The term *anaphylactoid reaction* has been used to describe a clinically indistinguishable syndrome, probably involving similar mediators, but not mediated by IgE antibody and not necessarily requiring previous exposure to the inciting substance (Bochner and Lichtenstein, 1991; Watkins, 1979).

A variety of pathways and agents independent of antibodies may produce anaphylactoid reactions during anesthesia and in the intensive care unit, as outlined in Table 4.1. The coagulation, fibrinolytic, kinin, and complement pathways have important interactions. Activation of any one of these systems may recruit other pathways to provide surface-mediated host defense reactions. These processes have been called the *plasma contact activation system* and each of the component pathways will be reviewed. Nonimmunologic histamine release is considered separately in Chapter 5.

COMPLEMENT SYSTEM

The complement system consists of a series of at least 20 distinct plasma and cell-membrane proteins that can be activated by one of at least two triggering sequences (Ruddy et al., 1972). Complement activation proceeds in a sequential

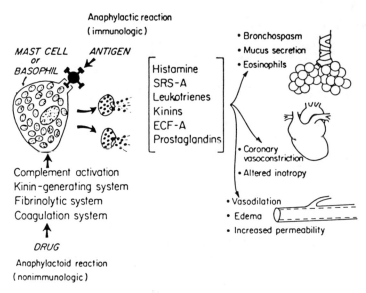

Figure 4.1 A summary of the pathophysiologic changes producing anaphylactic and anaphylactoid reactions. Top left: Anaphylactic reactions. The allergen enters the body and combines with IgE antibodies on the surface of mast cells and basophils. The mast cells and basophils are activated, releasing mediators (histamine, slow reacting substance of anaphylaxis—leukotrienes, kinins, eosinophilic chemotactic factor, prostaglandins, and others). The release of these substances is associated with the signs and symptoms of anaphylaxis—bronchospasm; pharyngeal, glottic, and pulmonary edema; vasodilation; hypotension; alterations in cardiac contractility and dysrhythmias, subcutaneous edema; and urticaria. Bottom left: Anaphylactoid reactions. The offending agent enters the body and works by nonimmunologically activating systems that cause degranulation of mast cells and basophils or activation of other humoral amplification systems. The systems that can be activated to cause release of mediators from basophils and mast cells include the complement system, the coagulation and fibrinolytic system, and the kinin-generating system. Activation of these systems can result in the release of the same mediators from basophils and mast cells, and can result in a syndrome that is clinically indistinguishable from anaphylaxis. *Reprinted with permission from Levy JH, Roizen MF, Morris JM. Anaphylactic and anaphylactoid reactions. Spine 1986;11:282–91.*

fashion comparable to the clotting cascade (Figure 4.2). After activation, the biologic effector proteins 1) lyse susceptible targets, 2) promote phagocytosis by coating targets with complement-derived protein fragments that interact with receptors on phagocytic cells, and 3) generate peptides that recruit the participation of other cellular and humoral effector systems of the inflammatory response (Frank, 1988). The humoral effects of antigen–IgG or antigen–IgM interactions are mediated through the complement system (Frank, 1988; Ruddy et al., 1972). Formation of the complete complement sequence on membranes of bacteria, fungi, red blood cells, or cells of other tissues produces lysis with loss of membrane integrity. Two pathways are known to activate the complement

Table 4.1 Pathogenesis of Anaphylactoid Reactions

Complement activation	Activation of humoral amplification systems
Activation of classical pathway	Coagulation
Heparin-protamine	Fibrinolysis
Plasmin	Kinin activation
Activation of alternative pathway	Direct histamine release
Radiocontrast media	Opioids
Drugs	Muscle relaxants
Protamine	Radiocontrast agents
Endotoxin	Vancomycin
Exotoxin	
Zymosan	

system; they are called *classical* and *alternative*. Each will be considered separately.

Classical Pathway

The classical pathway can be activated by the binding of IgG or IgM to antigens on cellular membranes or in circulation, forming immune complexes (see Figure 4.2). Immunologic activation during antigen–antibody interaction allows binding and assembly of the C1 complex to the tail portion (Fc region) of two IgG molecules or one IgM molecule (Ruddy et al., 1972). The C1 complex contains three individual subunits—C1q, C1r, and C1s—that cross-link with two IgG molecules or one IgM molecule. Once activated, the C1 complex, also called C1 esterase, is capable of interacting with and cleaving the next two proteins in the complement cascade, C4 and C2. The C1 esterase is regulated by the presence of a plasma regulatory protein called the C1 esterase inhibitor or C1 inhibitor (also abbreviated as C1 INH). People who lack a C1 esterase inhibitor or have a defective one have recurrent attacks of swelling called angioedema, especially with oral manipulation (intubation or oral surgery) (see the following section).

The classical complement pathway can be activated nonimmunologically by plasmin (Murano, 1978), heparin–protamine complexes in vitro and in vivo (Best et al., 1983; 1984; Rent et al., 1975), IgG aggregates (Frank, 1988), and activated factor XII (Ghebrehiwit et al., 1981).

Alternative Pathway

The alternative pathway (also called the properiden pathway) can be activated nonimmunologically independent of antibodies (Figure 4.2). Activation by lipopolysaccharides from gram-negative bacteria (endotoxin) (Fearon et al., 1975); by teichoic acid from gram-positive bacteria; by cell-wall products from fungi (zymosan); by drugs (Althesin, radiographic contrast media) (Laser et al., 1980; Watkins et al., 1976); by membranes (used for oxygenators of cardiopul-

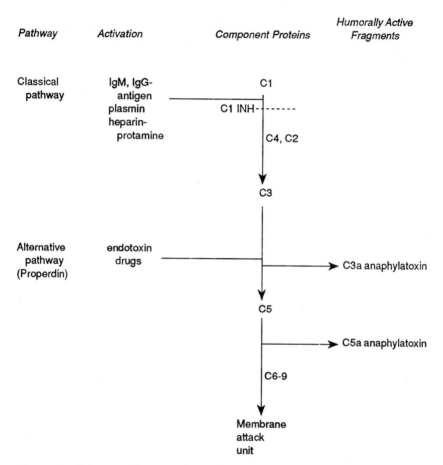

Figure 4.2 Schematic diagram of complement activation. The component proteins of the complement system can be activated by immunologic and nonimmunologic mechanisms to liberate humorally active fragments and generate a membrane attack unit for cell lysis. A circulating plasma inhibitor of the complement cascade, the C1 esterase inhibitor (C1 INH) is normally present.

monary bypass membranes or cellophane membranes of dialyzers) (Craddock et al., 1977); by perfluorocarbon artificial blood; and by interactions of polyanion–polycations (Fiedel et al., 1976; Rent et al., 1975) have been reported.

Complement Activation and Pathologic Effects

Complement activation by either pathway produces low-molecular-weight peptides of complement proteins C3, C4, and C5, which mediate cellular and humoral responses (Frank, 1988). These fragments, C3a, C4a, and C5a, are called *anaphylatoxins* because they stimulate mast cells and basophils to release mediators, contract smooth muscle, and increase vascular permeability (Table 4.2) (Glovsky et al., 1979; Grant et al., 1975, 1976). A fragment of C2 is thought to possess kinin activity, producing increased vascular permeability (Frank, 1989). The interaction of C5a with specific high-affinity receptors on neutrophils and platelets initiates cellular aggregation, an increase in adherence between cells and to endothelial surfaces, directed migration toward the source of complement activation (chemotaxis), and cellular activation. These activated neutrophils liberate arachidonic acid metabolites, oxygen-free radicals, and lysosomal enzymes (Weissman et al., 1980) to produce tissue inflammation (Jacob et al., 1980) and increase capillary permeability (Björk and Smedegard, 1984; Hammerschmidt, 1980). Both C3a and C5a release interleukin-1 from both macrophages and monocytes, which further promotes the adhesion of neutrophils and other inflammatory cells. Carboxypeptidases are enzymes responsible for inactivating complement anaphylatoxins.

Investigators have implicated C5a generation and neutrophil aggregation to explain the neutropenia and hypoxia of dialysis and adult respiratory distress syndrome (ARDS) (Hammerschmidt et al., 1980), the clinical manifestations of transfusion reactions (Latson et al., 1986), pulmonary vasoconstriction after protamine reactions (Morel et al., 1987), and serum sickness after streptokinase injections (Alexopoulos et al., 1984). Activation of complement by endotoxin is believed to be the mechanism of respiratory failure and vasodilation in gram-negative sepsis (Jacob et al., 1980).

Complement activation during anesthesia can occur as a result of reactions to blood products (Teissner et al., 1983), radiocontrast media (Best et al., 1983; 1984; Laser et al., 1980), perfluorocarbon administration (Vercellotti et al., 1981; 1982), protamine (Siegel et al., 1974), or other agents, as shown in Table 4.3. Complement activation is initiated after cardiopulmonary bypass (Chenoweth et al., 1981; Collett et al., 1984; Haslam et al., 1980). During extracorporeal circulation, the lungs are out of circuit, therefore C5a-activated leukocytes may accumulate in other target organs. Complement activation and generation of other inflammatory systems are implicated in causing multiorgan dysfunction after cardiopulmonary bypass (see the following section).

Table 4.2 Biologic Effects of Complement Anaphylatoxins

	C3a	C5a
Contract smooth muscle	+	+
Release histamine	+	+
Increase capillary permeability	+	+
Chemotactic for leukocytes		+
Aggregate leukocytes, platelets		+
Release interleukin-1	+	+

Table 4.3 Agents Producing Complement Activation During Anesthesia

Cardiopulmonary bypass	Protamine
Cremophor solubilized drugs	Radiocontrast agents
Dextrans	Transfusion reactions
Perfluorochemical derivatives	

INTERACTION OF THE COMPLEMENT, KININ, COAGULATION, AND FIBRINOLYTIC PATHWAYS: CONTACT ACTIVATION

Coagulation and fibrinolytic pathways have important interactions with the classical complement cascade. Activation of any of these separate plasma contact activation systems can generate kinins and other inflammatory mediators. Four proteins, Factor XII (Hageman factor), prekallikrein (Fletcher factor), high-molecular-weight kininogen (HMWK, Williams, Fitzgerald, Flaujeoc factor), and Factor XI (plasma thromboplastin antecedent), are the proteins required to initiate, amplify, and propagate surface-mediated defense reactions in humans (Colman, 1984).

Contact activation is initiated by Factor XII (Hageman factor) of the intrinsic clotting system, which can be activated to XIIa by nonphysiologic negatively charged surfaces such as glass, kaolin (clay), celite (diataumacious earth), or phospholipids (see Figure 4.3) (Kaplan and Austen, 1975; Murano, 1978). The physiologic activator is believed to be subendothelial vascular basement membrane (Colman and Schmaier, 1986). Activation of Factor XII by contact activation cleaves the parent molecule into two Hageman factor fragments, called XIIa (also called α-factor XIIa or HFa) and XIIf (also called β-factor XIIa or HFf), in the presence of prekallikrein and its cofactor, high-molecular-weight kininogen (Griffin and Cochrane, 1976; Revak and Cochrane, 1976; Revak et al., 1974; 1977). Factor XIIa fragment converts Factor XI and XIa to activate the intrinsic coagulation cascade (Bouma and Griffin, 1977; Cochrane and Griffin, 1982; Kurachi and Davie, 1977; Wiggins et al., 1979).

Both Hageman factor fragments convert prekallikrein to kallikrein. Kallikrein leads to further activation of the parent Hageman factor (Factor XII) to have a positive feedback mechanism and **amplify** the reaction, and also generates bradykinin by the cleaving of high-molecular-weight kininogen (Cochrane et al., 1972; 1973; Griffin and Cochrane, 1976; Meier et al., 1977). Kallikrein also cleaves plasminogen to generate the fibrinolytic enzyme plasmin (Bouma et al., 1980; Colman, 1969; Kaplan and Austen, 1975; Murano, 1978). Plasmin is capable of triggering the classical complement pathway by activating the C1s component of C1 esterase (Kaplan and Austen, 1975; Murano, 1978). Hageman factor fragments can also activate the classical complement pathway (Colman and Schmaier, 1986).

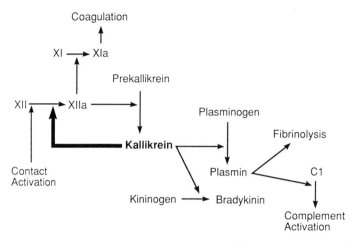

Figure 4.3 Relationship between contact activation of Hageman factor (XII) and activation of the coagulation, kinin, fibrinolytic, and complement systems.

Regulation

The plasma contact activation systems have similar structures and inhibitors (the C1 inhibitor complement protein, α_2-macroglobulin, and α_1-antitrypsin). The C1 inhibitor also inactivates proteases of the Hageman factor-dependent pathways, including Factor XII and its fragments, kallikrein, factor XIa, and plasmin, as shown in Table 4.4 (Forbes et al., 1970; Ratnoff et al., 1969; Schrieber et al., 1973). The C1 inhibitor is thus capable of influencing activation of intrinsic clotting, kinin generating, and fibrolytic pathways. Studies of C1 inhibitor-deficient sera from patients with hereditary angioedema (see the following section) have suggested that, in the absence of the C1 inhibitor, antithrombin III is the major inhibitor of both types of Hageman factor fragments (Revak and Cochrane, 1976). Antithrombin III is a poor inhibitor of factors XIIa, XIa, and kallikrein, however. Heparin, which markedly accelerates inactivation of factor Xa and thrombin by antithrombin III, exhibits minimal enhancement of the inactivation of the contact enzymes.

Investigators examining plasma kallikrein inactivation by plasma protease inhibitors suggest that the C1 inhibitor is the principal inactivator of kallikrein (von der Graaf et al., 1983; Schapira et al., 1982). Schapira and coworkers also noted that α_2-macroglobulin, antithrombin III, and α_1-antitrypsin inhibit kallikrein activation (Schapira et al., 1981; 1982). Factor XI is activated to Factor XIa primarily by Factor XIIa, but Factor XIIf can also activate Factor XI (Cochrane, 1982). Like other contact system proteases, Factor XIa can be inactivated by the C1 inhibitor. Plasmin's major inactivator is α_2-antiplasmin and, to a lesser extent, C1 inhibitor (see Table 4.4).

Table 4.4 Plasma Inhibitors of Contact Activation Proteases

Inhibitor	MWT	C1	XIIa	Kallikrein	XIa	Plasmin
C1 inhibitor	96–105	+++	+++	++	++	±
α_2-antiplasmin	65–70	–	+	–	–	+++
Antithrombin III	58	+	+	+	+	–
α_1-antitrypsin	53	–	–	+	+++	–
α_2-macroglobulin	725	–	+	++	–	–

MWT = molecular weight, kilodaltons.
Data from Cochrane CG, Griffin JH. The biochemistry and pathophysiology of the contact system of plasma. Adv Immunol 1982;33:241–306; Prograis LJ, Brickman CM, Frank MM. C1-inhibitor. In Murano G. ed. Protease Inhibitors of Human Plasma: Biochemistry and Pathophysiology. New York: PJD Publications Ltd., 1986;303–50; Schapira M, Scott DF, Colman RW. Protection of human plasma kallikrein from inactivation by C1 inhibitor and other protease inhibitors: the role of high molecular weight kininogen. Biochemistry 1981;20:2738–43.

Clinical Significance
Contact Activation and Cardiopulmonary Bypass

The importance of contact activation or amplification pathways can be confusing to the clinician. During cardiopulmonary bypass, blood contacts foreign surfaces of the tubing, oxygenator, or venous reservoir to generate XIIa and activate the intrinsic coagulation system (Figure 4.4). The intrinsic coagulation cascade is inhibited by giving heparin to activate antithrombin III and inhibit thrombin, but heparin–antithrombin III has minimal effects on the contact activation of blood interfacing with the nonendothelial surfaces of the extracorporeal circuit tubing and membrane oxygenator (Pixley et al., 1985). Contact activation also generates Factor XIIa to produce kallikrein, plasmin, and, indirectly, complement activation that is not inhibited during cardiopulmonary bypass by heparin (Figure 4.5). Royston and coworkers first demonstrated that administering aprotinin, a protease inhibitor with a wide range of inhibitory activity analogous to the C1 esterase inhibitor, during cardiopulmonary bypass prevents this inflammatory response and significantly decreases bleeding and the need for blood transfusion (Bidstrup et al., 1989; Royston et al., 1987). A proposed hypothesis for the preserved platelet function is that by inhibiting the proteases activated during cardiac surgery, the glycoprotein 1b receptor responsible for adhesion on platelet surfaces is preserved when aprotinin is administered (van Oevren et al., 1987). Horrow and coworkers have also demonstrated that inhibiting plasmin alone with tranexamic acid decreases bleeding after cardiopulmonary bypass (Horrow et al., 1990).

When heparin is administered to patients receiving aprotinin, the activated clotting time or activated partial thromboplastin time is greatly prolonged. This finding does not represent a heparin-sparing effect, but rather is a reflection of the ability of aprotinin to inhibit kallikrein and its amplying effect on in vitro

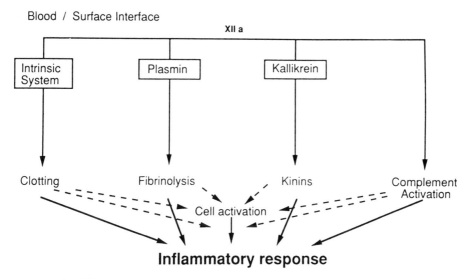

Figure 4.4 Effects of contact activation by blood/surface interactions on generation of the intrinsic coagulation cascade, kallikrein, and plasmin to produce cell activation and humoral inflammatory responses. *Reprinted with permission from Royston D. Aprotinin in open heart surgery: background and results in patients having aortocoronary bypass grafts. Perfusion 1990;5(S):63–72.*

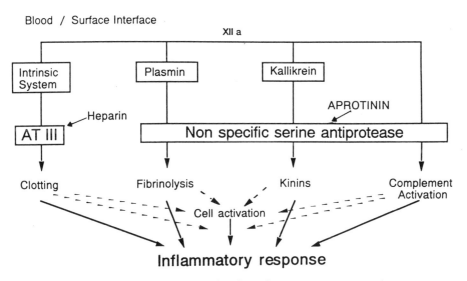

Figure 4.5 Effects of drugs used to inhibit the inflammatory responses that occur after blood/surface interfacing. *Reprinted with permission from Royston D. Aprotinin in open heart surgery: background and results in patients having aortocoronary bypass grafts. Perfusion 1990;5(S):63–72.*

contact activators (i.e., celite or kaolin) (Levy and Salmenpera, 1991). In an analogous manner, the baseline activated clotting time or activated partial thromboplastin time of a Factor XII-deficient patient is greatly prolonged without any clinically evident bleeding abnormality.

Contact Activation and Sepsis

Kallikrein can also convert kininogen to bradykinin, producing hypotension (Ellison, 1978). Serum levels of Hageman factor and prekallikrein decrease, whereas bradykinin increases during hypotension associated with gram-negative bacteremia (Mason et al., 1970). Acute endotoxemia or gram-positive bacteremia in humans is associated with depletion of prekallikrein, decreased peripheral resistance, and in some instances, complement activation (Robinson et al., 1975). Vasodilation and increased capillary permeability occur during disseminated intravascular coagulation from the activation of the different kinin pathways.

Contact Activation and Hereditary Angioedema

The C1 esterase inhibitor or C1 inhibitor is a plasma glycoprotein that inhibits the enzymatic activity of the C1 complement protein to prevent its spontaneous activation (Fearon, 1975; Frank et al., 1976; Frank, 1988). It interacts with both activated C1r and C1s to destroy their functional enzymatic activity by forming a tightly linked complex with the molecules. There are 105,000 and 96,000 molecular weight forms of the C1 inhibitor (Malbran et al., 1988). Most of the current information about the C1 inhibitor has come from studies of hereditary angioedema (Frank et al., 1976). The prevalence of the disease is unknown, but may be as high as 1:20,000 (Frank et al., 1976).

The classic form of hereditary angioedema, also called angioneurotic edema, is an autosomal dominant disorder in which the function of the C1 inhibitor is markedly reduced. Because of the spectrum of C1 inhibitor activity, hereditary angioedema also affects the kinin-generating and fibrinolytic systems. The cardinal symptoms of hereditary angioedema are edema of the extremities, face, and airway, and recurrent abdominal pain, which may be seen alone or in combination (Whaley, 1987). Patients often attribute their first episode to an identifiable traumatic event, such as a tonsillectomy, dental manipulation, or accidental trauma (Wall et al., 1989). Attacks of edema involving the airway present the greatest danger to patients with this disorder. Pharyngeal edema is usually precipitated by dental or oral pharyngeal manipulation. Airway obstruction occasionally occurs in the course of the attack and may progress to total obstruction.

Studies have defined two major forms of C1 esterase deficiency. The predominant form (type 1, common form) is characterized by reduced levels of C1, the esterase inhibitor protein, caused by a decreased synthetic rate of functional protein (Whaley, 1987). People affected with the variant form of the disease (type 2) have a normal or raised C1 esterase inhibitor concentration but synthesize a functionally defective protein. Both types of hereditary angioedema are further characterized by low levels of the complement proteins C2 and C4, low

CH_{50}, the presence of a family history of attacks, and the onset of symptoms in childhood or early adolescence (Whaley, 1987). The pathogenesis of edema formation is not clearly understood. The reduced levels of functional C1 inhibitor can lead to uncontrolled classic complement pathway activation, potentially releasing a C2 kinin fragment, or contact system activation with the release of bradykinin (Frank, 1988; Whaley, 1987). These kinin mediators have been assumed to be the cause of the increased vascular permeability responsible for the clinical symptoms.

A new type of acquired C1 esterase inhibitor deficiency has been reported as well. Acquired angioedema includes lower or absent levels of C1 inhibitor, C1q, C1, C4, and C2, a low CH_{50}, a lack of heredity, and the onset of symptoms in middle age (Bork and Witzke, 1989). In contrast to hereditary angioedema, synthesis of the C1 esterase inhibitor is normal or slightly elevated. Bork and Witzke suggest that increased activation of C1 accelerates catabolism of the C1 esterase inhibitor in this type of acquired angioedema. In all cases, benign or malignant lymphoproliferative disorders or B cell abnormalities with autoantibody production have been implicated. An additional type of acquired C1 esterase inhibitor deficiency has been reported that differs in that it is not associated with other lymphoproliferative diseases but with large amounts of antibodies to the inhibitor (Malbran et al., 1988).

In patients with hereditary or acquired angioedema, swelling is only treated if it is life-threatening or likely to become so. For this reason, only patients who develop edema in the region of the head, which may progress to glottic edema, or those patients who suffer severe edema of the internal organs require treatment (Frank et al., 1976).

Management of the Surgical Patient with Hereditary Angioedema

Patients who are undergoing surgical procedures are at increased risk for attacks and require special consideration (Abada and Owens, 1977; Gibbs et al., 1977; Poppers, 1987). The therapies of choice in an acute attack or for prophylaxis include fresh frozen plasma or the C1 inhibitor concentrates, which are not available in the United States (Bork and Witzke, 1989). In life-threatening cases, intubation or other intensive procedures may become necessary depending on the symptoms and location of the edema. In patients who suffer from frequent attacks or those undergoing pretreatent for surgery, the medication of choice is danazol, using dosages of 50 to 600 mg daily (Bork and Witzke, 1989). Danazol is an anabolic steroid that potentially increases synthesis of the C1 inhibitor protein. Stanazol, a more potent anabolic steroid, has also been tried successfully. Other prophylactic therapies include treatment with antifibrinolytic agents, such as epsilon aminocaproic acid or tranexamic acid (Sheffer et al., 1977).

Patients undergoing surgery, especially oropharyngeal surgery, or those who require intubation are at high risk for attacks. These patients should be transfused with 2 units of fresh frozen plasma on the day before the procedure, and every effort should be made to minimize oral airway manipulation since it may precipitate airway edema. If the patient develops a life-threatening attack of hereditary angioedema, treatment with fresh frozen plasma should be considered. One objection to this therapy is that fresh frozen plasma contains both C1 esterase inhibitor and complement components. Because the complement proteins are often very low or exhausted in the surgical patient, it is theoretically possible that the sudden availability of complement components in a patient suffering an attack may transiently make matters worse.

Wall and coworkers have reviewed their experiences with 25 patients with hereditary angioedema who required surgery (Wall et al., 1989). Their anesthetic management of these patients and all those who require airway manipulation includes the administration of 2 units of fresh frozen plasma on the evening before surgery. Long-term prophylactic therapy that includes antifibrinolytic drugs (epsilon aminocaproic acid, tranexamic acid, or anabolic steroids) should be continued both preoperatively and postoperatively. Patients not receiving any prophylactic therapy should undergo short-term treatment with epsilon aminocaproic acid, danazol, or other antifibrinolytic or anabolic steroids. These recommendations are based on other anesthetic cases and experiences reported in the literature. Replacement therapy with C1 inhibitor concentrate has been used in Europe. In cases of life-threatening edema, 500 to 1000 units are injected, with remission of edema within 2 to 3 hours of injection and complete resolution within 24 hours (Bork and Witzke, 1989). The biologic half-life of C1 esterase inhibitor in healthy subjects appears to be approximately 2 to 3 days (Bork and Witzke, 1989). Therefore, replacement with a C1 esterase inhibitor concentrate the night before, or the morning of, surgery should provide adequate protection in the immediate perioperative period. In severe trauma, however, additional C1 esterase inhibitor concentrates or fresh frozen plasma may be required if edema occurs postoperatively.

5

Nonimmunologic (Pharmacologic) Histamine Release

Although human mast cells from skin, lung, heart, adenoids, and tonsils differ in their secretory responses to antigens, anti-immunoglobulin-E (IgE), and calcium ionophore, they differ most strikingly in their nonimmunologic responses to certain drugs and neuropeptides, which cause them to release histamine but not other mediators (Figure 5.1) (Caulfield et al., 1990). A variety of different drugs and agents administered intravenously have the ability to release histamine. Studies suggested that only mast cells from human skin release histamine when exposed to nonimmunologic stimuli (Church et al., 1989a; 1989b; Lowman et al., 1988; Pearce et al., 1985; Tharp et al., 1987). Recent data have shown that isolated mast cells from human lung and heart also release histamine, however (Stellato et al., 1991). Basophils do not release histamine after nonimmunologic stimulation (Ebertz et al., 1986; Hermens et al., 1985; Stellato et al., 1991).

Molecules that cause the release of histamine from mast cell granules produce vasodilation and flushing along the vein of administration, or a wheal and flare response when injected intradermally. The mechanisms of nonimmunologic histamine release are poorly understood, but indicate a dose-dependent and reproducible noncytotoxic reaction that is complete within 15 seconds and is not dependent on extracellular calcium (see Figure 5.1) (Caulfield et al., 1990; Morrison et al., 1975). Previous exposure to a given agent is not necessary for histamine release to occur. The agents reported to cause histamine release include a diverse group of drugs and peptides, including such molecules as benzylisoquinoline-derived muscle relaxants (atracurium, doxacurium, d-tubocurarine, mivacurium, and metocurine), opioids (morphine, codeine, and meperidine), thiobarbiturates, glycopeptide antibiotics (vancomycin), and peptides (Table 5.1).

Most of the initial studies evaluating the histamine-releasing potential of various drugs have measured plasma levels using radioenzymatic or fluorometric assay after intravenous injection. Human skin and other tissues have also been used to evaluate mast cell degranulation and nonimmunologic histamine release by different methods that include 1) intradermal drug injection, measuring wheal and flare responses; 2) measuring histamine release in vitro from enzymatically

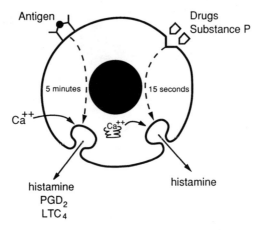

Figure 5.1 Schematic diagram of mediator release from human skin mast cells stimulated immunologically by antigens or nonimmunologically by drugs or substance P. Immunologic activation with an immunospecific antigen initiates the release of histamine, prostaglandin D_2 (PGD_2), and leukotriene C_4 (LTC_4) by a mechanism that takes 5 minutes to reach completion and requires influx of extracellular calcium. Nonimmunologic activation with substance P or drugs releases histamine, but not PGD_2 or LTC_4, through a mechanism that is complete within 15 seconds and uses calcium mobilized from intracellular stores. *Modified with permission from Caulfield JP, El-Lati S, Thomas G, Church MK. Dissociated human foreskin mast cells degranulate in response to anti-IgE and substance P. Lab Invest 1990;63:502–10.*

isolated or whole-tissue sections of mast cells; and 3) microscopic evaluation of skin specimens from wheal responses or isolated mast cells. Intradermal drug administration provides an important method of evaluating and comparing drugs for their relative histamine-releasing potency and cutaneous vascular reactions

Table 5.1 Agents that Produce Nonimmunologic Histamine Release

Antibiotics: vancomycin

Barbiturates: thiamylal, thiopental

Benzylisoquinoline-derived muscle relaxants: atracurium, *d*-tubocurarine, doxacurium, metocurine, mivacurium

Calcium ionophores

Complement peptides: C3a, C5a

Hyperosmotic agents: ionic radiocontrast media, mannitol

Opioids: morphine, meperidine, codeine

Peptides: gastrin, substance P, somatostatin, vasoactive intestinal peptide

Polybasic compounds: 48/80, protamine

(Casale et al., 1984; Levy et al., 1989c; 1991; North et al., 1987; Robertson et al., 1983; Saucedo and Erill, 1985; Stellato et al., 1991). Because different classes of drugs release histamine, the specific groups will be considered separately. Antibiotics and hyperosmotic agents are considered in more detail in Chapter 6.

PHARMACOLOGIC AGENTS
Antibiotics

Vancomycin causes histamine release from isolated human cutaneous mast cells (Levy et al., 1987). Elevations in plasma histamine levels have also been demonstrated after rapid intravenous administration, as shown in Figure 5.2 (Levy et al., 1987). The glycopeptide structure and high pKa of vancomycin may account for its ability to induce histamine release.

Barbiturates

Hirshman and coworkers demonstrated that both thiopental and thiamylal cause histamine release from human cutaneous mast cells (Figure 5.3) (Hirshman et al., 1985). Mechanisms proposed for these findings include potential histamine

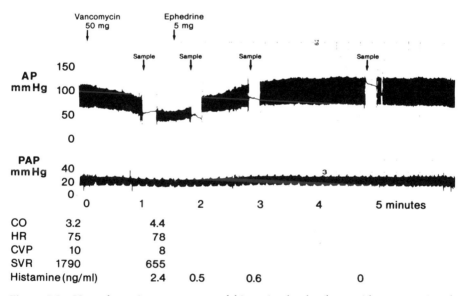

Figure 5.2 Hemodynamic parameters and histamine levels after rapid vancomycin administration. Hypotension was associated with an increased cardiac output, decreased calculated systemic vascular resistance, and elevated plasma histamine levels. The patient was given ephedrine, 5 mg, to treat the hypotension. *Reprinted with permission from Levy JH, Kettlekamp N, Goertz P, Hermens J, Hirshman CA. Histamine release by vancomycin: a mechanism for hypotension in man. Anesthesiology 1987;67:122–5.*

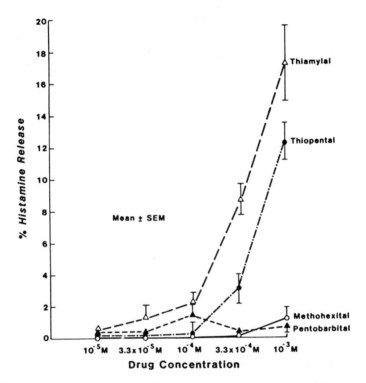

Figure 5.3 Comparison of percent histamine release from human skin in the presence of increasing concentrations of thiopental, thiamylal, methohexital, and pentobarbital. Both thiopental and thiamylal produced significant dose-related histamine release. Histamine release by thiamylal was significantly greater than by thiopental, from 3.3×10^{-5} to 10^{-3} M ($P < 0.05$). *Reprinted with permission from Hirshman CA, Edelstein RA, Eastman CL. Histamine release by barbiturates in human mast cells. Anesthesiology 1985;63:353–6.*

displacement from binding sites, or biophysical changes in mast cell granules or cell membranes. Histamine release caused by barbiturates does not depend on high lipid solubility, since methohexital, which is far more lipid-soluble than thiopental, did not release histamine (1000 vs. 580, $CH_2Cl_2:H_2O$ partition coefficient). Furthermore, histamine release caused by barbiturates does not reflect a nonspecific effect of barbituric acid or an ionized form of the drug. Rather, the sulfuration on the barbituric acid molecule has been suggested to be important in barbiturate-induced histamine release (Hirshman et al., 1985).

Muscle Relaxants

Muscle relaxants used in clinical practice include molecular derivatives of benzylisoquinoline (atracurium, doxacurium, *d*-tubocurarine, mivacurium, me-

Table 5.2 Structure of Muscle Relaxants in Current Use or Under Clinical Investigation

Benzylisoquinoline Derivatives	Steroid Derivatives	Acetylcholine Homologues
d-tubocurarine	Pancuronium	Succinylcholine
Metocurine	Vecuronium	
Atracurium	Pipecuronium	
Mivacurium	Rocuronium	
Doxacurium		

Modified from Levy JH, Adelson DM, Walker BF. Wheal and flare responses to muscle relaxants in humans. Agents Actions 1991;34:302–8.

tocurine), steroids (vecuronium, pancuronium, rocuronium), and acetylcholine (succinylcholine) molecules (Table 5.2). Only benzylisoquinoline-derived muscle relaxants degranulate human cutaneous mast cells and release histamine at clinically used concentrations (Figure 5.4). Numerous in vivo studies have also examined histamine release caused by the benzylisoquinolone-derived muscle relaxants that are known to produce adverse hemodynamic reactions. Moss and coworkers first demonstrated hypotension with d-tubocurarine that was directly correlated with increases in plasma histamine (Figure 5.5) (Moss et al., 1981). Gallo and coworkers also demonstrated a statistically significant decrease in blood pressure at 2 minutes and a decrease in systemic vascular resistance at 2, 5, and 10 minutes after a bolus of 0.5 mg/kg of atracurium (Gallo et al., 1988). They noted that the hemodynamic changes correlated directly with increases in plasma histamine levels as measured by radioenzymatic assay (Figure 5.6). Barnes and coworkers also found elevated plasma histamine levels of 2.6 ± 1.2 ng/mL (mean ± SD) using fluorometric analysis 1.5 minutes after a 0.6 mg/kg bolus of atracurium (Barnes et al., 1986). This was associated with cutaneous signs in 23 of 41 patients and decreases in mean arterial pressure greater than 10% of control values in 9 patients, but no correlation was shown between plasma histamine levels and decreases in blood pressure. Scott also noted an increase in plasma histamine levels from 715 ± 93 to 1415 ± 203 pg/mL that was associated with a decrease in mean arterial pressure to 82% ± 4% of baseline value blood pressure in 9 patients given 0.6 mg/kg over 5 seconds (Scott et al., 1985). Increases in plasma histamine and decreases in blood pressure were prevented by administering the drug over 75 seconds, or pretreating with H_1 and H_2 receptor antagonists. Similar studies evaluating mivacurium and doxacurium have developed protocols for administering the drug over several minutes to decrease histamine release.

Investigators have used in vivo and in vitro studies to compare the relative ability of different benzylisoquinoline-derived muscle relaxants to cause histamine release at multiples of ED_{95} (dose that results in 95% paralysis). Equipotent

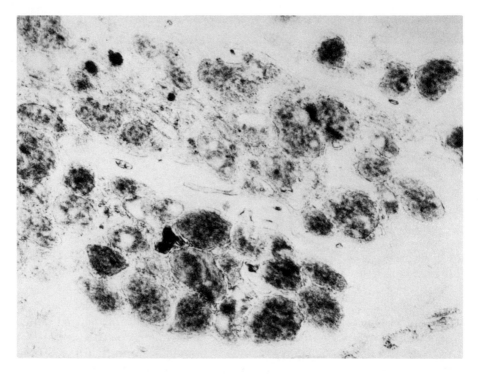

Figure 5.4 Electron micrograph of a degranulating mast cell after biopsy of an atracurium-induced wheal. Most cytoplasmic granules are swollen and fused to each other, demonstrating varying degrees of decreased density and loss of organization consistent with ongoing degranulation. *Reprinted with permission from Levy JH, Adelson DM, Walker BF. Wheal and flare responses to muscle relaxants in humans. Agents Actions 1991;34:302–8.*

ED_{95} doses show neuromuscular blocking potential but not the relative histamine-releasing potential. Furthermore, studies of histamine release based on increased plasma concentration after IV injection of these drugs may be less sensitive because plasma histamine is rapidly metabolized.

Using intradermal testing, Levy and coworkers noted no significant differences in wheal and flare responses among d-tubocurarine, metocurine, and atracurium, all structurally similar benzylisoquinoline derivatives (Figure 5.7) (Levy et al., 1991). Using isolated mast cells from skin and lung, Stellato and coworkers reported that only high concentrations of d-tubocurarine (10^{-3} M) caused histamine release, whereas atracurium produced a concentration-dependent release of histamine to a maximum of 46.2% ± 15.1% (skin) and 30.6% ± 6.0% (lung) (Stellato et al., 1991). Although Stenlake and coworkers have suggested that atracurium and metocurine cause less release of histamine than d-tubocu-

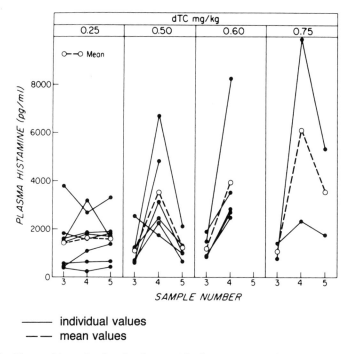

Figure 5.5 Plasma histamine levels after rapid administration of intravenous doses of *d*-tubocurarine. The samples were collected as follows: sample 3, before administration; sample 4, after 2 minutes; and sample 5, 5 minutes after *d*-tubocurarine administration in intubated, anesthetized patients. *Reprinted with permission from Moss J, Rosow CW, Savarese JJ, Philbin DM, Kniffen KJ. Role of histamine in the hypotensive action of d-tubocurarine in humans. Anesthesiology 1981;55:19–25.*

rarine because of the methoxy group substitutions and also, in atracurium, because of the incorporation of carboxyl groups in the side-chain and altered steriochemistry of the benzylisoquinoline structure, this appears unlikely (Stenlake et al., 1983). Increasing drug potency allows less drug to be administered, exposing mast cells to lower concentrations.

Levy and coworkers reported that the wheal and flare responses to *d*-tubocurarine, metocurine, and atracurium were significantly smaller than those of morphine and histamine (Levy et al., 1991). These findings suggest that equimolar displacement of histamine by known mast cell degranulators may not occur as previously reported (Levy et al., 1989c). Rather, the wheal and flare responses to opioids are related to both direct and indirect vascular responses and histamine release.

Papaverine, a benzylisoquinoline structure that closely resembles the side-groups of atracurium and one of the major alkaloids in opium, has also been

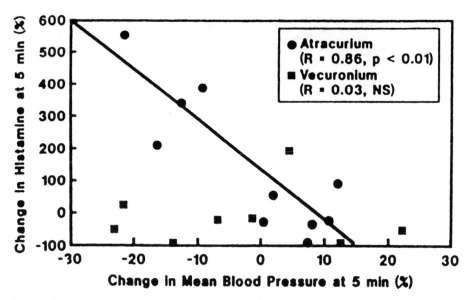

Figure 5.6 Relationship between changes in histamine levels and changes in blood pressure after atracurium at a dose of 0.5 mg/kg or vecuronium at a dose of 0.12 mg/kg in cardiac surgical patients. There is a direct correlation between changes in histamine release and decreases in blood pressure with atracurium but not with vecuronium. *Reprinted with permission from Gallo JA, Cork RC, Puchi P. Comparison of effects of atracurium and vecuronium in cardiac surgical patients. Anesth Analg 1988;67:161–5.*

evaluated for its ability to degranulate human cutaneous mast cells. Papaverine is a potent vasodilator, and this effect may be produced in part by histamine release. The benzylisoquinoline moiety of atracurium may represent the specific molecular configuration responsible for histamine release by atracurium. Atracurium's structure combines succinylcholine with two quarternary benzylisoquinoline moieties. Papaverine's flare (but not its wheal) was statistically smaller than that of atracurium and there was no evidence of degranulation on microscopic analysis of papaverine-induced wheals. Succinylcholine does not produce cutaneous responses when injected, nor does it release histamine in vitro (Levy et al., 1991; Stellato et al., 1991). An explanation for the cutaneous responses to atracurium and degranulation of mast cells may lie in the differences in the benzylisoquinoline moiety. The benzylisoquinoline–nitrogen ring of papaverine contains double bonds, whereas the nitrogen ring present in atracurium is saturated. The benzylisoquinoine side-chains of metocurine and *d*-tubocurarine share these characteristics with atracurium and both are mast cell degranulators, suggesting that a hydrogenated, benzylisoquinoline–nitrogen-containing ring represents the molecular structure responsible for mast cell degranulation by atracurium (Levy et al., 1991).

Atracurium produces in vitro histamine release and cutaneous responses at

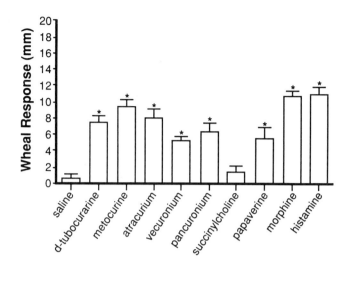
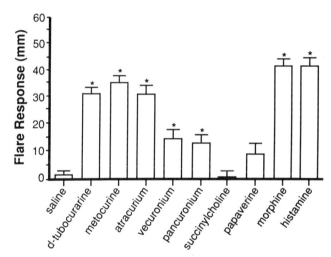

Figure 5.7 Wheal and flare responses to 5×10^{-4}M concentrations of muscle relaxants, morphine, papaverine, and histamine. Data are expressed as mean ± SEM. *$P < 0.05$ compared with saline controls. Reprinted with permission from Levy JH, Adelson DM, Walker BF. *Wheal and flare responses to muscle relaxants in humans. Agents Actions 1991;34:302–8.*

concentrations of $\geq 10^{-4}$ M (Figure 5.8) (Levy et al., 1991; Stellato et al., 1991). In clinical practice, however, IV injection of a 10 mg/mL stock solution of atracurium along a peripheral vein adjacent to mast cells transiently exposes them to a solution of approximately 10^{-2} M, which exceeds the threshold of 10^{-4} M for cutaneous responses. Even with slow IV administration of atracu-

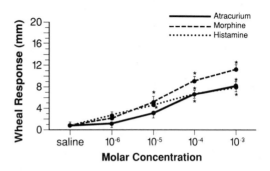

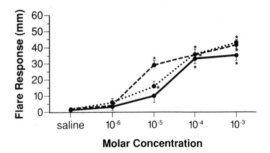

Figure 5.8 Wheal and flare responses to different concentrations of atracurium, morphine, and histamine. Data are expressed as mean ± SEM. *$P < 0.05$ compared with saline controls. *Reprinted with permission from Levy JH, Adelson DM, Walker BF. Wheal and flare responses to muscle relaxants in humans. Agents Actions 1991;34:302–8.*

rium, the cutaneous mast cells along the vein are transiently exposed to high concentrations. These findings further emphasize the work of Lorenz and Doenicke, who suggested that drug dilution and slow administration minimized histamine release at the injection site (Lorenz et al., 1990).

Figure 5.9 Individual values of human histamine release after large doses of fentanyl and morphine administered for cardiac surgery. Morphine was administered at a rate of 100 μg/kg/min and fentanyl at 5 μg/kg/min. Hemodynamic measurements and blood samples for histamine were obtained after administration of one third and after the total dose of narcotic, then 5 and 10 minutes later. *Reprinted with permission from Rosow CE, Moss J, Philbin DM, Savarese JJ. Histamine release during morphine and fentanyl anesthesia. Anesthesiology 1982;56:93–6.*

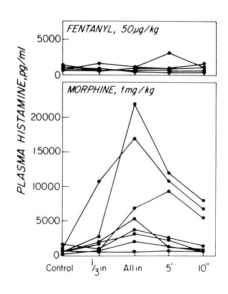

Injection of the steroidal muscle relaxants intradermally can also produce wheal and flare responses, but they are not of the same magnitude as those of the benzylisoquinoline-derived drugs (Booij et al., 1980; Levy et al., 1991). These changes are not associated with mast cell degranulation at 5×10^{-4} M. Stellato and coworkers demonstrated marked differences among the effects of muscle relaxants on mast cells from different anatomic sites (Stellato et al., 1991). They reported that vecuronium can liberate histamine in a dose-dependent fashion from dispersed and isolated human lung (7.2% ± 2.1%) and cutaneous mast cells (4.9% ± 1.4%) at 10^{-3} to 10^{-2} M, concentrations that are never achieved in vivo (Stellato et al., 1991). These findings suggest a potentially cytotoxic effect of drugs at nonphysiologic concentrations because release was seen from both mucosal (lung) and connective (skin) tissue mast cells. These authors noted that atracurium was a more potent histamine releaser from lung (46.2% ± 15.1%), skin (30.6% ± 6.0%), and cardiac mast cells.

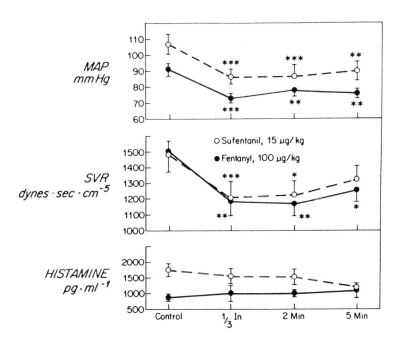

Figure 5.10 Histamine release in humans after fentanyl and sufentanil administration. Mean arterial pressure (MAP), systemic vascular resistance (SVR), and plasma histamine concentration are included. Fentanyl was infused at a rate of 400 μg/min and sufentanil at a rate of 60 μg/min intravenously. Hemodynamic measurements were made, and blood samples for histamine were obtained after one third of the narcotic dose had been administered, and at 2 and 5 minutes after completion of the narcotic infusion. *Reprinted with permission from Rosow CE, Philbin DM, Keegan CR, Moss J. Hemodynamics and histamine release during induction with sufentanil or fentanyl. Anesthesiology 1984;60: 489–91.*

Opioids

Morphine, meperidine, and codeine are the only clinically available opioids that can cause histamine release (Casale et al., 1984; Levy et al., 1989c). After high-dose morphine administration (1 mg/kg) for cardiac surgery, histamine concentrations of 20 ng/mL have been reported (Figure 5.9) (Rosow et al., 1982). Alfentanil, sufentanil, and fentanyl do not cause histamine release (Figures 5.9 and 5.10) (Levy et al., 1989c; Rosow et al., 1984). Although the mast cell and basophil represent major sources of histamine in humans, morphine releases histamine from cutaneous mast cells but not from basophils (Figure 5.11) (Hermens et al., 1985).

Levy and coworkers demonstrated significant wheal and flare responses after intradermal injections of morphine, meperidine, fentanyl, and sufentanil at equimolar concentrations of 5×10^{-4} M (Figure 5.12) (Levy et al., 1989c). Similar wheal responses to meperidine and morphine suggest that equimolar concentrations of these two histamine-releasing opioids may displace equivalent amounts of histamine from cutaneous mast cells. Fentanyl and sufentanil, but not alfentanil, were noted to produce wheals and flares, however, but not of the same magnitude as those of morphine and meperidine. Opioids showed variable effects in their ability to produce wheal and flare responses unrelated to their relative mu-receptor order of potency. These findings may be due to direct opioid-mediated capillary vasodilation, because naloxone antagonizes fentanyl-induced flare responses (Figure 5.12). Both naloxone and antihistamines only partially antagonize the wheal and flare responses to morphine (Figure 5.13). Antagonism of fentanyl wheal and flare responses by naloxone and partial antagonism of

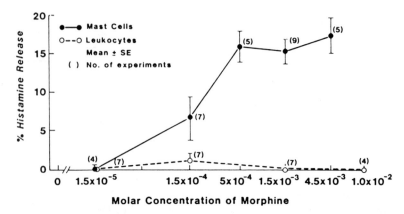

Figure 5.11 Percent histamine release from plasma leukocytes and human skin at increasing concentrations of morphine sulfate. Morphine sulfate induces dose-related histamine release from skin mast cell preparations but not from leukocyte preparations. *Reprinted with permission from Hermens JM, Ebertz JM, Hanifin JM, Hirshman CA. Comparison of histamine release in human skin mast cells by morphine, fentanyl, and oxymorphone. Anesthesiology 1985;62:124–9.*

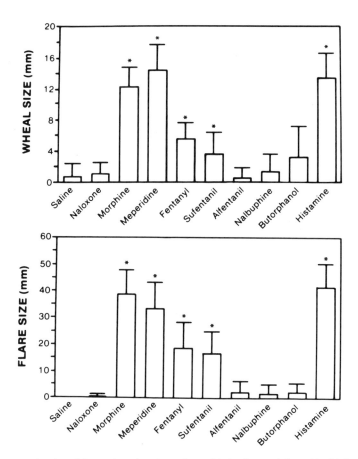

Figure 5.12 Wheal and flare size after intradermal injections of 5×10^{-4} M concentration of opioids, histamine, and normal saline in 16 volunteers. Data are expressed as mean ± SD. * $P < 0.05$ compared with saline controls. *Reprinted with permission from Levy JH, Brister NW, Shearin A, et al. Wheal and flare responses to opioids in humans. Anesthesiology 1989;70:756–60.*

morphine-induced flare by naloxone suggest direct opioid-mediated capillary vasodilation as an important mechanism in producing cutaneous responses. Naloxone was more effective at decreasing the size of the wheal and flare response to fentanyl because morphine's effect is related to both histamine release and direct opioid effects, whereas fentanyl-induced effects appear to be related to direct vascular responses only. This has important implications, since any attempts to antagonize the adverse hemodynamic effects of rapid intravenous morphine injection with H_1 and H_2 receptor antagonists may not completely attenuate these effects because of direct opioid-mediated vasodilation. Opioids may also regulate vascular tone by direct vascular effects (Fuerstein and Siren, 1987; Hanko and Hardebo, 1978). Data suggest that sufentanil produces neu-

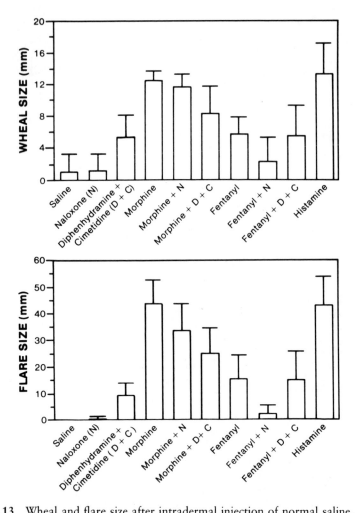

Figure 5.13 Wheal and flare size after intradermal injection of normal saline, naloxone (N), diphenhydramine and cimetidine (D + C), morphine alone and with antagonist, fentanyl alone and with antagonist, and histamine in 12 volunteers. All drug concentrations are 5×10^{-4} M in their injected form. Data are expressed as mean ± SD. D + C produced significant wheal and flare response compared with saline and attenuated the wheal and flare response to morphine ($P < 0.05$). N attenuated the wheal and flare response to fentanyl and the flare response to morphine ($P < 0.05$). *Reprinted with permission from Levy JH, Brister NW, Shearin A, et al. Wheal and flare responses to opioids in humans. Anesthesiology 1989;70:756–60.*

rogenic vasodilation that can be antagonized by α_1-adrenoreceptor blockade (O'Keefe et al., 1987). These findings emphasize that attempts to antagonize the adverse hemodynamic effects of histamine-releasing opioids with antihistamines will not be completely successful because of direct vascular responses.

The mechanism of nonimmunologic histamine release by opioids is unknown. Five types of opioid receptors or binding sites have been identified in mammalian tissues including the μ, δ, κ, σ and ϵ receptors. Casale and coworkers performed intradermal skin tests with dynorphin (κ-agonists), [D-Ala,^{2}-D-Leu^5] enkephalin (σ-agonist), morphiceptin (μ-agonist) and β-endorphin (which has a reasonably high affinity for μ and σ-opioid receptors) (Casale et al., 1984). All four compounds in nanomole quantities produced wheal responses of more than 7 mm; however, dynorphin was far more potent than either the μ-receptor agonists (morphiceptin) or σ-receptor agonists, ([D-Ala,^{2}-D-Leu^5] enkephalin). Since β-endorphin elicited a larger wheal response at equimolar concentrations than morphiceptin and [D-Ala,^{2}-D-Leu^5] enkephalin, Casale and associates postulated that β-endorphin effects could be from interaction with multiple opioid receptors, including those for dynorphin (κ-agonist), as well as the μ-receptor stimulated by the pharmacologic opiates. Stimulation of a naloxone-inhibitable μ-opioid receptor on mast cells with the most potent agonists, sufentanil or fentanyl, does not induce histamine release, however. Opiate effects on mast cells may be produced by nonopiate-specific binding sites or nonspecific drug-induced effects. Although dynorphin was the most potent of the compounds tested, enkephalin, morphiceptin, and β-endorphin also elicited wheal and flare responses, suggesting that nonopioid receptors are involved in opioid-induced mast cell degranulation.

Peptides

A variety of different peptides can cause histamine release from cutaneous mast cells. The presence of a cluster of basic amino acids, usually lysine and arginine residues, at the terminal end is essential for activity, together with a blocked carboxyl group at the C-terminal end (Foreman and Piotrowski, 1984). In addition, many of the active peptides have hydrophobic residues, including phenylalanine and tryptophan, in the C-terminal portion of the molecule. The peptides implicated include the neuropeptides (substance P and others), vasoactive intestinal peptide, anaphylatoxins (C5a, C3a), gastrin (Tharp et al., 1984), and protamine (Sauder et al., 1990). Although protamine releases histamine in vitro, these concentrations are not achieved clinically and protamine is administered only to reverse circulating heparin, never alone. Histamine release from human lung was not demonstrated by protamine or protamine–heparin (Levy et al., 1989e).

Neuropeptides are synthesized within the cell body of sensory nerves and preferentially migrate towards peripheral sensory endings, where they concentrate (Church et al., 1989a; 1989b). The peptide first associated with sensory neurons, the undecapeptide substance P, has been shown to induce a wheal and

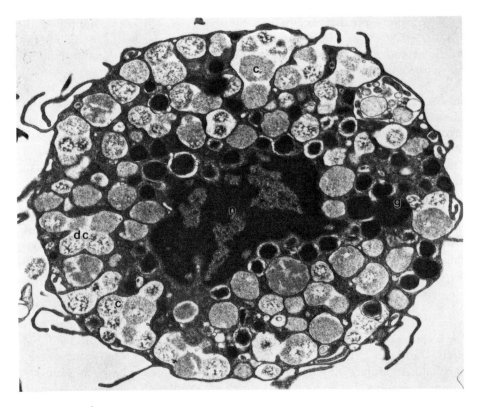

Figure 5.14 The effects of substance P on isolated human cutaneous mast cells. Substance P produces nonimmunologic mast cell degranulation with fusion of granules and loss of electron density. The granules are fusing with the outer mast cell membrane and releasing their histamine-containing constituents. *Reprinted with permission from Caulfield JP, El-Lati S, Thomas G, Church MK. Dissociated human foreskin mast cells degranulate in response to anti-IgE and substance P. Lab Invest 1990;63:502–10.*

flare reaction when injected into human skin, to trigger histamine release in human cutaneous mast cells, and to degranulate mast cells, as shown in Figure 5.14 (Caulfield et al., 1990; Church et al., 1989a; 1989b; Ebertz et al., 1986). Substance P, somatostatin, and vasoactive intestinal polypeptide all induce wheal and flare reactions when injected into human skin and cause histamine release from human cutaneous mast cells. Substance P is an undecapeptide in which the N-terminal amino acids arginine–proline–lysine–proline constitute a positively charged area of the molecule, whereas the remaining residues and the amide-substituted C-terminal methionine provide a lipophilic area. Substance P is 100 times more potent than histamine in producing a wheal and flare reaction when injected into human skin. Church found that a step-by-step removal of the N-terminal amino acids led to a progressive loss of activity. The molar ratios of histamine:prostaglandin D_2:leukotriene C_4 generated by substance P have a ratio of 1000:1:0.1 in comparison with the anti-IgE ratio of 1000:25:2. Similar results were obtained by Church with the other neuropeptides (Church et al., 1989a; 1989b). The ability of skin mast cells to release mediators in response to neuropeptide stimulation suggests that a neuroimmune interaction exists within human skin. Human cutaneous mast cells are in close proximity to a variety of sensory nerves and blood vessels. Capsaicin depletes the substance P and neuropeptides from primary sensory afferents and reduces the flare produced by subsequent histamine injection.

CLINICAL SIGNIFICANCE

Cardiovascular responses to drugs in patients can be complex, since many drugs have diverse effects on myocardial function and the systemic vasculature in addition to causing histamine release. Morphine, for example, may directly dilate the venous capacitance bed, decreasing both venous return and cardiac output (Figure 5.15). In addition, morphine causes histamine release from cutaneous mast cells, producing both arterial and venous dilation; however, histamine may increase contractility. Morphine may also decrease the heart rate and sympathetic tone to produce variable effects on both arterial pressure and cardiac output. Because of these diverse effects, the net effect of morphine on calculated systemic vascular resistance and myocardial function can be unpredictable, depending on the intravascular volume, resting sympathetic tone, and ventricular function.

Hirshman and coworkers further noted that, although administration of

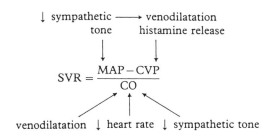

Figure 5.15 The effects of a drug such as morphine on calculated systemic vascular resistance (SVR) are complex and depend on multiple factors that vary from patient to patient. Morphine administration both directly and indirectly affects mean arterial pressure (MAP), central venous pressure (CVP), and ultimately cardiac output, through changes in filling pressures, heart rate, and sympathetic tone. The net effect on calculated SVR depends on intravascular volume, resting sympathetic tone, and ventricular function. *Reprinted with permission from Levy JH, Hug CC. Cardiopulmonary bypass as a method of assessing the effects of anesthetics on myocardial function. Br J Anaesth 1988;60:35S–7S.*

H_1 and H_2 receptor antagonists (diphenhydramine and cimetidine) attenuates changes in systemic vascular resistance, pretreatment does not completely attenuate the hypotensive response associated with morphine (Hirshman et al., 1982). The vascular effects of morphine and other opioids are related to both histamine release and direct opioid-mediated effects (Levy et al., 1989c). Attempts to antagonize the adverse hemodynamic effects of histamine-releasing opioids with antihistamines is not completely successful because of direct vascular responses (Levy et al., 1989c).

Nonimmunologic mast cell degranulation represents a variable biologic response partly dependent on the relative molar concentrations of histamine-releasing drugs (Levy et al., 1989c; 1991; North et al., 1987; Stellato et al., 1991). The ability of atracurium to degranulate mast cells may result from the saturated nitrogen-containing rings of the benzylisoquinoline molecule; further modifications of the benzylisoquinoline-containing muscle relaxants to produce different potencies or durations of action probably still result in molecules that, on an equimolar basis, degranuate mast cells (Levy et al., 1991). In addition, some patients may be histamine releasers, responding to small doses of thiopental, morphine, or atracurium with profound urticaria and hypotension. There is tremendous variability in histamine release after intravenous administration of a known degranulator (see Figures 5.5 and 5.7) (Levy et al., 1989c; 1991; Moss et al., 1981; Rosow et al., 1982). Unfortunately, there is at present no way to predict which patients will release histamine excessively.

PART **II**

Management of Anaphylaxis

6

Common Anaphylactic and Anaphylactoid Reactions Seen by the Anesthesiologist

The incidence of perioperative anaphylactic reactions has been suggested to be increasing (Laxenaire et al., 1985). A national survey in France that included 200,000 general anesthetics indicated an incidence of anaphylactic reactions of 1 in 4500 with a mortality of 6% (Hatton et al., 1983). Fisher has reported that the incidence in Australia rose from 1 in 28,000 in 1970 to 1 in 5000 in 1981 (Fisher, 1982). In Germany and in the Netherlands, Langrehr and associates reported an incidence of 1 in 600 (Langrehr et al., 1982), whereas in France, Laxenaire and coworkers reported an incidence of 1 in 1500 (Laxenaire et al., 1982).

The apparent increase in the incidence of anaphylaxis attributable to drugs administered perioperatively may not be an actual increase in occurrence, but may reflect an increased awareness and recognition of these reactions when they do occur. Most of the information regarding anaphylactic reactions to drugs administered during anesthesia and in the intensive care units in the United States is from case reports and, to a lesser extent, retrospective studies. Their relative propensity to produce an allergic reaction is therefore not reflected in these reports. Protamine is the only drug that has been studied in a relatively large series for the incidence of anaphylaxis (Levy et al., 1986a; 1989d). Reactions to induction agents or muscle relaxants may be more frequently reported because these drugs are administered more often. The clinical manifestations of actual allergic reactions often may be mistakenly attributed to predictable adverse drug reactions and may often go unreported. Most anesthetic agents cause hypotension and dose-related cardiovascular depression by direct and indirect mechanisms. Bronchospasm may occur during laryngoscopy and intubation under light planes of anesthesia. Urticaria and hypotension can occur after rapid administration of thiobarbiturates, morphine, meperidine, benzylisoquinoline-derived muscle relaxants, or vancomycin.

An immunologic mechanism for most clinically suspected immediate hypersensitivity reactions occurring perioperatively has not been demonstrated. An allergic cause is suspected because the reaction occurs after the administration of a drug. Although some agents are more frequently responsible for anaphylactic reactions than others, any drug can cause an allergic, potentially fatal reaction. Fortunately, most allergic reactions from drugs are not serious or life-threatening and subside promptly when the drug is discontinued or therapy is initiated. Why some patients' allergic responses are confined to isolated, localized cutaneous reactions or bronchospasm, whereas others exhibit cardiovascular collapse or a full-blown syndrome, is not clear.

The agents most likely to cause an anaphylactic/anaphylactoid reaction during anesthesia or in the intensive care unit are histamine-releasing drugs (see Chapter 5), blood products, antibiotics, latex (rubber), induction agents, muscle relaxants, protamine, or chymopapain. The Boston Collaborative Drug Surveillance Program recorded 8 cases of anaphylaxis in a series of 11,526 consecutively monitored medical inpatients (Jick, 1984). Although the incidence of anaphylaxis was 0.06%, reactions were most common after infusions of protein-containing solutions such as blood or its derivatives (0.24%) and antibiotics such as injectable aqueous penicillin and sodium cephalothin (0.13%). The mortality rate from anaphylaxis was 12.5%, or 1 of 8 patients.

A variety of parenterally administered drugs and agents have been reported to cause anaphylactic/anaphylactoid reactions intraoperatively and in the intensive care unit (Table 6.1). A review of the French and English language literature from 1964 to 1984 revealed 975 cases of immediate-type hypersensitivity reactions due to parenterally administered anesthetic drugs. Reports included hypnotic agents, 411 cases (42.3%); muscle relaxants, 500 cases (50%); opioids, 32 cases (3.2%); benzodiazepines, 22 cases (2.3%); and neuropleptic agents, 10 cases (1.0%). Reactions to specific drugs and blood products administered intraoperatively and in the intensive care unit have been reported as incidences, therefore information about the individual drugs is often sparse. Any drug has the potential to produce an immediate hypersensitivity reaction. The occurrence of anaphylactic or anaphylactoid reactions to specific parenterally administered drugs and blood products a patient may receive intraoperatively and in the intensive care unit will be reviewed.

ANESTHETIC AGENTS
Induction Agents

All intravenous induction agents have been implicated in producing life-threatening allergic reactions. Early studies indicated that reactions were most common with cremophor-solubilized drugs, propanidid (Epontol, Bayer), and alphaxalone/alphadolone (Althesin, Glaxo), but these agents have been removed from clinical use in most countries. Reactions to the barbiturates methohexital and thiopental were less common. Only eight cases of ketamine reactions have

Table 6.1 Agents Implicated in Anaphylactic/Anaphylactoid Reactions

Anesthetic Drugs

Induction agents
  Barbiturates, benzodiazepines, etomidate, propofol, cremophor solubilized drugs

Local anesthetics
  Para-aminobenzoic ester agents, amides (?)

Muscle relaxants
  Atracurium, doxacurium, *d*-tubocurarine, gallamine, metocurine, mivacurium, pancuronium, succinylcholine, vecuronium

Opioids
  Meperidine, morphine, fentanyl

Other Agents Implicated

Antibiotics
  Aminoglycosides, cephalosporins, penicillin, sulfonamides, vancomycin

Antihistamines

Aprotinin

Atropine

Blood products
  whole blood, packed red blood cells, fresh frozen plasma, cryoprecipitate, fibrin glue, gamma globulin, platelets

Colloid volume expanders
  Dextrans, protein fractions, albumin, hydroxyethel starch

Chymopapain

Corticosteroids

Cyclosporin

Droperidol

Drug additives/preservatives

Furosemide

Insulin

Latex (rubber)

Mannitol

Methylmethacrylate

Nonsteroidal antiinflammatory drugs

Protamine

Radiocontrast dye

Streptokinase

Vascular graft material

Vitamin K

been reported (Laxenaire and Moneret-Vautrin, 1990; Mathieu et al., 1975). The induction agents will be considered separately.

Barbiturates

Over 290 cases of anaphylactic or anaphylactoid reactions to the barbiturates have been reported (Laxenaire et al., 1983). Of the 268 reported cases of thiopental reactions, detailed case presentations were available for only 185. Cutaneous manifestations occurred in 65% of cases, cardiovascular in 56%, respiratory in 36%, and gastrointestinal in 0.04%. Of the 22 cases of methohexital reactions, 20 cases are detailed in the literature. Cutaneous manifestations were present in 85% of cases, cardiovascular in 85%, respiratory in 55%, and gastrointestinal in 25%. Thiopental is most often implicated, accounting for 268 cases.

Harle and coworkers have demonstrated immunospecific immunoglobulin-E (IgE) antibodies to thiopental in patients after reactions (Harle et al., 1986; 1987). They demonstrated that there is more than one allergenic determinant on the thiopental molecule and cross reactivity can occur to other barbiturates. IgE-mediated reactions to thiobarbiturates are rare (1 in 22,773 cases) (Beamish and Brown, 1981). Hirshman and associates have also demonstrated dose-related histamine release from human cutaneous mast cells by thiamylal and thiopental, but not methohexital or pentobarbital at thiobarbiturate concentrations from 10^{-5} to 10^{-3} M, drug levels that can be observed in clinical use (Hirshman et al., 1983). Although seemingly high, the incidence of reported anaphylactoid reactions to methohexital is 1 in 1630 (Beamish and Brown, 1981).

Benzodiazepines

Boileau and coworkers reported 25 cases of reactions to diazepam over the past 20 years (Boileau et al., 1985). Individual case reports of anaphylaxis have also appeared in the literature (Falk, 1977; Ghosh, 1977; Padfield and Watkins, 1977). Reactions to diazepam, prepared with cremophor as the solvent, have also been described (Huttel et al., 1980). Moneret-Vautrin and coworkers reported 2 cases of anaphylactic shock probably caused by sensitization to a solvent of flunitrazepam (Moneret-Vautrin et al., 1986). Benzodiazepines do not release histamine after intravenous administration (Laxenaire and Moneret-Vautrin, 1990). Because benzodiazepine reactions are rare, these drugs represent important alternatives for the patient with a history of allergy to other induction agents.

Cremophor EL Solubilized Drugs

The agents Althesin (alphaxalone and alphadolone) and propanidid have been removed from use in most parts of the world because of their inordinately high incidence (1 in 608 to 1 in 900) of anaphylactoid reactions. Both drugs are solubilized in the vehicle Cremophor EL (polyoxyethelated castor oil, BASF, Aktiengesellschaft), which may account for their ability to activate both the alternative and classical complement pathways (Radford et al., 1982; Watkins et al., 1976). The initial formulation for propofol included Cremophor EL, but the emulsion was changed because of the risk of adverse reactions (see section on propofol).

Etomidate

Etomidate is an imidazole derivative solubilized in propylene glycol; it is one of the anesthetic drugs that does not cause release of plasma histamine after intravenous administration. Between 1978 and 1982, 5 cases of possible etomidate reactions, involving immediate widespread cutaneous flushing or urticaria only were investigated without conclusive findings (Watkins, 1983). In 1982, 2 additional cases involved hypotension. In both succinylcholine or alcuronium had been used. The first case was repeated uneventfully when etomidate was used with pancuronium; the other was again thought to be caused by the muscle relaxants. Etomidate has also been implicated in producing urticaria and severe bronchospasm sufficient to cause a hypoxic cardiac arrest in a 13-year-old girl (Fazackerly et al., 1988), and erythema, hypotension, and tachycardia in a patient undergoing cardiac surgery (Sold and Rothhammer, 1985). Despite the rare reports of reactions, Watkins recommends the use of etomidate in high-risk patients, such as those with allergy or atopy, and in those who have previously exhibited severe anaphylactoid responses.

Propofol

Propofol, 2,6-diisopropylphenol (Diprivan) is an intravenous anesthetic agent chemically unrelated to the barbiturate, steroid (althesin), imidazole (etomidate), or eugenol (propanidid) derivatives. Propofol is an alkyl phenol, one of the hindered phenolic compounds that exist as oils at room temperature, and can be administered intravenously only with a solubilizing agent such as polyoxyethylated castor oil (Cremophor EL) or similar substance. The initial studies evaluating propofol used a 2% formulation in 10% Cremophor EL, and subsequently a 1% solution in 16% Cremophor EL. Because of a high incidence of pain on injection, the association between Cremophor EL and anaphylactoid reactions (Clarke et al., 1975; Dye and Watkins, 1980), and 1 reported case of an anaphylactoid reaction (Briggs et al., 1982), propofol was subsequently emulsified in a 1% aqueous solution of 10% soybean oil, 2.25% glycerol, and 1.2% purified egg phosphatide (Intralipid). Anaphylaxis, with documented evidence of IgE involvement, has also been attributed to propofol with the different formulation (Laxenaire et al., 1988). Propofol is an important new intravenous anesthetic induction agent for the patient with allergy to other induction agents.

Local Anesthetics

Although a patient may report a history of allergy to local anesthetics, true allergic reactions to these agents are rare. A careful review of the signs and symptoms occurring after alleged allergic reactions is useful in distinguishing false and true allergy. In a series of 71 patients who had a history of local anesthetic allergies, only 15% had a history of clinical manifestations that indicated a hypersensitivity response (i.e., urticaria, wheezing, or diffuse facial swelling) (Incaudo et al., 1978).

Clinical manifestations of local anesthetic reactions have also been consistent with IgE-mediated reactions, presenting as urticaria, bronchospasm, and shock. Documentation of IgE-mediated reactions to local anesthetics in such patients is almost totally lacking, however (deShazo and Nelson, 1989). IgE-mediated sensitivity has also been reported, although rarely, to parabens, preservatives used in local anesthetics (Nagle et al., 1977). Local anesthetic reactions are often predictable adverse drug reactions, the result of vasovagal changes, toxic reactions due to overdosage (inadvertent intravenous injection), side-effects from epinephrine, or psychomotor responses, including hyperventilation. The toxic effects of local anesthetics involve the central nervous and cardiovascular systems and may produce slurred speech, euphoria, dizziness, excitement, nausea, emesis, disorientation, or seizures (Schatz, 1989). Vasovagal reactions are usually associated with bradycardia, sweating, pallor, and rapid improvement in symptoms when the patient is supine. Sympathetic stimulation, either from epinephrine or anxiety, may result in tremor, diaphoresis, tachycardia, or hypertension. Unilateral facial swelling after dental procedures or oral surgery most likely results from direct surgical or needle trauma.

Although rare, allergic reactions to amide drugs have also been reported (Brown et al., 1981). Multidose vials of local anesthetics contain methyl or propylparaben, a para-aminobenzoic acid derivative used as a preservative, which can act as an allergen (Nagle et al., 1977). Allergic reactions to local anesthetics can also be due to sulfiting agents used as vasopressor antioxidants (see the section on drug additives) (Schwartz and Sher, 1985). Bisulfite or metabisulfite is present in solutions of procaine, chlorprocaine, bupivacaine, lidocaine, mepivicaine, tetracaine, and etidocaine with vasopressors (Simon, 1984). Concentrations of the sulfites may range up to 2 mg/mL.

Although complement activation during an anaphylactic reaction to lidocaine has been demonstrated, the scientific evidence implicating allergic mechanisms for any local anesthetic reaction is unclear (Tannenbaum et al., 1975). Nonetheless, skin testing along with incremental drug challenge is recommended to identify cross-reactivity and to identify which agents may be safely employed (Schatz, 1984). If the local anesthetic agent to which a patient reacted is unknown, then lidocaine or another amide derivative should be considered. This method is a direct challenge test, also called provocative dose testing. The techniques and doses for performing local anesthetic testing have been described previously (see also Chapter 7) (Schatz, 1984) (Table 6.2).

Evaluation of a patient with a history of a local anesthetic reaction should include a complete history of the episode and skin testing, along with incremental drug challenge. A protocol for local anesthetic testing is shown in Table 6.2. The local anesthetic tested should be one that is appropriate for the proposed

Table 6.2 Protocol for Local Anesthetic Testing

Step*	Route	Volume (mL)	Dilution
1	Prick	–	1:100
2	Prick	–	Undiluted
3	Intradermal	0.02	1:100
4	Subcutaneous	0.1	1:100
5	Subcutaneous	0.1	1:10
6	Subcutaneous	0.1	Undiluted
7	Subcutaneous	0.5	Undiluted
8	Subcutaneous	1.0	Undiluted

* Administer local anesthetic without preservative at 15-minute intervals starting with step 1. See Chapter 7 for additional details on skin testing.

procedure and that would not be expected to cross-react with the drug implicated in the previous reaction. If the previous drug is unknown, an amide anesthetic (probably lidocaine) should be chosen (Table 6.3). In a patient with a history suggestive of either an IgE-mediated reaction or possible paraben sensitivity, preparations without paraben should be used for testing, challenge, and treatment. Preparations without epinephrine should be used for skin testing because epinephrine may mask a positive skin test (De Swarte, 1989).

Table 6.3 Classification of Local Anesthetics

Group I. Benzoic Acid Esters	Group II: Amides (Others)
Amydricaine (Alypin)	Bupivcaine (Marcaine)
Butacaine (Butyn)	Dibucaine (Nupercaine)
Benzocaine	Dicycloine (Dyclone)
Chlorprocaine (Nesacaine)	Lidocaine (Xylocaine)
Cyclomethycaine (Surfacaine)	Mepivicaine (Carbocaine)
Isobucaine (Kincaine)	Oxethazine (Oxaine)
Meprylcaine	Phenacaine (Holocaine)
Metabulethamine	Promoxine (Tronothane)
Pipercocaine (Metycaine)	
Procaine (Novocaine)	
Tetracaine (Pontocaine)	

Modified from Weiss ME, Levy JH: Allergic and transfusion reactions Chapter in Speiss BD, Vender JS: *Acute Postoperative Care*. W.B. Sanders, In Press.

Muscle Relaxants

The benzylisoquinilone-derived muscle relaxants, including atracurium, *d*-tubocurarine, doxacurium, metocurine, and mivacurium have the potential to produce nonimmunologic histamine release (see Chapter 5). IgE-mediated anaphylaxis to muscle relaxants has also been demonstrated by investigators in Australia, France, and the United Kingdom (Assem and Ling, 1988; Baldo and Fisher, 1983a; 1983b; 1983c; Moneret-Vautrin et al., 1985; Vervloet et al., 1985) (Table 6.4). Evidence supporting an IgE mechanism includes positive Prausnitz-Künster tests, basophil histamine release studies, inhibition of basophil degranulation after desensitization, and the demonstration of drug-specific IgE antibodies in sera from patients after suspected anaphylaxis to muscle relaxants (Baldo and Fisher, 1983a; 1983b; Harle et al., 1984; Vervloet et al., 1983; Withington et al., 1987).

Investigators using radioallergosorbent testing (RAST) inhibition studies have shown a frequent cross-reactivity in vitro and potentially in vivo among most of the muscle relaxants in patients who have IgE antibodies (Baldo and Fisher, 1983a; 1983b; 1983c). Moneret-Vautrin and associates have also evaluated cross-reactivity to the muscle relaxants in vivo with cutaneous testing and in vitro by basophil degranulation. When comparing one or two other muscle relaxants, cross-reaction was found in 84% of patients sensitized to one muscle relaxant (Moneret-Vautrin et al., 1984; 1985; 1988). It has been estimated that 10% to 50% of patients with muscle relaxant allergies cross-react with other quaternary ammonium molecules of similar structure (Harle and Baldo, 1986; Harle et al., 1985a; 1985b; Moneret-Vautrin et al., 1984; 1985). The use of choline, functioning as a hapten inhibitor, prevents the in vitro activation of IgE molecules directed against muscle relaxants (Vervloet et al., 1985). The IgE

Table 6.4 Anaphylactoid Reactions to Muscle Relaxants Reported in the English and French Literature from 1964 to 1984

Drug	Cases Reported	Cases Tested	Percent IgE Mediated
Succinylcholine	265	207	61
Alcuronium	83	75	88
Gallamine	65	47	78
d-tubocurarine	40	27	96
Pancuronium	29	12	46
Atracurium	18	NA	

Data from Boileau S, Hummer-Sigiel M, Moeller R, Drouet N. Reevaluation des risques respectifs d'anaphylaxie et d'histaminoliberation avec les substances anesthesiologiques. Ann Fr Anesth Reanim 1985;4:195–204.
NA = not available.

molecules directed against muscle relaxants can also cross-react with a variety of different structures that contain a quaternary ammonium ion, such as antihistamines, neostigmine, and morphine (Baldo and Fisher, 1983a; 1983b; 1983c; Harle et al., 1985a). The cross-reactivity has established that the binding epitope on the antibody molecule is the quaternary ammonium molecule. This molecular configuration occurs widely in many drugs and also in foods, cosmetics, disinfectants, and industrial materials. Multiple opportunities exist for people to come into contact with these molecular structures and synthesize IgE antibodies to the unusual antigenic determinants. Therefore, sensitization to a cross-reacting quaternary ammonium molecule may occur without actual previous exposure to muscle relaxants.

Most drugs are low-molecular-weight molecules incapable of producing a reaction without acting as a hapten. Succinylcholine is a small divalent molecule capable of inducing antibody formation, however, and it can bridge IgE antibodies on the surface of mast cells and basophils through their quaternary ammonium determinants (Baldo and Fisher, 1983a; 1983b; 1983c). Since all muscle relaxants contain two ammonium ions, they are functionally divalent, capable of cross-linking cell-surface IgE and initiating mediator release from mast cells and basophils without binding or haptenizing to larger carrier molecules (Vervloet et al., 1985). In addition, Adkinson has suggested that mirror molecules such as succinylcholine and atracurium, which contain symmetrical repeating subunits, are recognized as foreign (NF Adkinson, personal communication, 1989).

All muscle relaxants are molecules with biquaternary ammonium ions spaced 1.0 to 1.1 nm apart. Biquaternary ammonium ions spaced $\leq$ 0.4 nm apart appear incapable of inducing histamine release; whereas the optimal length for cross-linking cell-surface IgE appears to be $\geq$ 0.6 nm (Didier et al., 1987a). Succinylcholine is also considered to be the most immunogenic of all the muscle relaxants (Didier et al., 1987a). The flexibility of the molecule linking the quarternary ammonium ion allows for structural movement to bridge two IgE antibodies on mast cells and basophils and produce anaphylaxis. Didier and coworkers suggest that compounds with a rigid backbone (such as vecuronium or pancuronium) are less active than flexible molecules (such as succinylcholine or atracurium) in bridging IgE antibodies and triggering mediator release (Didier et al, 1987a). The maximum chain length between the ammonium groups of succinylcholine (1.16 nm) is not very different from that of vecuronium (1.18 nm), but the molecular structures are different. The steroid derivatives all possess assymetrical ammonium groups.

Muscle relaxants are most often implicated in epidemiologic studies of *anesthetic* drug-induced anaphylaxis. Fisher and Munro evaluated 134 consecutive patients after anaphylactoid reactions (Fisher and Munro, 1983). The clinical manifestations included cardiovascular collapse, bronchospasm, and angioneurotic edema, occurring individually or together. Patients with rashes, tachycardia, or transient hypotension were excluded. Using intradermal, passive transfer (Prausnitz-Küstner), or subsequent exposure criteria, 67 patients (50%)

had reactions to muscle relaxants. Of the 67 patients reacting to the muscle relaxants 54 were women, and the incidence of allergy, atopy, and asthma was significantly greater in patients studied than in nonreacting patients. Alcuronium was responsible for 23 cases, succinylcholine for 21 cases, d-tubocurarine for 6 cases, and gallamine for 10 cases, and combinations of relaxants were responsible for an additional 5 cases.

Epidemiologic data from France suggest that muscle relaxants are responsible for three of four perioperative anaphylactic reactions (Laxenaire and Moneret-Vautrin, 1990). In a retrospective study from France, Laxenaire and Moneret-Vautrin evaluated 100 patients with suspected intraoperative anaphylactic reactions. Clinical manifestations included cardiovascular collapse (79%); bronchospasm (23%); flushing (55%); and edema (26%). Using intradermal, human basophil degranulation, and Prausnitz-Küstner testing (see Chapter 7), the diagnosis of anaphylaxis was confirmed when two of the tests were positive on a second (and even a third) follow-up study. These authors found that 42 of the 100 patients demonstrated true IgE-mediated reactions, in which succinylcholine was responsible for 20 cases, gallamine for 2 cases, and pancuronium for 2 cases (Laxenaire et al., 1982).

The Center of Allergy and Anesthesia in Nancy, France, has detected approximately 40 anaphylactic reactions to muscle relaxants each year since 1982 (Laxenaire and Moneret-Vautrin, 1990). Succinylcholine was the muscle relaxant most often responsible; however, other agents have also been reported as the frequency of use has changed over the years. In addition, it is noted that the reactions occur most commonly in women, with a ratio of 8:1 (Youngman et al., 1983). Sensitization to ammonium ion epitopes in cosmetics has been postulated to explain the predominance of reactions in women.

Previous studies show conclusively that patients who are sensitive to muscle relaxants and who have not been exposed to the newer agents may still have drug-reactive IgE antibodies in their serum that are capable of binding to the newer agents. Although the newer agents may be structurally different, they still contain two quarternary ammonium groups accessible to antibody binding. Once a patient has been sensitized to a neuromuscular blocking agent, subsequent exposure may still precipitate anaphylaxis, necessitating immunologic evaluation to determine which muscle relaxants may be safe to administer.

Opioids

Morphine, meperidine, and codeine release histamine from cutaneous mast cells in a dose-dependent fashion (see Chapter 5). Bronchospasm, noncardiogenic pulmonary edema, and angioedema, manifestations of true allergic reactions, have not been reported after morphine administration, even when large doses (1.5 to 3.0 mg) were administered to patients with heart disease undergoing cardiac surgery (Lowenstein et al., 1969). Heroin may cause pulmonary edema and death in drug addicts; however, this could result from a hypersensitivity reaction to injected impurities, such as talc or casein, to which the addict has been sensitized. Meperidine was the first opioid to which true anaphylaxis and IgE antibodies have been demonstrated by radioallergosorbent testing (see Chapter 12) (Levy and Rockoff, 1982). Several cases of fentanyl anaphylaxis have been reported with skin tests positive to fentanyl (Bennett et al., 1986; Zucker-Pinchoff and Ramanathan, 1989). One such case involved an anesthesiologist who received epidural fentanyl during a cesarean section and developed periorbital itching, edema, and cardiovascular collapse (Zucker-Pinchoff and Ramanathan, 1989). Harle and coworkers also reported a case of anaphylaxis to papaveretum, the whole extract of opium that contains 47.5% to 52.5% morphine, 2.5% to 5.0% codeine, 16.0% to 22.0% narcotine, and 2.5% to 7.0% papaverine (Harle et al., 1989). Using hapten inhibition studies, they noted that IgE antibody cross-reacted with morphine (72% inhibition), nalorphine (46% inhibition), and meperidine and methadone (31% inhibition). There was minimal cross-reactivity with fentanyl (3%) (Harle et al., 1989). Harle and coworkers suggest that the structural features of morphine–IgE binding are the cyclohexenyl ring with a hydroxyl group at C-6, and a methyl substituent attached to the N-atom.

OTHER AGENTS
Antibiotics

Antibiotics are routinely administered for wound prophylaxis or in the intensive care unit to treat infection. Penicillin, its derivatives, vancomycin, and sulfonamides are the antibiotics most commonly administered and most often implicated in anaphylactic or anaphylactoid reactions. Although aminoglycosides are often administered, they rarely produce life-threatening allergic reactions (Kraft, 1983).

Penicillin

Penicillin antibiotics are the medications most likely to cause allergic drug reactions. Patients with a negative history of penicillin allergy experience a 1% to 10% reaction rate; however, a history of previous reactions increases the risk to 6% to 40% (Sogn, 1984). Idsoe and coworkers reported allergic reactions in 0.7% to 8% of patients receiving penicillin, whereas anaphylactic reactions occur in 0.004% to 0.015% of penicillin treatment cases (Idsoe et al., 1968). Fatality from penicillin anaphylaxis occurs about once in every 50,000 to 100,000 treatment cases, or a total of about 400 to 800 deaths per year (Idsoe et al., 1968; Sheffer, 1985). Penicillin accounted for 75% of all fatal anaphylactic reactions in a retrospective study evaluating postmortem findings (Delage and Irey, 1972). A history of penicillin allergy is not required for a life-threatening reaction. A study of 15 anaphylactic fatalities after penicillin administration showed that 14% of these patients had a history of nonpenicillin allergy, 70% had received penicillin previously, and 33% had previous allergic reactions to penicillin (Idsoe et al, 1968). The symptoms leading to death occurred within 15 minutes after exposure in 54% of patients.

All four types of immunopathologic reactions described by Gell and Coombs have been seen with penicillin, including anaphylaxis (type I), hemolytic anemia (type II), serum sickness (type III), and contact dermatitis (type IV). The pathogenesis of some penicillin reactions, including the common maculopapular rash, is uncertain and has been labeled *idiopathic*. For reasons presently unknown, ampicillin induces rashes with much greater frequency than penicillin (Shapiro et al., 1969). Pseudoanaphylactic reactions after inadvertent intravenous injection of procaine penicillin are most likely due to a combination of toxic and embolic phenomena from procaine (Galpin et al., 1974).

Penicillin is a small molecule (molecular weight 356 daltons) that is incapable of eliciting an immune response by itself (Weiss and Adkinson, 1988). Penicillin must first covalently bind to tissue macromolecules (presumably proteins) to produce multivalent hapten–protein complexes required for both the induction of an immune response and the elicitation of an allergic reaction (Eisen, 1959). Levine showed that the beta-lactam ring in penicillins spontaneously opens under physiologic conditions, forming the penicilloyl group (Levine, 1965), which may be facilitated by low-molecular-weight molecules in serum (Sullivan, 1989). The penicilloyl group has been designated the major determinant because about 95% of the penicillin molecules that irreversibly combine with proteins form penicilloyl groups (Levine, 1966). This reaction occurs with the prototype benzylpenicillin and virtually all semisynthetic penicillins. Benzylpenicillin can also be degraded by other metabolic pathways to form additional antigenic determinants (Levine, 1969). These derivatives are formed in small quantities and stimulate a variable immune response, and thus have been termed the minor determinants. Therefore, for penicillin and other beta-lactams, IgE antibodies can be produced against a number of haptenic derivatives of the major and minor determinants. Anaphylactic reactions to penicillin are usually mediated by IgE antibodies directed against minor determinants, although some anaphylactic reactions have occurred in patients with only penicilloyl-specific IgE antibodies (Levine et al., 1966; Levine and Redmond, 1969). Accelerated and late urticarial reactions are generally mediated by penicilloyl-specific IgE antibody (major determinant) (Levine, 1966).

Parenteral administration of penicillin produces more allergic reactions than does oral administration of penicillin (Sullivan, 1982). Recent evidence suggests that this may be related more to dose than to route of administration. When equivalent doses of penicillin are given orally, the incidence of allergic reactions is comparable with that of intramuscular procaine penicillin (Sogn, 1987). People with a history of previous penicillin reactions have a 4- to 6-fold increased risk of subsequent reactions to penicillin compared with those without previous histories (Sogn, 1987). Most serious and fatal allergic reactions to penicillin and beta-lactam antibiotics occur in people who have never had a previous allergic reaction, however. Sensitization of these people may have been caused by their last therapeutic course of penicillin or, less likely, by occult environmental exposures.

Approximately 10% to 20% of hospitalized patients claim a history of penicillin allergy; however, studies have shown that many of these patients have been either incorrectly labeled as allergic to penicillin or have lost their sensitivity to it. The most useful single piece of information in assessing a person's potential for an immediate IgE-mediated reaction is his or her skin test response to major and minor penicillin determinants. For patients who require penicillin but whose histories suggest an IgE-mediated anaphylactic reaction, referral to an allergist is advised. RASTs have been developed to detect IgE antibodies against the penicilloyl determinant (Wide and Juhlin, 1971). At present, there is no in vitro RAST for minor determinant antibodies. Therefore, RAST and other in vitro analogues have limited clinical use.

When therapeutic doses of penicillin are given to patients with histories of penicillin allergy but with negative skin tests to minor determinants, IgE-mediated reactions occur very rarely and are almost always mild and self-limited (Weiss and Adkinson, 1988). About 1% of skin-test-negative patients develop accelerated urticarial reactions and approximately 3% develop other mild reactions (Weiss and Adkinson, 1988). Anaphylaxis to penicillin has not been reported in skin-test-negative patients. Therefore, negative skin tests indicate that penicillin antibiotics may be given safely. A limited number of patients with positive skin tests have been treated with therapeutic doses of penicillin. The risk of an anaphylactic or accelerated allergic reaction ranges from 50% to 70% in such patients (Weiss and Adkinson, 1988). Therefore, if skin tests are positive, equally effective, noncross-reacting antibodies should be substituted when available. Protocols have been developed for penicillin desensitization using both the oral and the parenteral route (Adkinson and Wheeler, 1983; Sullivan et al., 1982). Approximately one third of patients undergoing desensitization have a transient allergic reaction either during desensitization or in the course of subsequent treatment (Sullivan et al., 1982). These reactions are usually mild and self-limited in nature, but may be severe. Once desensitized, the patient's treatment with penicillin must not lapse or the risk of an allergic reaction will increase.

Cephalosporins

Like penicillins, cephalosporins possess a beta-lactam ring, but the five-membered thiazolidine ring is replaced by the six-membered dihydrothiazine ring. Shortly after the cephalosporins came into clinical use, allergic reactions including anaphylaxis were reported and the question of cross-reactivity between cephalosporins and penicillins was raised (Blanca et al., 1989). Studies in both animals and humans using immunoassays and bioassays to evaluate immunoglobulin-G (IgG), immunoglobulin-M (IgM), and IgE antibodies have demonstrated cross-reactivity between penicillins and cephalosporins (Abraham et al., 1968; Petz, 1978; Shibata et al., 1966). In vitro experimental studies are difficult to interpret however, and may overestimate the risk (Blanca et al., 1989). Primary cephalosporin allergy in nonpenicillin-allergic patients has been reported but the exact incidence is not clear (Abraham et al., 1968; Ong and Sullivan, 1988). Studies have been limited because the haptenic determinants involved in cephalosporin allergy are unknown. The exact incidence of clinically relevant cross-reactivity between the penicillins and the cephalosporins is unknown, but probably small, life-threatening anaphylactic cross-reactivity can occur.

New Beta-Lactam Antibiotics

Two new classes of beta-lactam antibodies are the carbapenems (imipenem) and monobactams (aztreonam). Initial studies suggest significant cross-reactivity between penicillin determinants and imipenem, indicating the prudence of withholding carbopenems from patients with positive penicillin skin tests (Saxon et al., 1987). Initial investigations suggest weak cross-reactivity between aztreonam and other beta-lactam antibiotics and indicate that aztreonam may be administered safely to most, if not all, penicillin-allergic subjects (Adkinson et al., 1984).

Sulfonamides

Anaphylactic shock has been induced by oral administration of trimethoprim–sulfamethoxazole (Sher et al., 1986). Although the immunochemistry of sulfonamide allergy in humans is not completely understood, recent evidence suggests that some sulfonamide reactions are mediated through IgE antibody (Carrington et al., 1987) and hepatic metabolism is required to convert the native sulfonamide into its immunogenic metabolite (Rieder et al., 1989). Sulfonamides are frequently responsible for drug-induced skin eruptions (usually exanthematous) and drug fever, often appearing between the 7th and 10th day of treatment. Less common reactions include vasculitis, pulmonary difficulties, the Stevens-Johnson syndrome, and urticaria. The introduction of trimethoprim–sulfamethoxazole, which is effective in treating a variety of infections, has been responsible for resurgence of the widespread use of sulfonamides. The incidence of reactions from trimethoprim–sulfamethazole in hospitalized patients is 3% to 6% (Jick, 1982). The incidence of reactions is approximately 10 to 15 times higher among patients with the acquired immunodeficiency syndrome (AIDS) (Gorden et al., 1984), although the reason for this is unknown.

Vancomycin

Vancomycin, the only glycopeptide antibiotic in clinical use, is reported to produce life-threatening anaphylactoid reactions after rapid intravenous administration in humans (Cook and Farrar, 1978; Dajee et al., 1984; Miller and Tausk, 1977). Investigators have shown that administration of 1 gram of vancomycin in 10 mL of crystalloid over 10 minutes was associated with a 25% to 50% decrease in systolic blood pressure, lasting 2 to 3 minutes in 11 of 56 patients (Newfield and Roizen, 1979). Hypotension was not observed in patients receiving the drug over 30 minutes.

A mechanism suggested for hypotension after vancomycin administration is myocardial depression, because vancomycin and other antibiotics produce in vitro myocardial depression (Cohen et al., 1970). Levy and associates reported hypotension associated with an increased cardiac output, increased stroke volume, decreased systemic vascular resistance, and elevated plasma histamine levels in patients receiving vancomycin after rapid administration, as shown in Figure

5.2 (Levy et al., 1987). They also demonstrated the ability of vancomycin to release histamine from isolated human cutaneous mast cells. Verburg and associates also demonstrated transient histamine release related to the concentration of the drug used and the infusion rate (Verburg et al., 1985). The red man syndrome observed after vancomycin use appears to be related to nonimmunologic histamine release from cutaneous mast cells (Levy et al., 1987). To avoid hypotension with vancomycin administration, the drug should be given slowly in a dilute solution (1 g in 200 mL) to prevent adverse hemodynamic effects.

Antihistamines

Rare but documented anaphylactic reactions to antihistamines (H_2 receptor antagonists) including cimetidine (Knapp et al., 1982; Whalen, 1985) and ranitidine (Greer and Fellows, 1990) have been reported. Although relatively rare, these drugs can produce hypersensitivity reactions despite their widespread use.

Aprotinin

Aprotinin (Trayslol) is a basic polypeptide with 16 different amino acids and a molecular weight of 6511. Aprotinin is obtained commercially as an isolate from bovine lung and its biologic activity is expressed as kallikrein inactivator units (KIU). Aprotinin inhibits human trypsin, plasmin, plasma kallikrein, and tissue kallikreins by binding to the active site of the enzyme to form reversible stoichiometric enzyme-inhibitor complexes (Verstraete, 1985). When administered during cardiopulmonary bypass, aprotinin dramatically decreases the need for transfusion requirements by 70% to 88% (Bidstrup et al., 1989; Royston et al., 1987). Aprotinin is currently available in most parts of the world.

Because aprotinin is a polypeptide derived from bovine lung, it has the potential to cause anaphylaxis after intravenous administration (Dorn et al., 1976; Gregori, 1967; Levy, 1974; Schuler et al., 1987); however, reactions are probably more likely to occur after repeated use of the drug (Vashuk, 1971). Aprotinin has never been available for use in the United States, so previous exposure in most patients is unlikely. In a previous clinical trial, 15 patients received repeated doses of aprotinin at 6-week intervals and no allergic phenomena were detected (Freeman et al., 1983). Specific IgE antibodies to aprotinin have been demonstrated using radioallergosorbent testing in 10 of 18 patients who manifested hypersensitivity reactions to aprotinin, but also in 14 of 44 patients without any history of aprotinin allergy. After aprotinin administration in cardiac surgical patients, 2 of 902 patients (0.22%) developed allergic reactions with IgM and IgG antibodies (Dietrich et al., 1990).

Aprotinin's low molecular weight and probable similarity to endogenous protease inhibitors suggest that the allergenic potential of aprotinin in humans is limited, and although anaphylactic reactions have been reported, they are relatively rare. Furthermore, few patients in the United States have ever received aprotinin. The risk of transfusion reactions (both allergic and delayed) after multiple transfusions or protamine administration in high-risk groups exceeds the risks of aprotinin administration. In patients who have previously received aprotinin, prick testing before administering a therapeutic dose is recommended. An intravenous test dose is recommended for all patients receiving aprotinin.

Atropine

Atropine is a low-molecular-weight alkaloid that is an organic ester. An anaphylactic reaction after atropine has been reported in a 38-year-old woman who developed cardiovascular collapse, tachycardia, generalized urticaria, and severe facial edema after the administration of 0.7 mg of atropine. She required resuscitation with epinephrine and volume. She was noted to have a positive skin test and Prausnitz-Küestner test, suggesting the presence of IgE antibodies (Aguilera et al., 1988).

Blood Products

Blood products, packed red blood cells, whole blood, platelets, fresh frozen plasma, cryoprecipitate, and fibrin glue contain a mosaic of cellular antigens, plasma antibodies, and immunocompetent cells that vary in their clinical effects following transfusion. Although red blood cells are matched to recipient ABO and Rh blood group antigens before transfusion, a variety of unmatched, minor erythrocyte antigens can also be transfused. Furthermore, many blood products contain antigens from polymorphonuclear leukocytes, lymphocytes, and platelets including the transplantation (human lymphocyte antigen [HLA]), granulocyte-specific, and platelet-specific antigens (Table 6.5). Donor blood also contains immunospecific blood group antibodies that are passively transferred to recipients, and immunocompetent donor lymphocytes (mostly T cells) that may cause transfusion-associated graft-vs.-host disease when transfused to immunocompromised patients (Thaler et al., 1989). The transfusion reactions involving the immune system are listed in Table 6.6. Transfusion reactions are classified as hemolytic or nonhemolytic and will be considered separately.

Hemolytic Transfusion Reactions

Hemolytic reactions can be defined as the occurrence of increased red blood cell destruction after transfusion (Webster, 1980). After transfusion of ABO incompatible red blood cells, IgG or IgM anti-A or anti-B antibodies in the recipient react with donor red blood cells and complement is fixed with lysis of the cells and liberation of complement anaphylatoxins (Klarkowski, 1980; Schreiber, 1982). These reactions are often acute and may lead to shock, renal failure (disseminated intravascular coagulation), and death. Other manifestations include hemoglobinuria, back and flank pain, restlessness, flushing, rigor, and dyspnea. Hypotension or bleeding may be the only signs in an intubated patient. Bleeding complications with disseminated intravascular coagulation are due to

Table 6.5 Leukocyte or Platelet Antigens

Transplantation antigens	Platelet-specific
ABO	PLA^1, PLA^2
HLA	PLE^1, PLE^2
Granulocyte-specific	Ko(a), Ko(b)
NA$_1$, NA$_2$	Duzo
NB$_1$	Red cell antigens on platelets and leukocytes
NC$_1$	P$_1$, M, N, I, i
ND$_1$	Lewis (absorbed from plasma)
9a	Jk^{a}Jk^b, U (not on lymphocytes)

Reprinted with permission from Bashir H. Adverse reactions due to leucocyte and platelet antibodies. Anaesth Intens Care 1980;8:132–8.

release of tissue thromblastins from the erythrocyte stroma and activation of the Hageman factor (Webster, 1980). Careful blood banking procedures, quality control, and patient identification when administering blood have made acute hemolytic transfusion reactions far less common.

Delayed Hemolytic Transfusion Reactions   Delayed hemolytic transfusion reactions have been reported in 1 of 4000 to 1 of 22,000 units transfused in typical patients (Cox et al., 1988) and can have severe consequences if not detected, serologically confirmed, and properly treated (Solanki and McCurdy, 1978). Alloantibodies due to immune response to unmatched minor antigens can decrease to undetectable levels over time and thus may not be noted during crossmatching (Bove, 1968). A rapid anamnestic antibody response to transfused red blood cells may ensue, leading to an acute (although delayed) transfusion reaction. Typically, the manifestations of a delayed hemolytic transfusion reaction are not as striking as in immediate hemolytic reactions, with an unexplained decrease in hematocrit as the only recognizable feature, although patients may have fever, back pain, arthritis, and hemoglobinuria. The diagnosis of a delayed hemolytic reaction is usually evident serologically. A positive direct antiglobulin test is a common finding, especially early in the course of the transfusion reaction. The therapy for acute hemolytic reactions is as follows.

1. Immediately stop the transfusion to prevent additional incompatible red blood cell administration. The compatibility of transfused blood must be reevaluated by the blood bank.
2. Rapidly assess severity. If the patient has developed shock, then therapeutic interventions, as described in Chapter 10, should be followed.
3. Maintain renal blood flow with intravenous fluids, furosemide, and mannitol after the patient has been resuscitated and is hemodynamically stable.
4. Replace coagulation factors if severe bleeding occurs.

Table 6.6 Transfusion Reactions Involving the Immune System

Reaction	Approximate Incidence*	Probable Mechanism	Treatment	Prevention
Alloimmunization	1 in 10	Immune response to foreign antigen	None, but may complicate subsequent crossmatching	Avoid transfusion
Febrile nonhemolytic	1 in 100	Donor leukocytes vs. recipient antibodies	Antipyretics	Pretransfusion antipyretics, leukocyte-poor components
Urticaria	1 in 100	Donor plasma proteins vs. recipient antibodies	Antihistamines	Pretransfusion antihistamine, washed RBCs, avoid plasma-containing components
Delayed hemolysis	1 in 2500	NonABO donor RBC antigen vs. recipient antibody	Follow Hct, renal function, coagulation	Avoid clerical errors Avoid incomplete crossmatch in high-risk recipients
Acute lung injury	1 in 10,000	Donor antibody vs. recipient leukocytes	Supportive ventilation, steroids, treatment of RV failure	Avoid plasma-containing components
Acute hemolysis	1 in 25,000	ABO incompatibility (recipient antibody vs. donor RBCs)	Supportive (shock), treat DIC, diuretics, corticosteroids	Avoid clerical errors
Anaphylaxis	1 in 150,000	Donor allergen vs. recipient IgE	Epinephrine, fluids, etc.	Donor screening for medications
Graft-vs.-host disease	?	Allogenic transfusion of immunocompetent T cells		Gamma irradiation before transfusion

* Per unit transfused.
DIC = disseminated intravascular coagulation; Hct = hematocrit; IgE = Immunoglobulin E; RBC = red blood cells; RV = right ventricular.

Nonhemolytic Transfusion Reactions

Nonhemolytic transfusion reactions are common and include febrile reactions and allergic, urticarial, anaphylactic, and transfusion-related acute lung injury. Rush and Lee reported 76 nonhemolytic reactions after 11,000 transfusions over a 1-year period (0.69%) (Rush and Lee, 1980). The types of reactions included urticaria (34 cases), fever (30 cases), dyspnea (6 cases), syncope (4 cases), and shock (2 cases). Allergic reactions to blood products can liberate a spectrum of inflammatory mediators, producing endothelial damage, increased capillary permeability, and resultant perivascular edema in the lung (Byrne and Dixon, 1971; Hammerschmidt, 1980). This section will discuss the pathophysiology of allergic mediated nonhemolytic transfusion reactions.

Febrile Transfusion Reactions Febrile transfusion reactions are common and due to donor leukocytes in the transfused product. Recipient IgG antibodies directed against an antigenic determinant on the surface of donor granulocytes are known as *leukoagglutinins* or *antileukocyte antibodies*. Leukoagglutinins can be demonstrated in patients who experience febrile transfusion reactions. The frequency with which leukoagglutinins develop increases with the number of transfusions (Barton, 1981). One third of patients (33 of 100) who had open heart surgery followed by massive blood administration developed leukoagglutinins (Pretty et al., 1968), but <1% had febrile reactions. Transplacental leakage of fetal blood after delivery may result in maternal sensitization to maternal leukocyte antigens (Barton, 1981). In a similar patient population, 52 of 54 patients developed either a leukoagglutinin, a lymphocytotoxic antibody, or both within 1 week of transfusion (Gleichmann and Breininge, 1975). Leukoagglutinins develop in 19% of women after their second pregnancy (Payne, 1962).

When leukoagglutinins against nonviable donor granulocytes are present in the recipient's plasma, a febrile reaction due to release of leukocyte pyrogens may ensue (Hammerschmidt and Jacob, 1982). A typical febrile reaction begins within 0.5 to 2 hours after the commencement of the transfusion (Barton, 1981). Clinically, the reaction is characterized by a sensation of cold with or without rigor or pallor, followed by tachycardia and an abrupt rise in temperature. Improvement follows in 2 to 24 hours. In severe reactions, hypotension, cyanosis, tachypnea, self-limited fibrinolysis, and transient leukopenia due to leukocyte margination may occur (Brittingham and Chaplin, 1957). Although leukoagglutinins in the recipient are responsible for most febrile transfusion reactions, other reactions, including bacterial contamination of the blood or hemolytic reactions, should be considered. Antipyretics and antihistamines have been administered to suppress the reaction; leukocyte-poor products should be transfused in critically ill patients with a history of febrile transfusion reactions. Whole blood and packed red blood cells can be rendered leukocyte-poor by differential sedimentation, filtration, or freeze-thawing after washing.

Transfusion-Related Allergic Reactions and Acute Lung Injury Allergic reactions to blood products are due to passively transfused plasma proteins that react with white blood cells, platelets, or recipient plasma proteins (Bashir, 1980; Heinrich et al., 1973). These reactions may range from urticaria, fever, and pruritis to life-threatening bronchospasm, hypotension, angioedema, and acute respiratory distress. Transfusion-associated respiratory distress may be due to fluid overload, especially in patients with ventricular dysfunction; however, pulmonary edema may be due to an allergic transfusion reaction (Lloyd et al., 1984).

If the donor blood contains leukoagglutinins directed against antigens on viable recipient granulocytes, then the leukocytes are metabolically active and capable of aggregating in the pulmonary microcirculation to produce direct lung injury (Andrews et al., 1976; Hammerschmidt and Jacob, 1982; Popovsky and Moore, 1985). The pathogenesis is presumed to be due to passive transfusion and reaction of donor granulocyte or lymphocyte antibodies with recipient granulocytes. In 36 transfusion-related episodes of acute lung injury, Popovsky and Moore demonstrated that 89% were correlated with the passive transfusion of donor granulocyte antibodies and 72% were associated with donor lymphocyte antibodies (Table 6.7). HLA-specific antibodies were identified in 65% of cases. In a minority of cases, however, the pathogenesis may have been due to reaction of recipient granulocyte antibodies with donor granulocytes (Swank and Moore, 1989).

The attachment of an IgG antibody to the granulocyte or lymphocyte surface may serve as a direct trigger to the cell, causing it to aggregate and thus generate inflammatory leukocyte products (Hammerschmidt and Jacob, 1982). Furthermore, the attachment of an antibody to the granulocyte or lymphocyte surface may create an antigen-antibody complex also capable of activating the complement cascade (Figure 6.1) (Hammerschmidt and Jacob, 1982). The sequestered, activated granulocytes in the pulmonary vasculature produce pulmonary leukostasis, characterized by microvascular occlusion from white cell emboli and vascular inflammation (Anuras, 1977; Hammerschmidt and Jacob, 1982;

Table 6.7 Laboratory Data from 36 Patients with Transfusion-Related Acute Lung Injury

Test	Cases	
	N	%
Granulocyte antibodies		
Patient (pretransfusion)	2	6
Donor	32	89
Lymphocytotoxic antibodies (donor)	26	72
HLA-specific antibodies	11*	65
HLA-antigen (patient)/antibody correspondence	10*	59

* Seventeen patients were tested.
Modified from Popovsky MA, Moore SB. Diagnostic and pathogenetic considerations in transfusion-related acute lung injury. Transfusion 1985;25:573–7.

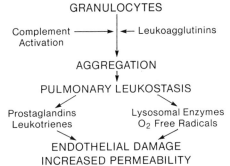

Figure 6.1 Sequence of events producing granulocyte aggregation in the lung, pulmonary leukostasis, and cardiopulmonary dysfunction.

Reed et al., 1984). Acute lung injury results from pulmonary endothelial damage after the release of leukocyte products, including arachidonic acid metabolites, oxygen-free radicals, and proteolytic enzymes (Reed et al., 1984; Weissman et al., 1980). The onset occurs within 30 minutes to 2 hours (Latson et al., 1986). Clinical findings include hypoxemia, noncardiogenic pulmonary edema, pulmonary hypertension with a pulmonary artery diastolic–pulmonary capillary wedge gradient, and acute lung injury with respiratory failure (Figure 6.2) (Dubois et al., 1980; Hashim et al., 1984; Latson et al., 1986; Ward, 1968; 1970). Fatal reactions have also been reported (Felbo and Jensen, 1962). This form of acute respiratory failure has been called noncardiogenic pulmonary edema, or transfusion-related acute lung injury (TRALI) (Carilli et al., 1978; Popovsky and Moore, 1985; Swank and Moore, 1989).

Popovsky screened 2799 multiparous blood donors and found that 197 (7%) had leukocyte antibodies (Popovsky et al., 1983). Leukoagglutinins may represent 1.9% of the blood donor pool (Popovsky et al., 1983). The incidence of pulmonary leukoagglutinin reactions has been suggested to be 0.02% per unit transfused and 0.16% per patient transfused (Popovsky et al., 1983). Although this represents an infrequent occurrence, it suggests an incidence higher than previously appreciated. In two of the five leukoagglutinin reactions reported by Popovsky, red cells were the transfused products, suggesting that even relatively small volumes of antibody-containing plasma may be capable of initiating pulmonary reactions (Popovsky et al., 1983). Any blood product containing plasma, i.e., fresh frozen plasma (Kernoff et al., 1972; O'Connor et al., 1981), cryoprecipitate (Burman et al., 1973), platelets, whole blood (Popovsky et al., 1983), and packed red blood cells (Popovsky et al., 1983), can produce such a reaction. Patients with a history of leukoagglutinin reactions should receive saline-washed red blood cells when subsequent increases in oxygen-carrying capacity are required (Goldfinger and Lowe, 1981).

The treatment of severe leukoagglutinin reactions is supportive, including mechanical ventilation with positive end-expiratory pressure and treatment of right ventricular dysfunction (see Chapter 10). Popovsky and coworkers reported that 81% of patients with TRALI have rapid resolution of pulmonary infiltrates

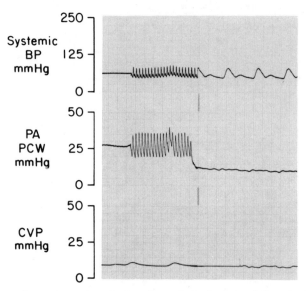

Figure 6.2 Hemodynamic tracings during the period of maximal elevation in pulmonary artery pressures after a transfusion-related acute lung injury reaction (leukoagglutinin). The PA–PCW gradient has increased to 14 mmHg. BP = systemic blood pressure; PA = pulmonary artery pressure; PCW = pulmonary capillary wedge pressure; CVP = central venous pressure. *Reprinted with permission from Latson TW, Kickler TS, Baumgartner WA. Pulmonary hypertension and noncardiogenic pulmonary edema following cardiopulmonary bypass associated with an antigranulocyte antibody. Anesthesiology 1986;64:106–11.*

and return of arterial blood gas values to normal within 96 hours of the initial respiratory insult (Table 6.8). In a minority of patients, however, pulmonary infiltrates persist for at least 7 days after the reaction (Popovsky and Moore, 1985; Popovsky et al., 1983). The mortality of TRALI was 6% (2 of 36 patients).

Immunoglobulin-Associated Reactions

IgG   Antibodies may potentially develop against the heavy-chain determinants of IgG (anti-Gm) after multiple transfusions (Barton, 1981). Sera obtained from 100 patients before and after open heart surgery and subsequent transfusions demonstrated that 34 of 100 patients developed antibodies to gamma globulin and 8 of 100 patients with preexisting antibodies developed new ones with different specificities (Pretty et al., 1968). The exact clinical importance of this is unclear. In patients receiving intravenous immunoglobulin, 20 of 70 had anaphylactic reactions and 15 of the 20 patients were hypogammaglobulinemic (Barandun et al., 1962).

IgA   One in every 700 to 850 people has relative immunoglobulin-A (IgA) deficiency (Ammann and Hong, 1971; Kolstinen, 1975; Vyas et al., 1975). This

Table 6.8 Morbidity of Transfusion-Related Acute Lung Injury in 36 Patients

	Cases	
Condition	N	%
Required oxygen support	36	100
Required mechanical ventilation	26	72
Pulmonary infiltrates		
Rapid resolution (<96 hours)	29	81
Slow resolution (±7 days)	6	17
Mortality	2	6

Modified from Popovsky MA, Moore SB. Diagnostic and pathogenetic considerations in transfusion-related acute lung injury. Transfusion 1985;25:573–7.

selective IgA deficiency is defined as 1) a serum IgA concentration below 0.05 mg/mL; 2) normal levels of other immunoglobulins; and 3) otherwise normal cell-mediated immune function (Ammann and Hong, 1971). Many of these people (20% to 25%) possess anti-IgA antibodies but have no history of blood product administration (Kolstinen, 1975). Often these antibodies are complement-fixing IgG (Barton, 1981) but can also be IgE (Burks et al., 1986). Anaphylactic reactions can occur when these patients are given only a few milliliters of whole blood, fresh frozen plasma, packed red blood cells, gamma globulin, cryoprecipitate, or fibrin glue that are replete with IgA (Leikola et al., 1973; Schmidt et al., 1969). Vyas and coworkers tested over 70,000 blood donors and found that IgA was completely absent in the serum of 83 (Vyas et al., 1975). Of these 83 subjects, 13 (16%) had high-titre class-specific anti-IgA antibodies that were complement-binding IgG and reacted with all IgA idiotypes (Vyas et al., 1975). IgE antibodies have also been reported to IgA (Burks et al., 1986). Therefore, frozen, washed, packed red blood cells or blood from other IgA-deficient donors should be administered when transfusions are required. A registry of IgA-deficient donors can be obtained from the Red Cross (Huestis, 1976). Collagen vascular disease and other autoimmune disorders, such as rheumatoid arthritis and systemic lupus erythematosus, are associated with IgA deficiency (Cassidy et al., 1969). IgA-deficient people are asymptomatic and may first present for evaluation of transfusion reactions.

IgM Multiparous women or multiply transfused patients may develop antibodies to IgM (Barton, 1981). There is no convincing evidence of the clinical significance of anti-IgM.

IgE The transfusion of IgE antibodies in blood products from atopic people may passively transfer reactively to a particular allergen. Thus, antibodies to penicillin, cephalothin, or potentially any agent can be passively transferred by transfusion and produce allergic reactions in the recipient (Branch and Houghton, 1979; Okuno, 1971). The incidence of this is low, however, and may be due to the short half-life of IgE (2.3 days intravascularly, 7 days on mast cells). Okuno screened 438 consecutive blood donors for antipenicillin antibodies and found the overall incidence was 3.2% (15 per 438 donors) (Okuno, 1971). This problem, although rare, can be avoided by using packed red blood cells when anemia is a problem (Branch and Houghton, 1979; Okuno, 1971).

Chymopapain

Chymopapain, a proteolytic enzyme injected to treat herniated nucleus pulposus, is associated with a 0.7% incidence of anaphylaxis (194 of 28,924 patients) (Smith Laboratories, 1984). Women are three times more likely to develop anaphylaxis than men (an incidence of 1.2% [121 of 10,443] compared with 0.4% [73 of 18,481]). In men, the incidence of anaphylaxis during general anesthesia is 0.5% (58 of 11,266) compared with 0.2% (10 of 4294) for local anesthesia, whereas in women, the incidence for general anesthesia is 1.4% (93 of 6535) compared with 0.7% for local anesthesia (17 of 2274). Although 96% of the reactions occurred within 20 minutes after enzyme injection, 83% occurred within the first 10 minutes.

Previous exposure to chymopapain in meat tenderizers, cosmetics, and beer may account for the high incidence of anaphylaxis. An in vitro assay has been developed to evaluate IgE antibodies to chymopapain (Chymodiactin) using an enzyme-linked immunosorbent assay (ChymoFAST). Preliminary information regarding skin testing for evaluation of chymopapain anaphylaxis suggests that this test is predictive (Grammer and Patterson, 1984). Chymopapain is unsuitable for intradermal testing because it is a proteolytic enzyme that produces false positive results and must be administered by prick testing, which delivers an estimated volume of 0.000003 mL (Squire, 1952). Pretreatment with histamine receptor antagonists, including diphenhydramine and cimetidine, before chymopapain administration does not inhibit or prevent anaphylaxis (see Chapter 12) (Bruno et al., 1984).

Colloid Volume Expanders

Anaphylactoid reactions to the volume expanders used clinically have been extensively studied. Ring and Messmer reported the incidence of reactions to these products in a multicenter prospective study involving 200,906 infusions. They noted an incidence of 0.033% for all colloid volume expanders with a specific incidence of 0.011% for human serum albumin, 0.115% for gelatin, 0.032% for dextran, and 0.085% for hydroxyethyl starch (Ring and Messmer, 1977). The mechanisms responsible for reactions to the different volume expanders involve both allergic and nonallergic pathway activation, and will be discussed in more detail. Gelatins, not approved for use in this country, will not be discussed.

Human Serum Albumin

Reactions to human serum albumin, although infrequent, are thought to represent (1) reactions to albumin aggregates formed after heating to 60°C for 10 hours to kill viruses (Ring et al., 1979); (2) reactions to the stabilizers sodium caprylate (octoic acid) and acetyltryptophane (Ring et al., 1979); or (3) ethylene-oxide-induced alterations in the albumin molecule (Grammer et al., 1984). Albumin aggregates are thought to combine nonspecifically with IgG and activate complement (Ring et al., 1979). Furthermore, added stabilizers may modify human serum albumin to produce sensitization and histamine release (Ring and Messmer, 1977; Ring et al., 1979).

Dextrans

Dextran-induced reactions have been studied extensively by Swedish investigators. Two types of dextran products are marketed in the United States: dextran 40 (molecular weight 40,000), prepared as a 10% solution; and dextran 70 (molecular weight 70,000), prepared as a 6% solution. Dextran 40 is approved for use as an intravascular volume expander, as a priming fluid during extracorporeal circulation, and for prophylaxis against venous thrombosis and pulmonary thromboembolic complications. Dextran 70 is approved only as a plasma volume expander. Over an 8-year period, 133 anaphylactoid reactions were reported to the Swedish Adverse Drug Reaction Committee, 113 of which were to dextran 70, and 20 to dextran 40 (Furhoff, 1977). Preformed dextran-reactive antibodies, primarily IgG and IgA, arise in response to dietary or bacterial polysaccharides. When dextrans are administered to these people, immune complexes are formed with complement activation and subsequent vasoactive mediator release (Ljungstroem et al., 1983). Recent data using the principle of antibody neutralization by haptens have demonstrated that administration of 20 mL of dextran 1 (Promit), a dextran with a molecular weight of 1000, significantly reduced the incidence of severe dextran reactions (Ljungstroem et al., 1983).

Hydroxyethyl Starch

Hydroxyethyl starch is a glucopyranose polymer designed as a volume expander, although it is used for granulocyte procurement and plasmapheresis. The 0.0085% incidence of hydroxyethyl starch reactions reported by Ring and Messmer represents 14 reactions in 16,405 infusions, only 1 of which was life-threatening (Ring and Messmer, 1977). Although life-threatening anaphylactoid reactions continue to be reported, the mechanism responsible is not clearly defined (Dutcher et al., 1984; Ring et al., 1976).

Plasma Protein Fractions

Plasma protein fractions may contain kinin contaminants or a Hageman factor, which function as prekallikrein activators to liberate bradykinin (Alving, 1978). Rapid administration of these products may produce hypotension, limiting the usefulness of these agents (Bland et al., 1973).

Corticosteroids

Anaphylactic reactions to corticosteroids have been reported (Freedman et al., 1981; Mansfield et al., 1986; Mendelson et al., 1974; Peller and Bardana, 1985; Pryse-Phillips et al., 1984). One such report involves an anaphylactic reaction to methylprednisolone hemisuccinate, which cross-reacted to hydrocortisone hemisuccinate but not to the acetate compounds. Mendelson and coworkers described a 17-year-old man with status asthmaticus who had an anaphylactic reaction after intravenous methylprednisolone with positive skin tests to methylprednisolone and hydrocortisone (Mendelson et al., 1974). Other cases have been reported with positive skin tests (Venkateswara, 1982). Anaphylaxis to the corticosteroids is extremely rare, despite sporadic case reports. Recognition of the potential for anaphylaxis caused by the agents used in treating anaphylactic reactions is especially important.

Cyclosporin (Sandimmune)

Cyclosporin, a cyclic polypeptide consisting of 11 amino acids, is an immunosuppressant of T-cell-derived lymphocytes used for renal, hepatic, or cardiac transplantation. The incidence of anaphylactic reactions to intravenous cyclosporin is estimated to be 1 in 1000 (Sandoz, Inc., 1984). It is believed these reactions are due to the Cremophor EL used as the vehicle for the intravenous preparation. Patients developing immediate-type hypersensitivity reactions to the intravenous formula may tolerate the oral form without effects (Chapuis et al., 1985). Reported reactions to intravenous cyclosporin include flushing of the face and upper thorax, acute respiratory distress with dyspnea and wheezing, and blood pressure changes (Kahan et al., 1984).

Droperidol

Two cases of anaphylaxis to droperidol have been reported in which the main clinical manifestation was bronchospasm (Ocelli et al., 1984). An allergic mechanism was demonstrated by positive skin and Prausnitz-Künster tests and basophil degranulation. Neither of the patients reported had ever received general anesthesia previously; however, one of the patients had been treated for an unknown psychiatric disorder during which the authors suggest that previous exposure to a similar butyrophenone such as haloperidol occurred.

Drug Additives

Anaphylactic or other adverse reactions to parenteral medications may be caused by additives used as preservatives. IgE-mediated reactions to parabens and sulfites are well documented.

Parabens are preservatives included in multidose vials of local anesthetics that can produce hypersensitivity reactions (Aldrete and Johnson, 1969; Nagle et al., 1977). They are aliphatic esters of parahydroxybenzoic acid and include methylethyl, propyl, and butyl parabens (Simon, 1984). Sodium benzoate, structurally related to the parabens, may cross-react.

Sulfiting agents are widely used as preservatives and antioxidants in solutions of medication (Simon, 1984; Simon et al., 1982). Sulfiting agents include sulfur dioxide, sodium or potassium sulfite, bisulfite, and metabisulfite. A variety of drugs can contain these preservatives, ranging from opioids (morphine, meperidine) to agents used in cardiopulmonary resuscitation (epinephrine, norepinephrine, procainamide, dobutamine, dopamine, dextrose) (Simon, 1984; Simon et al., 1982). In addition, catecholamine solutions used in the treatment of asthma may also contain sulfites (isoethrane, isoproterenol, racemic epinephrine) (Simon, 1984; Simon et al., 1982).

Any parenterally administered agent may produce a life-threatening allergic reaction because of preservatives that may be included in the solution and should be considered whenever evaluating patients with anaphylaxis. Some investigators consider it surprising that adverse reactions to drug additives are not more common (Simon, 1984; Simon et al., 1982).

Furosemide

Furosemide is probably the most commonly used intravenous diuretic. The molecule is a sulfa compound that is structurally related to the thiazide diuretics and sulfonamide antibiotics. Most of the commonly used intravenous diuretics share a common sulfonamide side-chain, which is present in furosemide, thiazides, bumetanide, and the sulfa-derived antibiotics (i.e., sulfamethoxazole). Anaphylaxis to furosemide, occurring 2 minutes after a 20-mg intravenous dose, has been reported (Hansbrough et al., 1987). The reaction was characterized by urticaria, periorbital edema, and hypotension (greater than 50% reduction of systolic blood pressure) and required treatment with subcutaneous epinephrine, intravenous saline, intravenous diphenhydramine, and intravenous methylprednisolone (Hansbrough et al., 1987). Allergy was confirmed by skin testing to furosemide and demonstrated cross-reactivity with chlorthiazide and sulfamethoxazole. Thiazide diuretics have also been reported to produce anaphylaxis (Gould et al., 1980). Noncardiogenic pulmonary edema consistent with an immediate hypersensitivity reaction has also been reported to thiazides but the exact mechanisms by which reactions occur is not clear. Although incomplete data suggest that allergy to sulfonamides, furosemide, or thiazides identifies a group of patients at increased risk of a reaction to other drugs in this group, the absolute risk of a reaction appears to be low (Sullivan, 1991).

Insulin

Insulin is a protein with a molecular weight of 5800 that consists of two polypeptide chains joined by disulfide bonds. Patients who receive daily injections of insulin can develop antibodies to the drug. Estimates of insulin allergy in patients receiving insulin range as high as 15% and usually present as local cutaneous reactions. Reactions can be life-threatening in 0.1% to 0.2% of patients (Ross, 1984; Ross et al., 1984). Anaphylaxis, although rare, can occur in patients receiving intravenous insulin (Ross et al., 1984).

Commercial insulin preparations are of animal or recombinant origin. Bovine insulin differs from human insulin in three amino acids; porcine insulin differs from human insulin in only one amino acid. These differences may account for the immunogenicity of commercial insulins. Changes in tertiary structure may also contribute to insulin immunogenicity. This alteration in tertiary structure is believed to be the cause, in part, of allergic reactions to recombinant human insulin (Grammer et al., 1984).

Mannitol

A 25% solution of mannitol (1600 mOsm/L) or other hyperosmotic agents (i.e., glucose 50%, 2523 mOsm/L) may have a direct, noncytotoxic effect on basophils and mast cells, triggering histamine release (Findlay et al., 1981), or interact to enhance IgE-mediated histamine release from basophils and mast cells (Eggleston et al., 1984; Hook and Siraganian, 1981). Findlay and coworkers have demonstrated that mannitol and other hyperosmolar solutions release histamine in vitro from human basophils at concentrations greater than 0.1 molar (Findlay et al., 1981). In addition, some patients may be abnormally sensitive to hyperosmolar stimuli. Therefore, all agents such as mannitol should be infused slowly whenever possible to avoid this problem.

Latex (Rubber)

Water-soluble proteins present in natural gum (rubber) are ubiquitous environmental antigens in the perioperative setting (Table 6.9). Patients have usually been exposed to latex in a variety of medical and nonmedical forms, including household rubber gloves, condoms, balloons, rubber dams, dental casts, urinary or intestinal catheters, and surgical gloves worn during gynecologic examination or surgical procedures (Spaner et al., 1989). Allergic reactions to latex have been well documented (Alexsson et al., 1987; Jancelowica et al., 1989). Turjanmaa and associates have reported the incidence of latent sensitization to latex to be 6.4% (Turjanmaa et al., 1989). Slater reported two cases of intraoperative anaphylactic shock in children with spina bifida (Slater, 1989). Others have reported anaphylaxis in patients with spina bifida or congenital urologic abnormalities and suggest that they are at greater risk for anaphylaxis to latex (Gold et al., 1991; Moneret-Vautrin et al., 1990). Gold reported 15 patients with documented anaphylaxis, all of whom had undergone multiple (2 to 26) operative procedures before the reactions, with an onset of 40 to 290 minutes after the induction of anesthesia.

Latex is a common component of equipment used in both anesthesia and surgery (Table 6.9). During operations, surgical gloves are in repeated and intense

Table 6.9 Medical Products That May Contain Latex

adhesive tape	hemodialysis equipment
airway devices	injection ports in intravenous tubing/injection adaptors
airway masks	
blood pressure cuffs	rubber dams
breathing circuits	rubber gloves
condom urinary collection devices	rubber tourniquets
electrode pads	tooth protectors/blocks
elastic bandages	urinary catheters
enema tubing	ventilator bellows
gastrointestinal tubes	wound drains
head straps	

contact with mucous membranes and open wounds. Tissue barriers are destroyed and blood and secretions provide an environment in which latex may be eluted from the gloves and absorbed (Moneret-Vautrin et al., 1990). This may explain why some patients develop localized cutaneous reactions when wearing rubber gloves but react with severe anaphylaxis during surgical, gynecologic, or dental procedures. The relative rarity of anaphylaxis to latex despite the presence of rubber products in daily life suggests that long-standing and repeated contact is necessary for sensitization to occur (Moneret-Vautrin et al., 1990).

Latex allergy should be suspected if unexpected anaphylactic reactions occur after the start of surgical procedures without obvious temporal relationships to drug or blood product administration (Gerber et al., 1989). In sensitized people, exposure can be prevented by using vinyl or neoprine surgical gloves and medical equipment made of synthetic plastic substitutes. Moneret-Vautrin and coworkers recommend avoiding all latex urinary catheters and other equipment sterilized with ethylene oxide in children with spina bifida. Ethylene oxide acts as an alkylating agent for sulfhydryl, carboxyl, hydroxyl, and amino radicals that can react with a variety of proteins to form a complete antigen (Moneret-Vautrin et al., 1990). Latex allergy may explain some of the cases of intraoperative anaphylaxis previously believed to be idiopathic.

Methylmethacrylate

Methylmethacrylate (bone cement) is used during total hip replacement surgery to attach prosthetic joints to raw bone surface. Supplied as a powdered partial polymer and a liquid monomer, it is mixed before injection into the femoral shaft, where polymerization occurs. Numerous cardiopulmonary complications have been reported after injection, including hypotension (Cohen and Smith, 1971), hypoxemia (Park et al., 1973), noncardiogenic pulmonary edema

(Safwat and Dror, 1982), and cardiac arrest (Cohen and Smith, 1971; Philips et al., 1971). Factors responsible for these physiologic changes include 1) vasodilation produced by intravascular absorption of the methylmethacrylate monomer (Safwat and Dror, 1982); 2) increased intramedullary pressure extruding emboli of fat, bone marrow, or methylmethacrylate from the femoral shaft into the circulation (Cohen and Smith, 1971; Kallos, 1975); and 3) methylmethacrylate-induced, dose-dependent increases in pulmonary hypertension and pulmonary microvascular permeability without polymorphonuclear leukocyte trapping in the pulmonary parenchyma (Fairman et al., 1984). These reactions are not immunologically mediated.

Nonsteroidal Antiinflammatory Drugs (NSAIDs)

The nonsteroidal antiinflammatory drugs (NSAIDs) (i.e., aspirin, ibuprofen, ketorolac) are cyclooxygenase inhibitors with analgesic and antiinflammatory effects. The NSAIDs are among the most frequent causes of adverse drug reactions (Szczeklik, 1987). Clinical manifestations of NSAID reactions include urticaria or angioedema or involve the respiratory system (bronchospasm, rhinitis, and sinusitis), and have been estimated to produce anaphylactoid reactions in approximately 1% of people (Stevenson, 1981). Bronchospasm after NSAID administration is rare in nonasthmatics but occurs in approximately 8% to 20% of asthmatics; in 30% to 40% of asthmatics with nasal polyps, rhinitis, and sinusitis; and in 60% to 85% of asthmatics who have a history of previous aspirin-induced or NSAID-induced reactions (Szczeklik, 1987; Stevenson, 1984). These reactions can be difficult to treat and can even be fatal. Patients may not report a history of a previous NSAID reaction. Reactions to the NSAIDs are not IgE-mediated, but the mechanism is incompletely understood at present. Stevenson suggests that, by inhibiting cyclooxygenase, NSAIDs shunt arachidonic acid metabolism through the 5-lipoxygenase pathway, producing increased amounts of the leukotrienes C_4, D_4, and E_4. Essentially all NSAIDs except benoxaprofen cross-react with aspirin and should be avoided in aspirin-sensitive asthmatics (Stevenson, 1984).

Ketorolac (Toradol) is the only injectible NSAID available in the United States and has been studied for its potential to produce anaphylactoid reactions. Eighty-four subjects with previous ketorolac exposure received 3 rechallenge doses of 30 mg spaced 2 to 6 hours apart. An additional 141 subjects without previous ketorolac exposure received the same 3-dose regimen on each of 2 dosing days with a 2-week drug-free interval between each dosing day. Among the 223 subjects who completed the rechallenge phase, none experienced anaphylactoid reactions (Toradol product monograph, 1990, Syntex Laboratories). An ongoing study has evaluated 200 subjects exposed to ketorolac administered either intramuscularly, orally, or topically 28 days or more before a rechallenge dose administered intravenously (Toradol product monograph, 1990, Syntex Laboratories). None of these subjects demonstrated evidence of hypersensitivity.

The design and models employed in these studies simulate the clinical circumstances associated with some zomepirac and tolmetin incidents of anaphylactoid reactions (i.e., rechallenge after variable drug-free periods). Zomepirac was removed from use because of its unusual propensity for anaphylactoid reactions. All the available data from studies to date indicate that there is no unusual propensity for ketorolac to cause hypersensitivity reactions.

Protamine

Protamine sulfate is a polycationic, strongly basic polypeptide (pkA, 11.5) with a molecular weight of 4500 to 5000 used medicinally to reverse heparin anticoagulation and retard the absorption of certain insulins, namely, neutral protamine Hagedorn (NPH) and protamine zinc insulin (PZI). The polypeptide, extracted from salmon milt in a protein purification process, consists of arginine-rich basic proteins (i.e., histones) occurring in fish cell nuclei (Horrow, 1985; Jacques, 1949; Ottensmeyer et al., 1975). The basic guanido groups of arginine are available for binding to the acidic heparin molecule (Toniolo, 1980). A spectrum of adverse reactions to intravenous protamine administration, including rash, urticaria, bronchospasm, pulmonary hypertension, or systemic hypotension leading at times to cardiovascular collapse and death, have been reported (Horrow, 1985; Levy et al., 1986a; 1989d). Multiple mechanisms for protamine reactions have been suggested and different groups of patients have been implicated to be at risk.

A spectrum of different hemodynamic effects has been described after protamine administration. The direct myocardial effects of protamine in humans are variable (Conahan et al., 1981; Fadali et al., 1976; Hines and Barash, 1986). Experimental data from animal studies demonstrate different thresholds to protamine in atrial and ventricular muscle (Caplan and Su, 1984). In addition, the cardiovascular effects of protamine administration may be dependent on the amount and type of circulating heparin (Fiser et al., 1985). Severe life-threatening cardiovascular dysfunction in humans after protamine administration is characterized by circulatory shock (Moorthy et al., 1980; Vontz et al., 1982), myocardial depression (Shapira et al., 1982), cardiac arrest (Chung and Miles, 1984), bronchospasm (Nordström et al., 1978), pulmonary hypertension (Levy et al., 1986a; Lowenstein et al., 1983), pulmonary edema with loss of capillary membrane integrity (Cobb and Fung, 1982; Holland et al., 1984; Olinger et al., 1980), and vasodilation with decreased systemic and pulmonary vascular resistance (Levy et al., 1989d).

Patients at risk for protamine reactions may be those who have been previously sensitized; this group of patients may be NPH insulin–dependent or PZI-dependent diabetics (Stewart et al., 1984). NPH insulin contains 0.5 milligrams of protamine per 100 units (Hagedorn et al., 1936); sensitization to protamine may occur during daily subcutaneous administration. Stewart and coworkers found that 4 of 15 patients (27%) had anaphylaxis after protamine administration in NPH diabetics after cardiac catheterization (Stewart et al., 1984). Although this figure seems high, they suggest that diabetic patients receiving daily subcutaneous injections of insulins containing protamine have a 30- to 50-fold increased risk for life-threatening reactions when given protamine intravenously. Levy and coworkers reported a much lower risk for anaphylactic reactions in NPH insulin-dependent diabetics undergoing cardiac surgery, that is, 0.6% (1 of 160) to 2% (1 of 50), which was 10 to 30 times greater than other patients (Levy et al., 1986a; 1989d). These studies were conducted using a much larger series of 4796 patients.

Another group reportedly at increased risk for protamine reactions are men who have undergone vasectomies, the theory being that they may develop antibodies to sperm (Samuel 1977; 1978; Samuel et al., 1978). The testis and sperm are immunologically isolated organs; however, interrupting the vas deferens and disrupting the blood–testis barrier exposes the tissues. A high percentage of men (55% to 73%) who have had vasectomies develop antibodies to sperm antigens (Hellema and Rumke, 1978; Samuel, 1977); of this group, 20% to 33% develop hemagglutinating autoantibodies against protaminelike compounds (Samuel et al., 1975). It has been postulated that these autoantibodies may cross-react with medicinal protamine, causing adverse reactions (Samuel, 1978). Although protamine reactions in vasectomized men have been reported (Watson et al., 1983), Levy and coworkers did not observe any clinical reactions in a prospective evaluation of 16 vasectomized patients undergoing cardiac surgery with protamine reversal of heparin (Levy et al., 1989d).

Fish-allergic people are also at theoretical risk for protamine reactions. Since protamine is produced from the matured testis of salmon or a related species of fish belonging to the family salmonidae or clupeidae, it has been suggested that those allergic to fish may have serum antibodies directed against protamine. Conversely, commercial protamine preparations may be contaminated with fish proteins that fish-allergic patients may react to. To date, evidence supporting the increased risk for protamine reactions in fish-allergic patients is lacking and is limited to case reports (Caplan and Berkman, 1976; Knape et al., 1981). Levy and coworkers did not observe any clinical reactions to protamine in 6 patients studied over a 3-year period who had a history of fish allergy (Levy et al., 1989d).

Previous exposure to intravenous protamine given for reversal of heparin anticoagulation may also increase the risk of a reaction on subsequent protamine administration. Patients undergoing repeat cardiac surgical procedures have not been shown to be at an increased risk, however. In other patients, Levy and coworkers noted the risk of protamine reactions in nonNPH-insulin-dependent diabetics to be 0.06% (Levy at al., 1989d). A much higher incidence of 10.7% (26 of 243) has been suggested by others (Weiler et al., 1990).

The exact mechanisms by which acute protamine reactions occur are not fully understood. Studies have implicated direct mast cell activation, complement activation, and antibody formation as the pathophysiology of protamine reactions. Animal studies initially suggested that protamine could cause direct, nonimmunologic release of histamine in hamster and rat peritoneal mast cells in vitro (Schnitzler, 1981). Studies using human basophils and human lung mast cells have not demonstrated significant histamine release from protamine or protamine–heparin complexes at concentrations of up to 100 μg/mL, however (Levy et al., 1986a; Levy et al., 1989e). Experimental evidence suggests protamine can degranulate human cutaneous mast cells in vitro to release histamine at concentrations not achieved clinically (Sauder et al., 1990). Protamine is never administered clinically without the presence of circulating heparin, however.

When protamine binds heparin, a polyanionic–polycationic complex is formed that can activate the complement system through the classical pathway to generate the anaphylatoxins C3a and C5a (Best et al., 1983; 1984; Chiu and Samson, 1984; Fehr and Rohr, 1983). Morel and coworkers have shown transient granulocyte sequestration in the pulmonary vasculature after rapid protamine administration (Morel et al., 1987). These mechanisms have been suggested to be responsible for some of the hypotensive reactions observed after protamine administration; however, there is conflicting evidence in the literature regarding the adverse hemodynamic effects of protamine in humans (Just-Viera et al., 1984). Pulmonary vasoconstriction after protamine has also been reported (Levy et al., 1986a; Lowenstein et al., 1983; McIntyre et al., 1986a). It is uncertain whether complement activation occurs by protamine–heparin interaction (Best et al., 1984; Cavarocchi et al., 1985; Rent et al., 1975), or through protamine and complement fixing and antiprotamine IgG antibody interaction (Lakin et al., 1978; Weiss et al., 1989). The pulmonary hypertension results from C5a-mediated thromboxane generation (Degges et al., 1987; McIntyre et al., 1986a; Morel et al., 1987). This has important implications for therapy (see Chapter 9). Evidence also suggests that protamine may inhibit the action of plasma carboxypeptidase N, which cleaves the C-terminal arginine residue from the complement anaphylatoxins and bradykinin, converting them to their less active *des arg* metabolites (Tan et al., 1989). Pulmonary vasoconstriction occurs as an occasional idiosyncratic reaction in humans, but can be consistently demonstrated in animals after reversal of heparin. If protamine–heparin activation of the complement cascade was the primary mechanism for hypotension or pulmonary hypertension, then the incidence of reactions should be more frequent. Although multiple pathways can be activated after protamine administration, life-threatening reactions are relatively rare (Levy et al., 1986a; 1989d). The only explanation of the predictably unpredictable nature of protamine reactions is that severe life-threatening reactions represent IgG- or IgE-mediated events.

Lakin and coworkers provided evidence that protamine-specific IgG antibodies could cause protamine reactions by activating complement (Lakin et al., 1978), whereas others have also reported the presence of protamine-specific IgG antibodies in small numbers of protamine reactors (Gottschlich, 1987). Weiss and coworkers, in a case-control study, showed that, in diabetic patients who had received previous protamine–insulin injections, the presence of antiprotamine IgE antibody was a significant risk factor for acute protamine reactions (relevant risk, 95), as was the presence of antiprotamine IgG (relative risk, 38) (Weiss et al., 1989). In patients without previous exposure to protamine–insulin injections, antiprotamine IgG antibody was also a risk factor for protamine

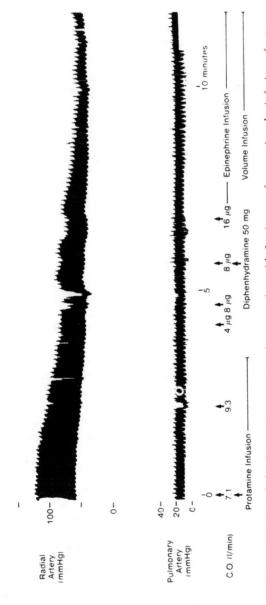

Figure 6.3 Anaphylactic reaction to protamine occurring with 2 minutes after starting the infusion of protamine in a patient with NPH-insulin-dependent diabetes after coronary artery bypass grafting. The patient was initially resuscitated with antihistamines, epinephrine, and volume administration, but later received an infusion of norepinephrine to return blood pressure to baseline. The initial cardiac output (CO) increased with the initial onset of the anaphylactic reaction. Pulmonary artery pressures did not increase, despite 2 to 3 L of volume infusion and epinephrine boluses and infusion. Reprinted with permission from Levy JH, Schwieger IM, Zaidan JR, Faraj BA, Weintraub WS. Evaluation of patients at risk for protamine reactions. J Thorac Cardiovasc Surg 1989;98:200–4.

reactions (relative risk, 25) (Weiss et al., 1989). It appears that in protamine–insulin-dependent diabetic patients, antibody-mediated mechanisms are the probable cause for the increased risk of protamine reactions. Complement-fixing IgG antibodies probably represent the mechanism of complement activation for the pulmonary hypertensive reactions (Weiss, personal communication, 1991). If IgE antibodies are present, then the clinical manifestations after protamine administration in these patients appear to be systemic vasodilation without increased pulmonary artery pressure, as shown in Figure 6.3. If complement activation occurs because of either IgG or direct activation, then pulmonary vasoconstriction occurs, as shown in Figure 6.4.

Preoperative screening of protamine–insulin-dependent diabetics for antiprotamine antibodies is not currently done because alternative heparin antagonists, such as hexadimethrine, are no longer available (Levy, 1989b). Skin testing with protamine does not appear to be useful in discriminating between subjects with significant serum antiprotamine IgE antibody and control subjects. Protamine may be an incomplete or univalent antigen that must first combine with a

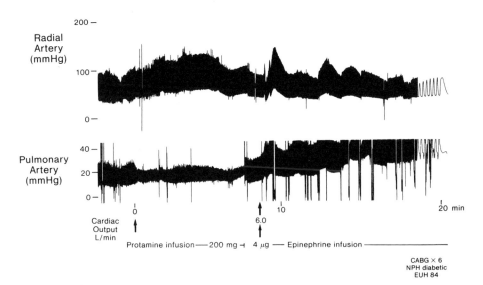

Figure 6.4 Hypotension and pulmonary hypertension after protamine administration in an NPH-insulin-dependent diabetic. Cardiac output obtained during the initial hypotensive episode was 6.0 L/min, and there were no ST–T wave changes indicative of myocardial ischemia. Epinephrine was subsequently administered as a 4-μg bolus, followed by a variable rate of infusion to restore hemodynamic stability. Pulmonary capillary wedge pressure measurements were 8 to 14 mmHg during the increases in pulmonary artery pressure with a wide pulmonary artery diastolic to pulmonary capillary wedge gradient. Isoproterenol was subsequently infused for persistent pulmonary hypertension. *Reprinted with permission from Levy JH, Zaidan JR, Faraj B. Prospective evaluation of risk of protamine reactions in NPH insulin dependent diabetics. Anesth Analg 1986;65:739–42.*

tissue macromolecule or possibly heparin to become a complete, multivalent antigen capable of eliciting mediator release.

Although suggestions have been made regarding the advantages of intraaortic injection of protamine after cardiopulmonary bypass, data suggest this route of administration may be associated with further hemodynamic instability (Milne et al., 1983). Particulate matter formed by the protamine–heparin complex not filtered in the lung may theoretically embolize to the coronary and cerebral circulation. Furthermore, cardiovascular dysfunction occurs even with left atrial administration when the lung is initially bypassed (Kronenfeld et al., 1987). If the patient has an immunospecific antibody to protamine, administration anywhere in the body can produce anaphylaxis.

Protamine is one of the few phylogenetically different proteins used therapeutically. Why more patients do not become rapidly sensitized to protamine after one administration is unclear. Perhaps these proteins structurally resemble basic human nuclear proteins (i.e., histones). Repeated protamine injections in rabbits, even with the administration of Freund's adjuvant, do not elicit an antibody response, suggesting protamine is not a potent allergen (Samuel, 1977). Furthermore, allergic reactions to NPH or protamine–zinc insulins are usually due to the insulin and not to protamine (Kern and Langner, 1938). Management of the patient with a history of protamine allergy is discussed in Chapter 7.

Radiocontrast Media

The incidence of reactions induced by ionic radiocontrast media (RCM) injections is between 5% and 8% (Greenberger, 1984). Vasomotor reactions (nausea, vomiting, flushing, or warmth) occur in 5% to 8% of patients (Greenberger, 1984). Anaphylactoid reactions (urticaria, angioedema, wheezing, dyspnea, hypotension, or death) occur in 2% to 3% of patients receiving intravenous or arterial infusions (Patterson et al., 1986). Fatal reactions after radiocontrast media administration occur in about 0.002% to 0.006% of intravenous procedures, and it has been estimated that as many as 500 deaths per year are due to reactions to radiocontrast media (Patterson et al., 1986). Most reactions begin 1 to 3 minutes after intravascular administration. Patients with a previous reaction to RCM have approximately a 33% (range, 17% to 60%) chance of a repeat reaction after reexposure (Patterson et al., 1986). Certain patients are at an increased risk for reaction. An allergic or atopic history increases the risk of a reaction 1.5 to 10 times (Ansell et al., 1980; Greenberger, 1984). Patients with a history of seafood or shellfish allergy have a 15% incidence of reactions, whereas patients with a history of asthma have an 11.2% incidence. Although a history of previous contrast reactions increases the risk of subsequent reactions 17% to 35%, repeat exposures are often without reactions (Greenberger, 1984).

A variety of immunologic and nonimmunologic mechanisms have been implicated in the pathogenesis of radiocontrast reactions, but the exact mechanism is unknown. Ionic radiocontrast media is hypertonic, with osmolarities of 1000 to 2100 mOsm/L (Goldberg, 1984). Hyperosmolar solutions may have significant hemodynamic effects on systemic vasculature or direct effects on mast cells and basophils. Perhaps the development of more sensitive assays and further investigation of arachidonic acid metabolites may demonstrate a role for these mediators in the pathogenesis of radiocontrast media reactions. A complete review of systemic reactions to intravascular contrast media has been described by Goldberg (Goldberg, 1984). Histamine liberation appears to be a feature of some reactions (Greenberger, 1984), although elevations in plasma histamine have occurred without hemodynamic changes or anaphylactic reactions (Greenberger, 1984). Activation of serum complement occurs after the intravascular injection of radiocontrast media (Goldberg, 1984), and may occur by the classical or alternative pathway. Therefore, it has been suggested that production of anaphylatoxins with subsequent mast cell and basophil mediator release is the cause of radiocontrast media reactions. The older agents are capable of inducing nonimmunologic histamine release from mast cells and basophils in the absence of complement activation, however (Greenberger, 1984). It has been suggested that the hypertonicity of radiocontrast media results in nonimmunologic mediator release from mast cells and basophils (Greenberger, 1984). Although it appears clear that the vasomotor reactions (pain, nausea, vomiting, and warmth) as well as histamine release in vitro are caused by hyperosmolarity, it is unclear if hyperosmolarity is the cause of all radiocontrast media reactions in humans. There is no evidence that IgE-mediated mechanisms play a role in radiocontrast media reactions.

Streptokinase

Streptokinase is a protein with a large molecular weight of 47,000 derived from group C β-hemolytic streptococci (McGrath et al., 1985). It is administered as a thrombolytic agent to lyse acute arterial thrombi and emboli, especially those obstructing coronary arteries. Anesthesiologists may see patients who have received streptokinase for emergency cardiac or vascular surgery. The incidence of allergic reactions to streptokinase is not yet clearly documented, with reports ranging from 1.7% to 18% (McGrath et al., 1985). Reactions range from anaphylaxis to serum sickness with crescentic glomerulonephritis, fever, purpura, myalgias, and arthralgias (Alexopoulous et al., 1984; Murray et al., 1986; Noel et al., 1987; Weatherbee et al., 1984). In vivo skin tests and in vitro immunoassays have been used to detect IgE antibodies to streptokinase. Protocols have been recommended for skin testing before streptokinase thrombolytic therapy, however, relatively few patients have been evaluated and the predictive value of these tests remains to be determined (Dykewicz et al., 1986). The use of recombinant tissue plasminogen activator as a thrombolytic agent may make the use of streptokinase less common.

Vascular Graft Material

Vascular graft material has been reported to produce adverse reactions characterized by persistent decreases in blood pressure associated with peripheral vasodilation, erythema, and clinically evident disseminated intravascular coagulation (Roizen et al., 1989). Two of three patients who had a vascular graft replaced had uneventful recoveries; however, the patients in whom the graft was not replaced died. Blood samples from two of the patients demonstrated elevations of plasma kallikrein levels and C3a. Although the authors reported an anaphylactoid reaction to vascular graft material, their reports probably represent contact activation of plasma by graft material, with subsequent kinin generation, activation of the complement system forming various lipid mediators, and disseminated intravascular coagulation. Most clinicians tend not to suspect an adverse reaction to graft material, because the substances used—woven or knitted Dacron—are historically inert. Although the matrix of the grafts used in the patients reported to have the reaction was Dacron, the combinations and identity of plasticizers used to bind and combine the Dacron are the proprietary information of each company and are believed to be different (Roizen et al., 1989). Although other clinical reactions can produce disseminated intravascular coagulation (sepsis, transfusion reactions, and massive tissue damage), this syndrome should be recognized when such a reaction occurs because survival depends on rapid replacement of the vascular graft.

Vitamin K (Phytonadione)

Vitamin K (phytonadione), a cofactor required for coagulation Factor II, VII, IX, and X synthesis, is administered both orally and intravenously to reverse warfarin. Several cases of cardiovascular collapse suggested to be produced by anaphylactic reactions after intravenous administration of vitamin K have been reported (Labatut et al., 1988; Lefrère and Girot, 1987; Rich and Drage, 1982). These reactions occur a few minutes after intravenous bolus infusions in people receiving undiluted drug for the first time. Vitamin K is solubilized in a polyoxyethylated fatty acid derivative similar to polyoxyethylated castor oil. Because of the relatively high risk of anaphylactoid reactions to intravenous polyoxyethylated castor oil (Cremophor EL), vitamin K injections should be given by the subcutaneous or intramuscular route.

7

Preoperative Considerations of the Allergic Patient

ALLERGY AND ADVERSE DRUG REACTIONS

Approximately 5% of adults in the United States are allergic to one or more drugs, and as many as 15% believe they may be or have been labeled as being allergic to one or more drugs (DeSwarte, 1986). Patients who state they have a specific drug allergy may be denied treatment with the medication when indicated. Unfortunately, a precise diagnosis of drug allergy can often be difficult to establish. Patients and physicians mistakenly refer to predictable adverse drug effects as being allergic (e.g., nausea after opiate administration). The Boston Collaborative Drug Surveillance Program has suggested that 30% of medical inpatients develop an adverse drug reaction at some time during hospitalization and that approximately 3% of all hospital admissions are due to adverse drug reactions. Drug-attributed deaths occurred in 0.01% of surgical inpatients and 0.1% of medical inpatients (Armstrong et al., 1976; DeSwarte, 1986). Allergic drug reactions account for 6% to 10% of all observed adverse drug reactions, and the risk of an allergic reaction is approximately 1% to 3% for most drugs (Borda et al., 1986; DeSwarte, 1986). Allergic drug reactions will therefore be reviewed within the context of predictable and unpredictable adverse reactions.

Predictable Adverse Drug Reactions

Predictable adverse drug reactions are summarized in Tables 7.1 and 7.2. They are dose dependent, related to the known pharmacologic actions of the drug, occur in otherwise normal patients, and account for approximately 80% of adverse drug effects. Most serious predictable adverse drug reactions are toxic in nature and directly related to either the amount of drug in the body (overdosage); inadvertent route of administration (e.g., lidocaine-induced seizures after accidental intravascular injection); impaired excretion or metabolism; or individual intolerance. Side effects are the most common adverse drug reactions, and are undesirable but often unavoidable pharmacologic actions of the drugs at the usual prescribed dosages (e.g., opioid-related nausea or respiratory depression).

Table 7.1 Characteristics of Predictable Adverse Drug Reactions

Dose dependent

Related to known pharmacologic drug actions

Occuring in normal patients

Account for 80% of adverse drug effects

Secondary effects are indirect consequences of the drug's primary pharmacologic action (e.g., nonimmunologic histamine release from mast cells [see Chapter 5]). Drug interactions are also a major source of predictable adverse reactions during anesthesia. Intravenous fentanyl, sufentanil, or alfentanil administration to a patient who has just received intravenous benzodiazepines or other intravenous sedative/hypnotic drugs can cause precipitous hypotension resulting from decreased sympathetic tone (Tomicheck et al., 1983).

Unpredictable Adverse Drug Reactions

Unpredictable adverse drug reactions are usually both dose independent and unrelated to the drug's pharmacologic actions, but are related to either intolerance, idiosyncratic effects, or the immunologic response (allergy) of the person (Table 7.3). Intolerance refers to a lowered threshold of reaction to a drug, which may have a genetic basis or may simply represent one extreme of a dose–response curve for pharmacologic effects. On occasion, adverse reactions can be related to genetic differences (e.g., idiosyncratic) occurring among susceptible people who possess an isolated genetic enzyme deficiency. Although drug intolerance suggests an increased pharmacodynamic effect occurring among susceptible people, idiosyncratic and allergic reactions are unrelated to the amount of drug in the body and cannot be explained by an understanding of the normal pharmacodynamics of the drug given in usual therapeutic doses (DeSwarte, 1986).

Allergic Drug Reactions

Allergic drug reactions are related to the person's immune response, that is, reactions in which the initiating event involves a reaction between the drug or drug metabolites and immunospecific antibodies or sensitized T cell-derived lymphocytes (i.e., an immunologic mechanism is present) (DeSwarte, 1986).

Table 7.2 Classification of Predictable Adverse Drug Reactions

Overdose/toxicity

Side effects

Secondary/indirect effects

Drug interactions

Table 7.3 Classification of Unpredictable Adverse Drug Reactions

Intolerance

Idiosyncrasy (pharmacogenetics)

Allergy

Unfortunately, a spectrum of other reactions may mimic immunoglobulin-E (IgE)-mediated reactions. DeSwarte suggests, even in the absence of direct immunologic evidence, diagnostic criteria that may distinguish an allergic drug reaction from other adverse effects are as follows:

1. Allergic reactions occur in only a small percentage of patients receiving the drug.
2. The observed clinical manifestations do not resemble known pharmacodynamics.
3. In the absence of previous exposure to the drug, allergic symptoms rarely appear after less than 1 week of continuous therapy. After previous sensitization, the reaction may develop rapidly on drug reexposure. Drugs that have been administered for several months or longer are usually not the agents responsible for an allergic reaction. In fact, this temporal relationship is often the most important factor in determining which of the different drugs administered may be the cause of the suspected allergic reaction.
4. The reaction may resemble other known immunopathologic responses, such as anaphylaxis, urticaria, asthma, and serum sickness. A variety of conditions, however, such as skin rashes, fever, pulmonary infiltrates with eosinophilia, hepatitis, acute interstitial nephritis, and a lupus syndrome, have been attributed to drug hypersensitivity.
5. The reaction may be reproduced by giving small doses of the suspected drug or an agent possessing similar or cross-reacting chemical structures.
6. Blood or tissue eosinophilia may be indicative of allergy.
7. Drug-specific antibodies or T cell-derived lymphocytes that are reactive with a specific drug can be identified.
8. The reaction usually subsides within days after discontinuing the drug (DeSwarte, 1986).

Even when an immune response to a drug can be demonstrated, it may not be associated with a clinical allergic reaction. For example, immunoglobulin-G (IgG) and immunoglobulin-M (IgM) antibodies to penicillin are present in virtually all patients who have received penicillin therapy, without adverse clinical reactions (DeSwarte, 1986). The immune responses to any drug can be diverse. For instance, penicillin has been associated with all of the hypersensitivity immune responses. Penicillin can produce different reactions in different patients, or even in the same patient. For example, penicillin can produce anaphylaxis and urticaria (Type I reaction, Coombs and Gell classification), hemolytic anemia (Type II), serum sickness reaction (Type III), and, with topical administration, contact dermatitis (Type IV) (DeSwarte, 1986).

MANAGEMENT OF THE ALLERGIC PATIENT

Patients with an allergic history have been suggested to have an increased risk for anaphylaxis. Packaging inserts for penicillin often contain a warning against the use of penicillin in atopic patients. Data obtained from medical inpatients show no increased frequency of adverse drug reactions in patients with atopy (hay fever, allergic rhinitis, asthma, or neurodermatitis), however (Ettlin et al., 1981). The study group of the American Academy of Allergy did not find any correlation between atopy and the frequency of allergic reactions to penicillin (Green and Rosenblum, 1971).

On the other hand, there appears to be a greater risk of anaphylaxis in patients with an allergic history or atopy receiving an intravenous anesthetic (Clarke 1981; 1982; Clarke et al., 1975; Fee et al., 1978; LaForest et al., 1980; Watkins et al., 1981). Clark noted that anaphylactoid reactions to barbiturates occurred frequently in patients with a history of allergy or atopy (asthma, eczema, hay fever), representing 14.9% of all reactors (Table 7.4) (Clarke et al., 1975). Dundee reported that the incidence of atopy in 10,000 surgical patients was 8.5% whereas the incidence of allergy was 13.5% from the United Kingdom (Fee et al., 1978). LaForest noted a history of allergy or atopy in 19% of 1000 Australian surgical patients studied (LaForest et al., 1980). In 85 patients LaForest evaluated for reactions, 46% noted a history of allergy or atopy. In the first North American study, Moscicki and coworkers reported the incidence of atopy in 27 patients evaluated for anaphylaxis was 44.4%; the reported incidence of atopy in the U.S. population was 5% to 22% (Moscicki et al., 1990). Although this group of patients represents an increased risk, Fisher and coworkers believe

Table 7.4 Incidence of Allergic History in Patients with Anaphylactoid Reactions During Anesthesia

Reference	Atopic History (%)	Drug Allergy (%)
Clarke et al., 1975	14.9	
Dundee et al., 1978	14.0	
Fisher and Roffe, 1984	38.8	
LaForest et al., 1980	46.0	
Laxenaire et al., 1985	31.0	16
Moscicki et al., 1990	44.4	
Vervloet et al., 1983	19.5	17

it is not sufficient to make pretreatment a reasonable prophylactic maneuver (LaForest et al., 1980).

The one factor known to increase the risk of allergic reactions is a history of previous reactions to that drug (Adkinson, 1984; Jick, 1984). Therefore, before any agent is given to a patient previously manifesting an allergic reaction to an anesthetic drug, several steps should be taken. A careful history should be obtained, and alternative drugs should be administered when possible. Desensitization by an allergist, which involves repeated incremental administrations of antigen or offending drug, has not been studied for anesthetic drugs and is impractical for anesthesiologists. This procedure favors univalent interaction with IgE antibodies and blocking of IgE crosslinking, rarely producing anaphylactic symptoms (Sullivan, 1984).

The approach to a patient with a history of an allergic reaction to an anesthetic drug should be as follows:

1. Obtain detailed history from the patient, with a careful review of the clinical manifestations and temporal sequence of the reaction. Previous anesthetic records or specific information from the patient's physicians should be obtained when possible.
2. If the history is consistent with an allergic reaction, or a high index of suspicion exists, those drugs should be strictly avoided.
3. If there is a history of a thiobarbiturate reaction, that class of induction agents should be avoided. If there is a history of a muscle relaxant reaction, then patients should be evaluated immunologically if they require subsequent general anesthesia where a muscle relaxant will be required.
4. If there is a history of a previous reaction to aspirin or nonsteroidal antiinflammatory drugs (NSAIDs), that class of drugs should be strictly avoided. If patients have rhinosinusitis (nasal polyps), NSAIDs should also be avoided. NSAIDs should be used cautiously in asthmatics because of the increased risk of bronchospasm.
5. If an anaphylactic reaction to one agent occurs, a Medic-Alert bracelet should be obtained for the patient.
6. If there is a question about what drug a patient is allergic to and the patient expects to undergo repeated operations, skin testing according to Fisher's protocol (see next section) may identify what drugs the patient may safely receive in the future. Careful observation and full resuscitation equipment must be available during skin testing.
7. Certain drug allergies pose a special problem because alternatives for providing the same function are unavailable. Protamine is the only clinically available drug for use as a heparin antagonist (Weiler et al., 1985). Although hexadimethrine (Polybrene), a polybasic compound, has been administered for protamine allergies, it is not available for use in the United States (Doolan et al., 1981; Weiss et al., 1958).

Therefore, alternative therapeutic regimens must be employed that include careful titration and not reversing the heparin (Castaneda, 1966); or administration of fresh frozen plasma or platelets as needed to treat bleeding (Campbell and Tabak, 1984). Heparinase, an enzymatic heparin antagonist, platelet Factor 4, an endogenous platelet protein that ionically binds heparin, and heparin-binding filters for removing heparin after cardiopulmonary bypass, are undergoing investigation but are not available for clinical use (Langer et al., 1982). Investigators are studying other polycations as possible substitutes for protamine in heparin neutralization (Fabian and Aronson, 1980). Protamine desensitization, reported in patients with previous reactions, is not clinically feasible, especially for patients with unstable cardiovascular disease requiring cardiac surgery (Stewart et al., 1984).

DETERMINING THE CAUSE OF ANAPHYLACTIC REACTIONS

Determining which agent is responsible for producing an anaphylactic reaction is difficult when more than one drug has been given. Often, the temporal sequence of the reaction after drug administration is the only clue. Specific allergen identification is not possible unless only one drug has been administered. After experiencing a life-threatening anaphylactic reaction, two priorities exist: 1) determine the drug responsible and avoid readministration in an uncontrolled setting, and 2) determine which drugs can be safely administered for subsequent anesthesia, because cross-reactions between anesthetic drugs can occur. Currently used tests to identify the allergen are described as well as other tests under investigation.

Skin Testing

Skin testing (intradermal and prick tests) is the most widely used, least expensive, and easiest technique for evaluating sensitivity to an allergen (Adkinson, 1986; Sage, 1981). Skin testing has an established role in the evaluation of immunoglobulin-E (IgE)-mediated penicillin allergy (Weiss and Adkinson, 1988), and has been reported in the evaluation of allergy to muscle relaxants (Fisher, 1979; Vervloet et al., 1983), barbiturates (Fisher, 1979; Moscicki, 1990), chymopapain (Grammer and Patterson, 1984), streptokinase (Dykewicz et al., 1986), insulin (Hamilton et al., 1980), and miscellaneous other drugs. Although evaluating anesthetic drug allergy is complicated by the unavailability of relevant drug metabolites or appropriate multivalent testing reagents, Fisher routinely performs skin tests for diagnosis in patients with a history of anaphylaxis during anesthesia (Fisher, 1979; Fisher, 1984). He has studied the problems of immediate-type hypersensitivity reactions to anesthetic drugs for over 15 years and has observed patients for subsequent drug exposures (Fisher and Munro, 1983; Fisher and Roffe, 1984). Using strict protocols, intradermal testing, as reported, provides reliable information as to the drug responsible. False-positive results may be produced by irritant effects of intradermal injection or direct histamine release by opioids and muscle relaxants. False-negative results have also been reported (Sellow et al., 1980). Skin testing may produce anaphylaxis by reexposure to an agent in a previously sensitized person (Royston and Wilkes, 1978). Skin testing is of no value in reactions to colloid volume expanders or radiocontrast media reactions, although in patients with a history of local anesthetic allergy it represents a method of incremental drug challenge to evaluate which drug a patient can safely receive.

Skin testing, using techniques described by Fisher, can be performed when patients request or have been referred by a physician or dentist for further evaluation regarding anesthetic allergies. Skin testing should be performed after informed consent and in a location where positive-pressure oxygen delivery system and full resuscitative equipment are available. A brief physical examination should be performed before drug administration. The author routinely places a blood pressure cuff and records vital signs before and during skin testing. The drug dilutions should be mixed according to protocols established by Fisher (Table 7.5) (Fisher, 1984). Drugs must be free of preservatives, additives, or antioxidants. The detailed methods described by Fisher are as follows (Fisher, 1979; 1984).

1. Patients are tested 1 month after a reaction, using all of the drugs administered when the patient developed the reaction. All muscle relaxants are tested because cross-sensitivity is common.
2. Patients should not be taking antihistamines, sympathomimetics, aminophylline derivatives, or disodium cromoglycate, which may interfere with or modify the responses to skin testing. A careful history should be obtained from the patient regarding current use of over-the-counter cough or cold formulas that may contain antihistamines and sympathomimetic agents.
3. The drugs are diluted in preservative-free normal saline immediately before testing, agitated, and left to stand for 5 minutes. The diluted drugs are drawn through a 19-gauge needle into 1.0-mL syringes, the needle replaced with a 25- or 26-gauge hypodermic needle, and air expelled from the syringe.
4. The patient is placed on a stretcher or seated in a chair with one forearm exposed. Skin is lightly cleaned with isopropyl alcohol while skin at a separate site is briskly rubbed with isopropyl alcohol to exclude sensitivity to the skin preparation. One-inch squares are then drawn with a marking pen and labeled on the forearm.
5. The drugs are injected intradermally into the center of the labeled square, introducing the needle bevel up and into the skin at a 10-degree angle until the central hole is covered. Approximately 0.01 to 0.02 mL solution should be injected to raise a 1- to 2-mm wheal.
6. If all tests are negative, the implicated drugs used as anesthetics

Table 7.5 Drug Dilutions Used for Intradermal Testing

Drug	Concentration	Dilution
Alfentanil	500 µg/mL	0.1 mL in 100 mL
Atracurium	10 mg/mL	0.1 mL in 1000 mL
Atropine	0.4 mg/mL	1.0 mL in 1000 mL
Bupivicaine	10 mg/mL	1.0 mL in 1000 mL
Cephalothin	50 mg/mL	1.0 mL in 100 mL
Droperidol	2.5 mg/mL	1.0 mL in 1000 mL
d-tubocurarine	3 mg/mL	0.1 mL in 1000 mL
Fentanyl	50 µg/mL	1.0 mL in 100 mL
Lidocaine	10 mg/mL	1.0 mL in 1000 mL
Meperidine	10 mg/mL	0.1 mL in 1000 mL
Mepivacaine	5 mg/mL	1.0 mL in 1000 mL
Methohexital	10 mg/mL	1.0 mL in 100 mL
Metocurine	2 mg/mL	0.1 mL in 1000 mL
Midazolam	1 mg/mL	1.0 mL in 1000 mL
Morphine	1 mg/mL	0.1 mL in 1000 mL
Neostigmine	1 mg/mL	1.0 mL in 1000 mL
Pancuronium	1 mg/mL	1.0 mL in 1000 mL
Prilocaine	10 mg/mL	1.0 mL in 1000 mL
Procaine	10 mg/mL	1.0 mL in 1000 mL
Propofol	10 mg/mL	1.0 mL in 1000 mL
Protamine	10 mg/mL	0.1 mL in 1000 mL
Sufentanil	50 µg/mL	1.0 mL in 100 mL
Succinylcholine	20 mg/mL	1.0 mL in 1000 mL
Thiopental	25 mg/mL	1.0 mL in 100 mL
Vancomycin	50 mg/mL	1.0 mL in 1000 mL
Vecuronium	1 mg/mL	1.0 mL in 1000 mL

Modified with permission from Fisher MM. Intradermal testing after anaphylactoid reaction to anaesthetic drugs: practical aspects of performance and interpretation. Anaesth Intensive Care 1984;12:115–20.

should be retested with the solution concentration increased tenfold. If any drugs are positive, drugs of similar structure are tested at the same dilutions (i.e., thiopental–methohexital, muscle relaxants).

7. Control drugs should also be tested. An injection of normal saline is used to exclude dermatographism, or during provocative dose testing for local anesthetic reactions, to exclude vasovagal reactions. In addi-

tion, a control injection of morphine (1.0 mg diluted in 100 mL of saline) or d-tubocurarine (1.0 mg diluted in 10 mL saline) will produce a wheal-and-flare response in all patients, and is used by Fisher to determine whether negative skin tests may be due to impaired responsiveness.

Interpretation

A positive response is a wheal greater than 10 mm, arising within 10 minutes and persisting for at least 30 minutes. False-positive responses to direct histamine release often arise more rapidly and fade within 20 minutes. Other abnormal responses observed by Fisher, which he considers valid and reliable criteria for a positive response, are

1. Wheals larger than 7.0 mm are considered significant if the patient is tested earlier or later than 1 month, if they persist in serial dilution, or if pseudopod formation occurs.
2. Large flares that persist for 30 minutes.
3. Generalized cutaneous responses (i.e., itching) occurring in the absence of a localized wheal-and-flare response, and if they can be demonstrated to occur with one drug.
4. Wheals larger than 0.8 mm that arise 3 to 4 hours after testing. Fisher has observed this with cremophor-related drugs only.

Passive Cutaneous Transfer (Prausnitz-Küstner)

Passive transfer of cutaneous reactivity (Prausnitz-Küstner) has been used by Fisher to diagnose immediate-type hypersensitivity reactions mediated by IgE (Fisher, 1980). Serum obtained from allergic patients is injected into multiple sites on the forearm of human volunteers, which are challenged 24 hours later with drugs. A positive test is a wheal and flare occurring within 20 minutes. This result indicates that either IgE or IgG antibodies have sensitized the volunteer's cutaneous mast cells. Antibodies responsible for the reaction can be determined by repeating the procedure after heating the serum to 56°C for 2 hours. This inactivates heat-labile IgE, leaving only IgG. Although easy to perform, this test exposes the volunteer to hepatitis; however, primates can be used instead of human volunteers.

Antibody Levels

IgE levels may decrease while complement level may be unchanged after an anaphylactic reaction (Fisher, 1980). Intravenous challenges of the suspected allergen have been attempted after which IgE levels have been measured (Etter et al., 1980). This procedure may be life-threatening and only suggests immunologic involvement; it therefore should be avoided altogether. Furthermore, the rapid loss of plasma necessitating intravascular volume expansion during anaphylactic reactions makes it impossible to interpret serum antibody levels.

Complement Levels

Total C3 and C4 levels have been followed during anaphylactoid reactions to suggest complement-mediated pathways (Fisher, 1980; Laxenaire et al., 1983). Laxenaire and Watkins suggest collecting blood samples into ethylene diamine tetracetic acid (EDTA)-containing glass tubes to measure complement conversion products 1, 6, 24, and 72 hours after anaphylactoid reactions (Laxenaire et al., 1983; Watkins and Thornton, 1982). Activation products of C3 (C3a and C3d) or C5 (C5a) are markers of complement-mediated pathways and are useful for suspected complement-mediated effects (Fisher et al., 1984). These levels are less dependent on dilutional changes and provide more sensitive markers of complement involvement than total C3 or C4 levels.

Although complement conversion measurements may be useful in sorting out mechanisms of reactions, they are often not helpful in deciphering the drug responsible. In addition, rapid plasma shifts during reactions make the interpretation of serum complement levels difficult.

In Vitro Leukocyte Histamine Release

Leukocyte histamine release can be observed using isolated granulocytes or whole blood preparations from the sensitized patient. Basophils, comprising 1% to 2% of the circulating polymorphonuclear leukocytes, have immunospecific IgE molecules on their surfaces, which degranulate and activate after antigenic stimulation. This test has been developed to explore underlying pathophysiologic mechanisms of immediate-type hypersensitivity reactions. The test represents an in vitro anaphylactic challenge and has been used to evaluate patients after suspected thiopental- (Hirshman et al., 1983), muscle relaxants- (Vervloet et al., 1983; 1985; Withington et al., 1987), penicillin- (Pienkowski et al., 1988), and protamine-mediated anaphylactic reactions.

The test is usually performed by combining a patient's blood with the suspected antigens. Histamine release is measured by either fluorometric or radioenzymatic assay. Total histamine is obtained from control samples for calculating the percent release. These techniques correlate well with skin testing and avoid exposing a potentially sensitive patient to the suspected antigen. Furthermore, they allow screening of multiple allergens without requiring the patient's presence. Leukocyte histamine release can provide accurate, confirmatory results when 1) positive skin tests do not correlate with case histories, 2) skin testing may be considered too hazardous or inconvenient, or 3) confirmation of negative or inconclusive skin tests is needed (Faraj et al., 1983).

Radioallergosorbent Test

Antigen-specific IgE antibody can be measured using the radioallergosorbent test (RAST) (Berg and Johansson, 1974; Wide, 1973). This technique is highly sensitive for detecting antibodies (Johansson, 1978). An antigen is complexed to an insoluble matrix (carbohydrate particle, paper disc, or the wall of polystyrene test tubes or plastic microliter wells); this complex is then incubated with the patient's serum and washed, eluting off unbound antibodies. The amount of immunospecific IgE antibody is determined by subsequent incubation of the complex with ^{125}I-labeled anti-IgE. Bound radioactivity reflects antigen-specific antibody and is compared with a reference system.

When performed appropriately, the RAST correlates well with skin-test endpoint titration, basophil histamine release, and provocation tests (Council on Scientific Affairs, 1987; Norman et al., 1973; Santrach et al., 1981). The results of the serum studied are compared with a positive reference serum and a negative control serum. Application of this test to diagnosing drug hypersensitivity due to IgE antibodies has been limited because of insufficient knowledge of the drug metabolite acting either as the antigen or the hapten. In 1971, a RAST was developed to measure IgE antibody to the major determinant of penicillin (Wide and Juhlin, 1971), and more recently RASTs have been developed to measure IgE antibody to insulin (Hamilton et al., 1980), chymopapain (Grammer and Patterson, 1984), muscle relaxants (Baldo and Fisher, 1983a; 1983b; Harle et al., 1984), thiopental (Harle et al., 1986), and protamine (Weiss et al., 1989). False-positive test results may be caused by high nonspecific binding, high total serum IgE levels, or poor technique (Dueck and O'Connor, 1984; Hamilton et al., 1980). False-negative results may occur due to interference of high levels of IgG "blocking antibodies" or the inability to maximize assay sensitivity (Zeiss et al., 1981). Although the sensitivity and predictive values of RASTs have been questioned, this test may offer new diagnostic potentials to determine the cause of anaphylaxis following multiple drug exposure. Unfortunately, the commercial availability of RASTs to drugs is limited.

Enzyme-Linked Immunoabsorbent Assay

Antigen-specific antibodies can also be measured by enzyme-linked immunoabsorbent assay (ELISA) testing (Roitt et al., 1989). As in the RAST, the antigen is complexed to an insoluble matrix, usually a plastic plate or tube. Patient serum is then added to the matrix and washed, eluting off unbound antibodies. The amount of immunospecific IgE is determined by addition of anti-IgE coupled to an enzyme such as peroxidase. Unbound enzyme-linked antibody is then washed away. A colorless substrate that is acted on by peroxidase, called a *chromogen,* is then added to the assay. The amount of antibody is determined by optical scanning of the colored end product.

The ELISA has been used to demonstrate IgE antibodies to chymopapain and protamine and has been developed to screen patients for other antibodies to diverse agents such as human immunodeficiency virus. The test can be performed in a relatively short time without the need for radioisotopes. There are no tests commercially available for evaluation of IgE antibodies to anesthetic drugs, but an enzyme-linked immunosorbent assay was developed for IgE antibodies to chymopapain (Chymodiactin, ChymoFAST, Smith Laboratories). A large prospective series of serum samples was obtained for ELISA testing before chymopapain injection for chemonucleolysis. Out of 3466 patients tested, 36 patients (1%) demonstrated Chymodiactin IgE concentration of ≥0.06 IU/mL. Of these 36 patients, only 11 underwent chemonucleolysis of their ruptured nucleus pulposus with Chymodiactin. Seven of these 11 patients (63.6%) developed anaphylaxis whereas only 8 of 3052 (0.26%) patients for whom clinical observation data were available developed reactions (Smith Laboratories, post-marketing survey). These findings indicate that patients with Chymodiactin IgE concentrations of 0.06 IU/mL should not undergo chymopapain injections.

Tryptase

Tryptase, a neutral protease stored in mast cell granules, is increased after mast-cell-related events such as anaphylaxis. Because the half-life of tryptase in plasma in approximately 2 hours and is not prone to rapid degradation, levels can be measured by radioimmunoassay in plasma, or serum in vitro (Tryptase RIACT, Pharmacia, Uppsala, Sweden). Tryptase represents an important alternative to histamine when sampling is delayed. Also, tryptase may represent a more specific marker for anaphylaxis. Matsson and coworkers reported two cases of anaphylaxis to anesthetic drugs in which tryptase levels were elevated (Matsson et al., 1991). Laroche and coworkers reported increases in plasma tryptase and histamine after perioperative anaphylaxis (Laroche et al., 1991). Schwartz recommends that plasma or serum tryptase be obtained as soon as possible after the anaphylactic episode and 1 hour after the onset to allow optimal sampling for tryptase levels. Normal tryptase levels in serum or plasma are less than 2.5 ng/mL, whereas levels greater than 10 ng/mL have been found in all patients with anaphylaxis and may reach as high as 1000 ng/mL (Schwartz et al., 1987; Schwartz, 1990). If tryptase levels are elevated, suggesting a true anaphylactic event has occurred, then definitive skin testing or additional tests can be performed to elucidate the causative agent of the reaction (see also Chapter 3).

USE OF TEST DOSES

Several factors make the clinical use of a test dose impractical. First, anaphylaxis is a dose-independent response. The smallest effective test dose for assessing an allergic reaction is difficult to determine. Minute doses, including those used for skin testing, have been reported to cause anaphylaxis. After a suspected anaphylactic reaction to succinylcholine, a patient was skin tested with 25 μg of the drug (1/4000th of the normal intravenous dosage) (Royston and Wilkes, 1978). A wheal and flare developed over the injection site and was followed by bronchospasm. A routine protamine "test" dose of 5 mg represents 6.02×10^{15} molecules, far too many molecules to administer for allergy testing. Another patient with a history of anaphylaxis on induction of anesthesia, after being given a thiopental "test dose" of 5 mg, suffered cardiovascular collapse (C.C. Hug, unpublished data). Intravenous test doses in patients with suspected drug allergies may be dangerous. Test doses that anesthesiologists administer assess pharmarcologic idiosyncratic effects and not allergy. When skin testing patients for penicillin allergy, 1×10^{-6} of the normal dose is administered. If intravenous test doses are to be used as a routine precaution in patients receiving drugs with a higher incidence of anaphylaxis (protamine or aprotinin), then very small quantities (i.e., 0.05 mL) of a highly diluted drug ($\mu g/mL$ or less) should be used.

PRETREATMENT FOR ANAPHYLACTIC/ANAPHYLACTOID REACTIONS

Sometimes a patient with a history of an anaphylactic or anaphylactoid reaction must receive a substance suspected of producing such a reaction (Greenberger et al., 1980). Certain patients may have a higher-than-average likelihood of having an anaphylactic reaction (e.g., an atopic woman who is to receive chymopapain). Clinicians may desire to pretreat these patients at risk with pharmacologic agents to attentuate potential reactions if they occur. The role or value of pretreatment needs to be considered.

Pretreatment of adult patients with a history of ionic radiocontrast media reactions is a well-established protocol and involves the use of diphenhydramine, 50 mg, an H_1 receptor antagonist by mouth or intramuscularly 1 hour before the procedure, and prednisone, 150 mg, in divided doses 13 hours before rechallenging (50 mg 13, 7, and 1 hour before the procedure) (Greenberger, 1984; Greenberger et al., 1981; Kelly et al., 1978). In addition, ephedrine, 25 mg, is administered orally unless angina, arrhythmias, or other contraindications exist (Greenberger, 1984). Although reactions are not completely prevented, pretreatment appears to decrease both the rate and severity of reactions (Kelly et al., 1978).

Greenberger and coworkers have reported the different pretreatment protocols for prophylaxis against 857 repeat contrast reactions (Greenberger et al., 1980; 1981; 1985). Pretreatment with prednisone-diphenhydramine in 415 procedures for patients with previous anaphylactoid reactions resulted in 45 reactions (10.8%) during which transient hypotension occurred in 3 patients (0.7%); the incidence of anaphylactoid reactions without pretreatment is 17% to 35% (Greenberger et al., 1985). The addition of ephedrine sulfate, 25 mg, orally 1 hour before the procedure to the prednisone-diphenhydramine protocol in 180 procedures was associated with only 9 reactions (5%) (Greenberger et al., 1985). The addition of an H_2 receptor antagonist, cimetidine, 300 mg, orally 1 hour before the procedure was not useful in 100 procedures in that 14 reactions (14%) occurred (Greenberger et al., 1985). Despite the protection obtained with pretreatment, it is important to realize these reactions are not immunologic and are considered anaphylactoid in nature (see Chapter 6) (Lalli, 1980).

On the other hand, pretreatment for true anaphylaxis has not been well established. The importance of administering β_2-adrenergic agents in the treatment of anaphylaxis is to stimulate intracellular $3',5'$-adenosine monophosphate both to act as a bronchodilator and to inhibitor mediator release in mast cells and basophils. Allergen-mediated histamine release can be inhibited in patients pretreated with terbutaline, a β_2-agonist that has been suggested to have an antianaphylactic effect (Radermacker and Gustin, 1981). The radiocontrast media pretreatment modifications using ephedrine, a catecholamine with both α- and β-adrenergic activity, may take advantage of these cellular effects.

Despite the lack of direct evidence proving the value of pharmacologic pretreatment for anaphylaxis, enough consistent thought recurs throughout the literature to justify proposing an approach to these problems. Predisposing factors should be sought, and the patient with multiple drug allergies should be suspected of being at increased risk. In these people, one might consider giving both H_1 and H_2 receptor antagonists for 16 to 24 hours before anesthesia or exposure to a suspected allergen (Doenicke and Lorenz, 1982; Halery and Altura, 1977; Kaliner et al., 1981; Lorenz et al., 1990; Owen et al., 1982). The H_1 receptor antagonist appears to need this much time to act on the receptor. The purpose of pretreatment with both H_1 and H_2 receptor blockers is not to prevent an anaphylactic reaction, but rather to alter the physiologic dose–response curve to histamine (Levy, 1985b). Although histamine release appears to produce the initial hypotension associated with anaphylaxis, antihistamines do not prevent secondary mediator release after mast cell or basophil activation.

Perhaps large doses of steroids in divided doses for at least 24 hours in combination with antihistamines should be administered to patients with multiple allergies or before exposure to agents associated with a high incidence of anaphylactic reactions (e.g., chymopapain) (Hammerschmidt et al., 1979; Schrieber, 1977). There are no data demonstrating the usefulness of corticosteroids in pretreatment for anaphylaxis, however. Dexamethasone does not completely inhibit mediator release from human lung tissue and purified mast cells after activation (Schleimer et al., 1983b). Further, anaphylactic reactions can occur despite the incidental use of a single dose of dexamethasone or methylprednisolone before drug administration (see Chapter 12) (Levy et al., 1986a).

Other considerations for pretreating patients for potential anaphylactic reactions include optimizing a patient's volume status before antigenic exposure—including replacement of a previous volume deficit for the surgical or critically ill patient. As important as pretreatment is the early recognition and therapeutic plan for severe, life-threatening reactions, as outlined in Chapter 10.

8

General Approach to Anaphylactic Reactions

A high index of suspicion is important in making the diagnosis of anaphylaxis. Anaphylaxis should always be considered after the immediate onset of hypotension with or without bronchospasm whenever a parenteral substance is administered intraoperatively or in an intensive care unit setting. Hypotension is *relative* to preexisting blood pressure, but can be typically defined as a systolic blood pressure less than 80 mmHg, a mean arterial pressure less than 60 mmHg, or a blood pressure less than 20% of control awake values. Shock is produced when tissue perfusion is inadequate to support organ function and cellular metabolism (e.g., obtundation, myocardial ischemia). Higher pressures may be consistent with shock in patients with chronic hypertension, whereas a blood pressure of 80/50 mmHg may be normal in a young healthy person.

A variety of clinical problems can produce cardiovascular collapse and respiratory dysfunction that may be confused with anaphylaxis (Kofke and Levy, 1986; Terr, 1985; Wasserman, 1983). A differential diagnosis of anaphylaxis should include consideration of the following (Table 8.1).

ADMINISTRATION OF SEDATIVE, HYPNOTIC, OR ANESTHETIC DRUGS

Precipitous hypotension often follows the administration of intravenous sedative, hypnotic, or anesthetic drugs in critically ill patients. This effect occurs typically in patients who are hypovolemic or require a high sympathetic tone to maintain perfusion pressure. Sedating these patients with any one or combination of agents (i.e. benzodiazepines or opioids) causes their basal catecholamine levels to fall and blood pressure to decrease as well (Tomicheck et al., 1983). Although this type of reaction represents a predictable adverse drug reaction, it may mimic anaphylaxis and require catecholamines and volume administration to correct. In addition, most opioids release histamine and directly produce vasodilation and decrease venous return. Intravenous anesthetic drugs can produce vasodilation and precipitous hypotension independent of allergic mechanisms.

Table 8.1 Differential Diagnosis of Anaphylaxis

Administration of sedative, hypnotic, or anesthetic drugs
Asthma
Cardiogenic shock
Disconnection or overdosage of vasoactive drug infusions
Dysrhythmias
Hereditary angioedema
Jarisch-Herxheimer reactions
Mastocytosis
Pericardial tamponade
Postextubation stridor
Pulmonary edema
Pulmonary embolus
Septic shock
Tension pneumothorax
Vasovagal reactions
Venous air embolism

ASTHMA

Bronchospasm and wheezing can develop after endotracheal intubation in patients with asthma. Although this may be confused with an anaphylactic reaction, patients with a history of asthma have airway inflammation and reactive airways sensitive to airway manipulation. Other causes of intraoperative wheezing should be considered, however (Table 8.2).

Table 8.2 Intraoperative Causes of Wheezing

Reactive airways
Pulmonary edema
Pneumothorax
Anaphylaxis
Aspiration
Endobronchial intubation
Airway obstruction
Endotracheal tube obstruction
Negative pressure expiration
Pulmonary emboli

CARDIOGENIC SHOCK

Cardiogenic shock occurs with acute ventricular dysfunction after myocardial infarction or valvular rupture. The signs and symptoms include cold clammy skin with poor capillary refill, hypotension, usually with high ventricular preload, dysrhythmias, dyspnea, orthopnea, tachypnea, rales, wheezing, pulmonary edema, and hypoxemia. Previous symptoms of chest pain and ischemic heart disease in association with acute electrocardiographic changes suggest cardiogenic shock.

DISCONNECTION OR OVERDOSAGE OF VASOACTIVE DRUG INFUSIONS

Inadvertent discontinuation of vasoconstrictor infusions in critically ill patients should always be considered as a cause of precipitous hypotension. Catecholamines should be infused into central venous catheters whenever possible to avoid this problem. In addition, inadvertent overdosage when sodium nitroprusside or nitroglycerin is administered intravenously can occur after accidental flushing. Infusion rates, sites of administration, and patency of intravenous cannulas should be reevaluated after precipitous hypotension in patients receiving vasoactive medications. A variety of different drugs administered intravenously can produce vasodilation and hypotension (Table 8.3).

Table 8.3 Drugs Administered Intravenously that Produce Vasodilation

Adenosine

Angiotensin-converting enzyme inhibitors: enalaprilat

α_2-adrenergic agonists: α-methyldopa, clonidine, prazosin

α_1-adrenergic blocking agents: phentolamine, tolazoline

Antipsychotic drugs: phenothiazines, butyrophenones

Arterial vasodilators: hydralazine

β_2-adrenergic agents: isoproterenol

Calcium channel blockers: diltiazam, isradipine, nicardipine, nifedipine, verapamil

Desmopressin

Ganglionic blockers: trimethapham

Opioids

Nitrates

Sedative/hypnotics: propofol, thiopental

Sodium nitroprusside

Phosphodiesterase inhibitors: amrinone, aminophylline, enoximone, milrinone, papaverine, dipyridamole

DYSRHYTHMIAS

Bradycardia, rapid ventricular rates, or sudden loss of sinus rhythm in patients with valvular heart disease (e.g., mitral or aortic stenosis) may seriously compromise left ventricular filling and decrease cardiac output to produce shock. The heart rate and rhythm should be evaluated in all patients in shock. Dysrhythmias can also occur secondary to anaphylaxis.

HEREDITARY ANGIOEDEMA

Hereditary angioedema is characterized by sporadic attacks of deep tissue swelling, often starting around the mouth and spreading to the larynx and face and producing airway obstruction. Patients usually have a history of this problem in response to stress, tissue trauma, or other factors. The diagnosis is made by decreased levels of C4 and an absent or defective C1 esterase inhibitor (see Chapter 4).

JARISCH-HERXHEIMER REACTIONS

Jarisch-Herxheimer reactions are classically described hours after therapy for infections such as syphilis. They are characterized by fever, shaking chills, neuralgia, and myalgias (Terr, 1985).

MASTOCYTOSIS

Mastocytosis is an uncommon condition that results from aberrant proliferation of tissue mast cells. The disease process may be confined to the skin (cutaneous mastocytosis) or may involve multiple organs (systemic mastocytosis). The most common form of cutaneous mastocytosis is urticaria pigmentosa, in which mast cells proliferate in the skin as multiple discrete hyperpigmentations occurring predominantly on the truncal regions (Greenblatt and Chen, 1990). After a variety of intraoperative stimuli, including extremes of temperature and histamine-releasing drugs, mast cell contents are released, possibly producing symptoms of urticaria, pruritis, flushing abdominal cramps, or episodes of cardiovascular collapse (Scott et al., 1983). The anesthetic management of these patients includes pretreatment with H_1 and H_2 receptor blockade and avoidance of drugs known to produce nonimmunologic mast cell degranulation (see Chapter 5). Additional premedication with aspirin, or other nonsteroidal antiinflammatory drugs that inhibit the production of prostaglandin D_2, the major prostaglandin released by mast cells, has been suggested (Greenblatt and Chen, 1990). Patients with mastocytosis may develop cardiovascular collapse after administration of histamine-releasing drugs if the syndrome is not previously recognized.

PERICARDIAL TAMPONADE

Pericardial tamponade may occur, especially with previous chest surgery, blunt chest trauma, or pericardial disease. The classic signs include hypotension, elevated central venous pressure (with neck vein distention), decreased heart tones, and pulsus paradoxus. In addition, the electrocardiogram may reveal decreased voltage and electrical alternans. Unless traumatic or surgical in origin, pericardial tamponade does not manifest itself as acute hypotension. Pericardiocentesis is required for both diagnosis and therapy.

POSTEXTUBATION STRIDOR

After extubation, patients may develop upper airway edema and have stridor, which can be confused with bronchospasm. Furthermore, acute pulmonary edema may result after relief of upper airway obstruction (Oswalt et al., 1977; Sofer et al., 1984; Travis et al., 1977). This mechanism of pulmonary edema can be explained by the sudden development of highly negative intrathoracic and pleural pressures in patients inspiring against an obstructed larynx, producing 1) increased venous return, leading to increased pulmonary vascular volumes, and 2) impairment of left ventricular ejection fraction (Sofer et al., 1984). These changes can raise transmural vascular pressures within the lung to produce fluid transudation. In addition, highly negative pleural pressures could produce highly negative pulmonary interstitial pressures, thus resulting in extravascular fluid formation. Although upper airway edema and pulmonary edema can occur after an anaphylactic reaction, this form of pulmonary edema is not related to drug or blood product administration, may not be associated with hypotension, and occurs after the relief of upper airway obstruction.

PULMONARY EDEMA

The most common causes of perioperative pulmonary edema include intravenous volume overloading, cardiogenic shock, exacerbations of underlying chronic congestive heart failure, and acute myocardial ischemia/infarction with left ventricular diastolic dysfunction. These causes of pulmonary edema are produced by ventricular dysfunction in patients with cardiovascular disease. Pulmonary edema can also occur because of increases in capillary permeability (noncardiogenic) after anaphylactic reactions (Levy and Rockoff, 1982; Maggart and Stewart, 1987). Noncardiogenic pulmonary edema can be associated with transfusion reactions, producing transfusion-related acute lung injury (see Chapter 6). There are other potential causes of noncardiogenic pulmonary edema, however (Table 8.4). Reperfusion pulmonary edema has been reported after lower-torso ischemia in humans. This form of noncardiogenic pulmonary edema has been postulated to be a reperfusion injury in which oxygen-free radicals and thromboxane A_2 mediate the altered lung permeability (Klausner et al., 1989).

Table 8.4 Causes of Noncardiogenic Pulmonary Edema

Anaphylaxis
Negative pressure pulmonary edema
Reperfusion pulmonary edema
Sepsis
Transfusion reactions (transfusion-related acute lung injury)

PULMONARY EMBOLUS

Acute hypotension and hypoxemia may result after a massive pulmonary embolus. The extent of obstruction by the pulmonary embolus determines the severity of the hemodynamic findings. Patients may have signs and symptoms that can be confused with anaphylaxis. These manifestations include sudden dyspnea, pleuritic chest pain, or severe substernal oppressive discomfort (Hurst, 1982). Physical examination reveals tachycardia as the single consistent finding. Massive pulmonary embolism may be associated with arterial hypoxemia, hypocapnia and acute right ventricular dysfunction. In contrast to anaphylaxis, this problem is not related to drug or blood product administration, usually occurs in patients at risk, and may be associated with pleuritic chest pain. Specific conditions associated with a high risk of pulmonary embolism include postoperative immobilization, pregnancy and the postpartum period, long bone injuries, chronic deep venous insufficiency of the legs, and carcinoma.

SEPTIC SHOCK

Septic shock occurs with acute gram-negative or gram-positive bacterial infection, and viral or fungal infections. The initial finding is usually hypotension in association with a high cardiac output. Endotoxin, exotoxin, cell wall products, or other factors may activate the complement cascade to liberate anaphylatoxins and other mediators (see Chapter 4). The initial manifestations of septic shock may appear similar to anaphylactic shock because of liberated mediators common to both syndromes. The signs and symptoms include fever spike, hypotension, tachycardia, warm skin, bounding pulses, decreased systemic vascular resistance, hypoxemia, and respiratory distress. Septic shock should be suspected in the critically ill febrile patient with a ruptured viscus, recent urinary tract instrumentation, infected prosthetic graft, or other predisposing factors or sources of infection.

TENSION PNEUMOTHORAX

A tension pneumothorax may appear as precipitous hypotension with or without wheezing during mechanical ventilation in the operating room or intensive care unit; it may be confused with anaphylaxis. Chest auscultation and clinical suspicion are important for diagnosing this reversible problem. Signs of tension pneumothorax include acute hypotension, hypoxemia, hyperresonance to percussion, decreased breath sounds on the affected side, and increased peak inspiratory pressure. Time should not be wasted obtaining a portable chest radiograph if life-threatening hypotension is present. Air should be immediately aspirated with a 14-gauge intravenous catheter placed in the second intercostal space over the midclavicular line on the affected side or with chest tube insertion.

VASOVAGAL REACTIONS

Vasovagal reactions classically occur during dental anesthesia and are often confused with allergic reactions. Patients develop a profound vagal-mediated cholinergic response to the fear of the dentist or needle, or other precipitating factors. Patients demonstrate pallor, sweating, nausea, and bradycardia, in contrast to the tachycardia and occasional flushing that characterize anaphylaxis (Terr, 1985).

VENOUS AIR EMBOLISM

Venous air embolism can produce precipitous hypotension intraoperatively or in the intensive care unit depending on the rate and volume of entrained gas (Albin et al., 1978). It occurs whenever a gravitationally generated negative pressure gradient exists between an open wound and the right atrium. Common clinical settings for venous air embolism include neurosurgery (especially in the sitting position), neck surgery, hepatic surgery, or disconnected central venous catheter. Patients with a high risk for air embolism who undergo surgical procedures are monitored with Doppler ultrasound or end-tidal carbon dioxide monitoring as early sensitive indicators of air embolism. With massive air emboli, air may pass directly through the pulmonary circulation or through small preexisting right-to-left shunts, reaching the coronary and cerebral circulation. Massive amounts of air in the pulmonary circulation block blood flow, producing acute pulmonary hypertension, right ventricular dysfunction, and hypotension. Therapy consists of closing the open vein, positioning the heart higher, turning the patient to the left lateral position with the head down, and attempting aspiration of intracardiac air through a central venous catheter.

9

Pharmacologic Therapy for Anaphylaxis

Drugs used in the therapy of anaphylactic reactions serve several purposes. They may 1) inhibit mediator generation and release of allergic mediators; 2) block tissue receptors interacting with released mediators; 3) reverse the end-organ effects of the physiologically active substances; or 4) inhibit the recruitment and migration of other inflammatory cells (Figure 9.1). Catecholamines, phosphodiesterase inhibitors, antihistamines, and corticosteroids represent the four major classes of drugs traditionally considered in the treatment of anaphylaxis and other immediate hypersensitivity reactions. The major drugs used to treat anaphylaxis are summarized in Table 9.1. Each of these classes of drugs will be discussed separately. Other drugs that may eventually be employed in the therapy of these reactions will also be considered. Because cardiovascular collapse represents the major manifestation of anaphylaxis during anesthesia and in the intensive care unit, the effects of currently available and experimental drugs used in its therapy will be emphasized.

CATECHOLAMINES

Catecholamines (epinephrine, norepinephrine, isoproterenol) are important therapeutic agents in the treatment of anaphylactic reactions. They each have varying effects on α_1-, β_1-, and β_2-adrenergic receptors, as shown in Table 9.2. The α_1-agonists are responsible for vasoconstriction. The β_2-agonists increase 3' 5'cyclic adenosine monophosphate (cAMP) in bronchial and vascular smooth muscle to produce bronchodilation and pulmonary vasodilation, and in mast cells and basophils to inhibit histamine release and arachidonic acid metabolite synthesis. The effects of catecholamines on α- and β-adrenergic receptors will be considered.

α-Adrenergic Receptor Stimulation

Vascular smooth muscle possesses receptor-operated calcium channels on membranes that can be activated by α_1-adrenergic agents to increase vascular

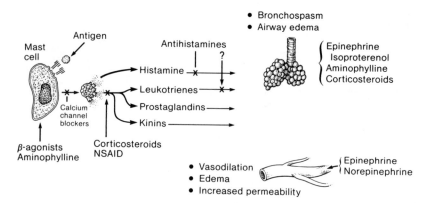

Figure 9.1 Therapeutic approaches to anaphylaxis. Drugs used in the treatment of anaphylaxis serve several purposes. They act to inhibit mediator release or synthesis, block tissue receptors interacting with the mediator's release, or reverse the end-organ effects. Epinephrine is an ideal drug acting to inhibit the reactions and reverse specific end-organ effects. Experimental drugs including calcium channel blockers, nonsteroidal antiinflammatory drugs (NSAID), and leukotriene antagonists have been studied in animal models of anaphylaxis and may have future therapeutic applications. *Modified from Frick OL. Immediate hypersensitivity. In: Stites DP, Stobo JD, Fudenberg HH, Wells JV, eds. Basic and Clinical Immunology, 14th ed. Los Angeles, Lange Medical Publications, 1982.*

tone and reverse systemic vasodilation. Agonists for the α_1-receptor (e.g., epinephrine, norepinephrine) contract smooth muscle by a mechanism that involves calcium release from intracellular stores (Lucchesi, 1989). It is not certain how the receptor-operated calcium channel is linked to the specific surface receptors in the smooth muscle cell, however. Lucchesi suggests that α_1-adrenergic receptor stimulation activates membrane phospholipase-C, resulting in the breakdown of inositol phospholipids. The hydrolysis of phosphoinositides in the plasma membrane forms inositol triphosphate, which enters the intracellular space and triggers calcium release from the sarcoplasmic reticulum (Lucchesi, 1989). In smooth muscle, the intracellular free calcium complexes with calmodulin to activate myosin light-chain kinase; the activated kinase phosphorylates myosin light-chain proteins, which results in smooth muscle contraction (Lucchesi, 1989).

A second component of the membrane phospholipid breakdown involves the formation of diacylglycerol that activates protein kinase C (Lucchesi, 1989). The turnover of membrane phospholipids might serve as the signal transduction process for the release of intracellularly bound calcium for the gating of calcium entry from the extracellular compartment. An alternative mechanism may rely on the influx of extracellular calcium in response to α_1-adrenergic receptor stimulation with the subsequent event being calcium-induced calcium release. In different vascular beds, multiple mechanisms might participate in the maintenance of smooth muscle tone (Levi et al., 1991; Lucchesi, 1989).

Table 9.1 Drugs Useful in the Therapy for Anaphylaxis

Drug	Receptor Effects	Pharmacologic Effects	Indication
Catecholamines			
Epinephrine	α-agonist β-agonist	Vasoconstrictor Bronchial dilator ↓ Mediator release	Initial therapy
Isoproterenol	β-agonist	Bronchial dilator ↓ Mediator release	Refractory bronchospasm Pulmonary hypertension Right ventricular dysfunction
Norepinephrine	α-agonist β-agonist	↑ Systemic vascular resistance	Refractory hypotension
Phosphodiesterase inhibitors			
Aminophylline		Bronchial dilator ↓ Mediator release	Persistent bronchospasm
Amrinone Enoximone Mirinone		Pulmonary vasodilator ↑ Inotropy	Pulmonary hypertension Right ventricular dysfunction
Antihistamines			
Diphenhydramine Chlorpheniramine	H_1 antagonist	Competitive inhibition of histamine at target cells	All forms of anaphylaxis
Cimetidine Ranitidine Famotidine	H_2 antagonist		Administer with an H_1 antagonist
Corticosteroids			
Hydrocortisone Methylprednisolone		↓ Arachidonic acid metabolites ↑ β-adrenergic effects	Refractory bronchospasm or hypotension Attenuate late phase reactions

Table 9.2 Pharmacologic Effects of Catecholamines

	Site of Action			
Drug	α	$β_1$	$β_2$	Mechanism of Action
Epinephrine	+	+ +	+ +	Direct
Isoproterenol	0	+ + +	+ + +	Direct
Norepinephrine	+ + +	+ +	0	Direct

0 = no change; + = slight stimulation; + + = moderate stimulation; + + + = marked stimulation. Epinephrine may have more α effects at higher doses. Modified from Stoelting RK, Miller RD. Pharmacology of the autonomic nervous system. In: Miller RD, ed. Anaesthesia. New York, Churchill Livingstone, 1981;539–60.

β-Adrenergic Receptor Stimulation

All β-adrenergic receptors stimulate adenylate cyclase by an interaction between the receptor and the enzyme that is mediated by various G-regulatory proteins. Stimulation of the receptor leads to increases in cAMP, activation of the cAMP-dependent kinases, and altered function of numerous cellular proteins as a result of their phosphorylation (Hoffman and Lefkowitz, 1990).

Stimulation of β$_1$-adrenergic receptors on the heart leads to positive inotropic and chronotropic responses. The increased intracellular concentrations of cAMP cause increased intracellular calcium with subsequent release from the storage systems. When released, calcium binds to inhibitory proteins to allow for actin and myosin to interact and increase contractility (Lucchesi, 1989).

Stimulation of β$_2$-adrenergic receptors on airway and vascular smooth muscle leads to the activation of adenylate cyclase and an increase in the intracellular concentration of cAMP (Stiles et al., 1984). This increase leads to the activation of protein kinase A, which inhibits the phosphorylation of myosin and lowers intracellular ionic calcium concentrations, resulting in relaxation (Barnes, 1989b; Lucchesi, 1989). The airway smooth muscle, airway epithelium, and vascular smooth muscle contain β$_2$-receptors exclusively (Carstairs et al., 1985). β$_2$-adrenergic agonists relax the smooth muscle of all airways, from the trachea to the terminal bronchioles, and relax the airway irrespective of the stimulus involved, thus protecting against all bronchoconstrictor challenges (Barnes, 1989b). β$_2$-adrenergic agonists may inhibit the release of mediators from mast cells in the airway and the release of acetylcholine from postganglionic cholinergic nerves in the airway but they do not inhibit either the late-phase response to allergens or the subsequent inflammatory cell-induced bronchial hyperresponsiveness (Butchers et al., 1980; Rhoden et al., 1988). β$_2$-adrenergic agonists do not have an inhibitory effect on macrophages in the human lung or eosinophils, inflammatory cells that have been implicated in both the late response and bronchial hyperresponsiveness (Barnes, 1989b).

Epinephrine

Epinephrine, one of the most potent vasopressors known, is a direct-acting catecholamine that stimulates α$_1$-, β$_1$-, and β$_2$-receptors. Because of its combined effects of inhibiting mediator release, supporting blood pressure during shock, and acting as a bronchodilator, epinephrine is a mainstay therapeutic agent for reversing cardiopulmonary collapse after anaphylactic reactions. Stimulation of the cardiac β$_1$-adrenergic receptors increases myocardial contractility, heart rate, automaticity, and myocardial oxygen consumption. β$_2$-adrenergic effects include aborting the degranulation process, bronchodilation, and producing pulmonary vasodilation (Barnes, 1989b; Beaven, 1976). The α$_1$-adrenergic effects produce vasoconstriction in many vascular beds including the smaller arterioles and precapillary resistance vessels of skin, mucosa, and kidney, along with venoconstriction (Hoffman and Lefkowitz, 1990).

The clinical effects of epinephrine are dose dependent. Intravenous doses of 1 to 2 µg/min in the adult stimulate primarily β-adrenergic receptors and can potentially produce a decrease in blood pressure; doses of 3 to 10 µg/min stimulate mixed α- and β-adrenergic receptors, producing a widened pulse pressure (i.e., a greater increase in systolic pressure than in diastolic), doses greater than 10 µg/min may produce primarily α_1 stimulation with varying degrees of pulmonary and systemic vasoconstriction (Curling et al., 1984). Epinephrine is routinely administered intravenously in cardiac surgical patients to treat cardiovascular dysfunction. Steen and coworkers studied cardiovascular effects during emergence from cardiopulmonary bypass (Steen et al., 1978). They found the intravenous infusion of epinephrine at a rate of 0.04 µg/kg/min elevated the cardiac index by 30%, the mean arterial pressure by 27%, and the pulse pressure by 75%. Dysrhythmias were noted only during direct cardiac manipulation. The authors suggested that at this dosage the α- and β-adrenergic effects were approximately equal. Earlier studies done with epinephrine infusions demonstrated a 40% increase in cardiac index with infusions of 0.1 to 0.18 µg/kg/min and a 78% to 98% increase in cardiac index with epinephrine infusions of 0.15 to 0.3 µg/kg/min (Barcroft and Star, 1951; Goldenberg et al., 1948).

Isoproterenol

Isoproterenol is a synthetic β_1- and β_2-specific adrenergic agonist that possesses almost no α-adrenergic activity. The β_2-adrenergic effects in the lung produce bronchodilation and stimulation of intracellular cAMP to inhibit mast cell and basophil activation. In the heart, it increases heart rate, contractility, automaticity, and myocardial oxygen consumption. The increase in oxygen demand can produce myocardial ischemia and ventricular dysrhythmias and therefore it must be used cautiously. Isoproterenol's β_2-adrenergic effects on skeletal, mesenteric, and renal vascular beds make it a potent vasodilator and it should be avoided in hypotensive or hypovolemic patients. Isoproterenol is a potent pulmonary artery and bronchial dilator used clinically for bronchospasm unresponsive to standard therapy or for pulmonary hypertension and right ventricular dysfunction.

Norepinephrine (Levarterenol)

Norepinephrine is a naturally occurring catecholamine normally stored and liberated by postganglionic adrenergic nerve terminals. Its major effects are mediated by both α_1- and β_1-adrenergic receptors with minimal effects on β_2-adrenergic receptors. Norepinephrine increases peripheral vascular resistance in most vascular beds, reducing splanchnic, renal, and hepatic blood flow by mesenteric vessel constriction (Hoffman and Lefkowitz, 1990). Unlike epinephrine, low-dose norepinephrine does not cause vasodilation because of its lack of β_2-adrenergic effects.

With small doses of 1 to 2 µg/min in adults, cardiac output increases, but at doses greater than 3 µg/min, systemic vascular resistance is increased (Curling et al., 1984). Norepinephrine is useful for refractory hypotension or in patients with a low systemic vascular resistance (i.e., hypotension with an increased cardiac output). Norepinephrine undergoes significant uptake by pulmonary vascular endothelium (Gillis and Pitt, 1982; Pitt, 1984). In patients with pulmonary hypertension, norepinephrine can potentially increase pulmonary vascular resistance and exacerbate right ventricular dysfunction especially with right atrial or central venous administration.

ANTIHISTAMINES

Antihistamines with H_1 receptor-specific effects act by occupying the same cellular H_1 receptor site on target organs as histamine, thus competitively inhibiting histamine binding to cell receptors (Reinhardt and Borchard, 1982; Simons, 1989; Woodward, 1990). They have minimal effects on the actual release of histamine. Most of the adverse effects of histamine are H_1 receptor-mediated; however, H_1 antagonists only partially antagonize many adverse effects of histamine. Although effective administration of antihistamines for pretreatment purposes includes the use of both H_1 and H_2 antihistamines, the role of H_2 receptor antagonism after anaphylaxis has not been demonstrated but may represent a useful adjunct to therapy.

A list of parenterally available antihistamines is included in Table 9.3. Diphenhydramine and other H_1 receptor antihistamines block cholinergic muscarinic receptors, which contributes to their antiemetic effects (Reinhard and Borchard, 1982). Promethazine and other antihistamines possess α-adrenergic receptor-blocking activity that may produce vasodilation when given by rapid intravenous injection (Simons, 1989).

Antihistamines do not completely reverse the adverse physiologic effects of anaphylaxis (Lorenz et al., 1990; Thornton and Lorenz, 1983). Two considerations may explain this response. First, a spectrum of anaphylactic mediators including leukotrienes and prostaglandins mediate the clinical syndrome while histamine is rapidly cleared from the body (Plaut, 1979). Second, the currently available antihistamines may not sufficiently block the receptors at the cardiopulmonary or cutaneous sites. Nonetheless, the initial manifestations of anaphy-

Table 9.3 Parenterally Available Antihistamines

Drug	Structure	Trade Name
H_1 Receptor Antagonists		
Diphenhydramine	Ethanolamine	Benadryl
Chlorpheniramine	Alkylamine	Chlor-Trimeton
Hydroxyzine	Piperazine	Vistaril
		Atarax
Promethazine	Phenothiazine	Phenergan
H_2 Receptor Antagonists		
Cimetidine	Imidazole	Tagamet
Ranitidine	Furan	Xantac
Famotidine	Thiazole	Pepsid

laxis appear to be partially histamine mediated, therefore antihistamines may be useful therapeutic agents (Smith et al., 1980).

PHOSPHODIESTERASE INHIBITORS

Phosphodiesterase inhibitors produce their effects by inhibiting the enzyme responsible for converting cyclic nucleotides (e.g., cAMP and cyclic guanosine monophosphate [cGMP]) to their inactive forms. The physiologic effects of drugs that inhibit phosphodiesterase depend on the ability of those drugs to inhibit the different molecular forms of the enzyme and the specific second messenger effects of cAMP on that tissue (Levy et al., 1990). Multiple molecular forms of cyclic nucleotide phosphodiesterase enzymes have been identified in several tissues and cell types (Gain and Appleman, 1978; Kukovetz et al., 1981; Weishaar et al., 1986). Cardiac muscle, vascular smooth muscle, platelets, liver, and lung all contain phosphodiesterase enzymes. Studies demonstrate heterogeneity regarding the number of phosphodiesterases present in various tissues as well as their substrate specificity (i.e., ability to metabolize cyclic nucleotides) (Weishaar et al., 1986). Fraction I is a cGMP phosphodiesterase that has a high affinity for cGMP; fraction II is a cyclic nucleotide phosphodiesterase that has a low affinity for both cAMP and cGMP; fraction III (also called type IV or IIIa and IIIb in revised terminology) is a cAMP phosphodiesterase that has a high affinity for cAMP (Gain and Appleman, 1978). Different drugs classified as phosphodiesterase inhibitors are listed in Table 9.4. Aminophylline, a nonspecific inhibitor, affects all phosphodiesterase fractions and is associated with a variety of adverse effects. Papaverine, a benzylisoquinoline derived from opium, inhibits all phosphodiesterase fractions and is primarily used clinically for its effect on vascular smooth muscle (Levy et al., 1990). The bipyridines—amrinone and milrinone—and the imidazolone derivatives—enoximone and piroximone—inhibit both cardiac and vascular phosphodiesterases. Zaprinast inhibits fraction I phosphodiesterase. Dipyridamole inhibits phosphodiesterase, primarily in platelets, to increase cAMP and prevent platelet aggregation. The currently approved phosphodiesterase inhibitors used clinically will be considered.

Aminophylline

Traditionally aminophylline was considered to inhibit phosphodiesterase, thus preventing the degradation of cAMP and decreasing histamine and arachidonic acid metabolite release and acting as a bronchodilator for antigen- or histamine-induced bronchospasm (Webb-Johnson and Andrews, 1977). New information has challenged the theory that bronchodilation is the major benefit produced by aminophylline (Isles et al., 1982). Aminophylline produces a variety of effects on respiratory function including central stimulation of ventilation, increased diaphragmatic contractility, and increased right and left ventricular ejection fraction (Matthay et al., 1978). At a cellular level, recent evidence suggests the aminophylline derivative theophylline blocks adenosine receptors

Table 9.4 Phosphodiesterase Inhibitors

Aminophylline
Amrinone
Dipyridamole
Enoximone
Milrinone
Papaverine

responsible for the central stimulant, diuretic, and tremorogenic effects (Isles et al., 1982). Micromolar concentrations of adenosine are effective in inhibiting histamine release from human basophils whereas higher concentrations cause inhibition in the human mast cell (Schleimer et al., 1984). Other possible modes of action for aminophylline include inhibition of intracellular release of calcium and stimulation of catecholamine release (Barnes, 1989b). In patients with acute asthma, aminophylline may represent a less effective bronchodilator than the sympathomimetic agents (Parker, 1982). Barnes suggests aminophylline may have an antiinflammatory action, possibly involving inhibiting submucosal edema (Barnes, 1989b).

Phosphodiesterase Fraction III Inhibitors

The newer cAMP-specific phosphodiesterase (fraction III) inhibitors have unique cardiovascular effects (Silver, 1989). Intravenous administration of amrinone, milrinone, or enoximone decreases left ventricular end-diastolic and pulmonary capillary wedge pressure and increases cardiac output in patients with congestive heart failure (Konstam et al., 1986; Levy et al., 1990). These drugs function as systemic and pulmonary arterial vasodilators, improving the inotropic state by increasing venous capacitance and decreasing venous return to the heart without increasing heart rate (Levy et al., 1990). Pulmonary vasodilation represents important and unique effects of the cAMP-specific phosphodiesterase inhibitors. The hemodynamic effects of the phosphodiesterase inhibitors closely resemble the cardiovascular effects of histamine, also a potent inodilator (Figure 9.2). Investigators have studied H_2 receptor agonists in congestive heart failure to evaluate the clinical usefulness of the unique H_2 receptor-mediated effect, which is independent of the β_1-adrenergic receptor and phosphodiesterase inhibitors, with limited success (Pelc et al., 1985).

CORTICOSTEROIDS

Corticosteroids are potent antiinflammatory agents but have little effect on the initial therapy of anaphylaxis. Evidence suggests that their effects are mediated by interactions with receptors in cell cytoplasm; these changes ultimately

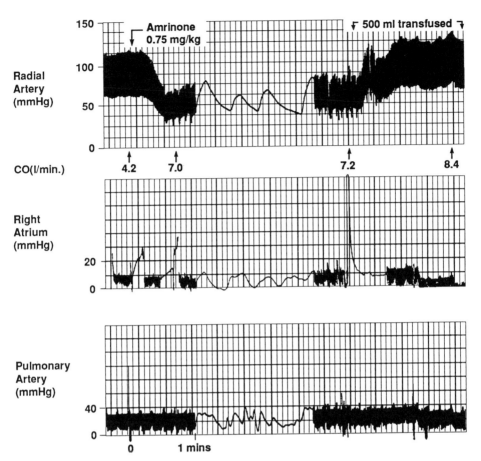

Figure 9.2 Hemodynamic effects of amrinone (a phosphodiesterase fraction III inhibitor) when given as a bolus of 0.75 mg/kg. The patient was a 53-year-old man who underwent 6-vessel coronary artery bypass grafting. The patient had an acute inferior wall myocardial infarction 3 days before surgery and the ejection fraction was noted to be 50% on cardiac catheterization. The patient was 85 kg with a body surface area of 2.2 m^2. After separation from cardiopulmonary bypass and with atrial pacing at a rate of 85, the cardiac output was 4.2 L/min (a cardiac index of 1.8 L/min/m^2). The right ventricle was noted to be dilated and hypokinetic. Amrinone was given as a rapid bolus of 0.75 mg/kg, cardiac output increased to 7.0 L/min, and right atrial and pulmonary artery pressures fell. A total of 500 mL of volume from the cardiopulmonary bypass reservoir was rapidly administered, with restoration of blood pressure and a cardiac output 8.4 L/min. Amrinone increases contractility and produces vasodilation in systemic, pulmonary, and venous capacitance beds.

lead to alterations in protein synthesis. Corticosteroids exert a variety of effects on allergic reactions; their capacity to limit and terminate allergic reactions is based on several mechanisms. Corticosteroids inhibit the breakdown of the phospholipid cell membrane to liberate free arachidonic acid (Hong and Levine, 1976). In addition, they induce the synthesis of specific nuclear regulatory proteins that inhibit phospholipase A_2 activity, limiting substrate available to both the cyclooxygenase and lipoxygenase pathways. These and other effects are not immediate and may require hours to days before they exert beneficial effects (Laser et al., 1977).

Other evidence suggests corticosteroids are useful adjuncts to therapy in anaphylactic reactions by 1) potentiating the effects of β-adrenergic agents on mast cells, basophils, and other cell membranes; 2) increasing vascular endothelial integrity and decreasing capillary permeability; 3) inhibiting the uptake and use of calcium ions; 4) restoring the microcirculatory perfusion back to normal; and 5) inhibiting the chemotaxis and chemokinesis of inflammatory cells during anaphylaxis (late phase responses). Large doses of corticosteroids, 30 mg/kg, have also been shown to inhibit polymorphonuclear leukocyte aggregation by C5a and to prevent microvascular leukostasis (Hammerschmidt et al., 1979). Both methylprednisolone and hydrocortisone inhibit aggregation whereas dexamethasone has no effect.

Conclusive studies of the clinical efficacy of corticosteroids in acute anaphylactic reactions are lacking. Corticosteroids are not first-line drugs but are important therapeutic adjuncts in persistent organ dysfunction, especially in patients with bronchospasm/asthma, and help attenuate secondary inflammatory responses.

EXPERIMENTAL DRUGS
Anticholinergic Drugs

Anticholinergic drugs antagonize acetylcholine at parasympathetic postganglionic sites (M_3 receptors) in airway smooth muscle, resulting in bronchodilation (Barnes, 1989b). Anticholinergic drugs inhibit only the component of bronchoconstriction caused by cholinergic nerves; they have no action against the direct effects of mediators on airway smooth muscle, in contrast to $β_2$-adrenergic agents, which inhibit bronchoconstriction irrespective of the stimulus used (Barnes, 1989a). Atropine, glycopyrolate, and ipratropium are anticholinergic agents most commonly used. Glycopyrolate and ipratropium are quarternary ammonium compounds that are poorly absorbed from the lung and produce minimal systemic effects when administered by aerosol (Gross, 1988). Anticholinergics are less effective than $β_2$-adrenergic agents in the treatment of asthma (Barnes, 1989b). Ipratropium has been used in patients with chronic obstructive pulmonary disease as an effective bronchodilator, however (Gross, 1988). The role of anticholinergics in the treatment of anaphylaxis is not known, but they may represent useful adjuncts to $β_2$-adrenergic drugs and corticosteroids in persistent bronchospasm.

Calcium Entry Blockers

Calcium entry blockers are used clinically to inhibit calcium entry into vascular smooth muscle. They act by binding with high-affinity receptors located on or near vascular calcium channels (Schwarz, 1988). Calcium channels are thought to be membrane-spanning glycoproteins with a water-filled pore that function like ion-selective valves, allowing calcium to move from extracellular space to the cytosol (Schwarz, 1988). The dihydropyridine analogues (i.e., isradipine, nicardipine, nifedipine) are relatively specific for vascular smooth muscle, whereas verapamil also affects conduction in sinoatrial and atrioventricular tissue (slow calcium channels), and depresses myocardial contractility.

The calcium entry blockers nifedipine and verapamil have been shown to inhibit the synthesis and release of leukotrienes in human lung tissues, thromboxane A_2 formation, platelet activating factor, and lysosomal enzymes from human neutrophils (Chand et al., 1985). Calcium entry blockers can alter the calcium uptake (influx) into mast cells but produce variable inhibitory effects on allergic and nonallergic histamine secretion in experimental models. Influences of calcium channel blockers on mediator release appears to depend on the cell source, species, nature, and the concentration of the secretory stimuli as well as on the composition and concentration of calcium entry blockers used. Chand and coworkers suggest a functional heterogeneity of calcium channels in leukocytes, mast cells, and basophils (Chand et al., 1985). Interference with the calcium-dependent steps involved in the formation or release of chemical mediators appears to be the primary mode of action for calcium channel blockers in these cells. The differential effects of calcium antagonists on calcium-dependent activation of phospholipase A_2, 5-lipoxygenase, and calmodulin (or other intracellular calcium-binding proteins) in different cell types (mast cells, basophils, leukocytes, and lung tissue) may explain their varying effectiveness in inhibiting the synthesis or release of chemical mediators and antagonizing bronchoconstriction in response to diverse stimuli (Chand et al., 1985). Chand and coworkers suggest that in immediate hypersensitivity, calcium homeostasis (uptake, mobilization, distribution, and relocation) may be altered in mast cells, basophils, and lung tissue. The altered calcium homeostasis could be responsible for the induction of airway hyperreactivity in asthmatics and for hyperreleasability of chemical mediators from mast cells and leukocytes. Nifedipine inhibits histamine release from human basophils (Bedard and Busse, 1983), and verapamil in animal models exhibits an antianaphylactic effect (Descotes et al., 1982).

Calcium entry blockers may have a potential role in pretreatment of anaphylactic reactions. They should not be administered acutely to treat anaphylactic reactions because they can potentially exacerbate arterial dilation. Calcium chloride, frequently administered intravenously to treat hypotension or myocardial depression in critically ill patients, should be avoided during suspected anaphylactic or anaphylactoid reactions. Calcium is essential to inflammatory cellular activation and mediator release, and may potentially exacerbate or hasten cardiovascular collapse (see Chapter 12). Experimental evidence demonstrating myocardial depression and decreased coronary blood flow when calcium is administered during anaphylaxis supports this recommendation (Tanz et al., 1985).

Drugs That Inhibit Complement Activation or Its Effects

As discussed in Chapter 4, complement is activated by immunoglobulin-G (IgG)-antigen or immunoglobulin-M (IgM)-antigen interaction, plasmin, or heparin–protamine complex (Figure 9.3). Blockade at one of several sites in the sequence of events shown in Figure 9.3 has been used both clinically and experimentally, and may underlie new clinical approaches to the management of complement-induced and leukoagglutinin-induced pulmonary vasoconstriction. There are three potential ways to inhibit complement activation or its effects, including 1) inhibiting complement activation by preventing activation of the C1 esterase; 2) inhibiting the synthesis of mediators after neutrophil and other inflammatory cell activation by steroidal and nonsteroidal antiinflammatory drugs or prostaglandin E_1; and 3) reversing pulmonary vasoconstriction pharmacologically (Table 9.5) (Hauptmann et al., 1985). Experimental approaches for inhibiting complement activation or reversing its effects will be considered.

Complement Inhibition

Heparin possesses antiinflammatory properties and can inhibit complement activation by increasing the rate and activation of complement enzyme C1s by the C1 inhibitor (Patrick and Johnson, 1980). Investigators are currently looking for heparin fragments that have a high specificity for complement-inhibiting effects (Patrick and Johnson, 1980). These findings may also explain the reversal of protamine-induced pulmonary vasoconstriction or hemodynamic instability after the acute readministration of heparin (Lock and Hessel, 1990).

Aprotinin and plasmin inhibitors prevent contact activation and plasmin-mediated initiation of the complement cascade. The plasmin inhibitors ϵ-aminocaproic acid and tranexamic acid block the ability of plasmin to activate the C1 esterase. These drugs have also been tried in prophylaxis of the patients with hereditary angioedema (see Chapter 4).

Using heparin–protamine-induced experimental models of complement activation and pulmonary vasoconstriction, nafamstat mesilate (FUT-175), a protease and complement pathway inhibitor, decreased both the elevation of arterial C3a and thromboxane B_2 levels and the rise in the pulmonary vascular resistance (Kreil et al., 1989).

Steroidal and Nonsteroidal Antiinflammatory Drugs

Corticosteroids in high doses can inhibit polymorphonuclear leukocyte aggregation, as previously discussed. Nonsteroidal antiinflammatory drugs act solely by inhibiting the synthesis of the prostaglandins from arachidonic acid through inhibition of the enzyme cyclooxygenase. These drugs may inhibit the synthesis of mediators because of the humoral activation of inflammatory cascades by anaphylatoxins. Specific thromboxane synthetase inhibitors or compet-

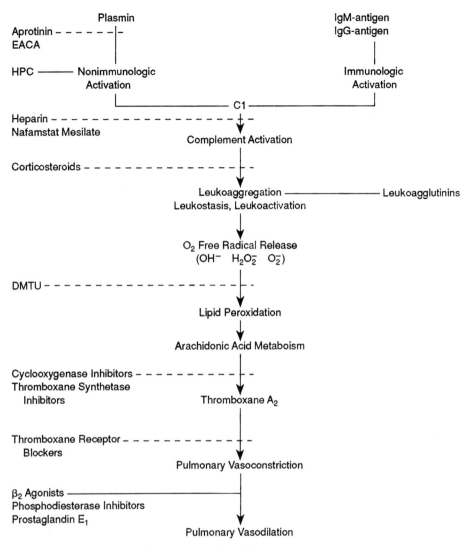

Figure 9.3 Therapeutic approaches to inhibit complement activation or its effects. Complement is activated immunologically by IgG-antigen or IgM-antigen interactions, or nonimmunologically by plasmin or heparin–protamine complexes (HPC) as shown. Blockade at one of the different sites in the sequence of activation has been used both clinically and experimentally to treat complement-induced pulmonary vasoconstriction. There are three potential ways to inhibit complement activation or its effects, including inhibiting either C1 initiation or activation, inhibiting mediator synthesis that antagonizes their effects, or reversing pulmonary vasoconstriction pharmacologically. Leukoagglutinins (IgG antibodies) directed against leukocytes can also initiate this cascade to produce acute pulmonary vasoconstriction. DMTU = dimethylthyourea; EACA = ε-aminocaproic acid. *Modified with permission from Morel DR, Lowenstein E, Nguyenduy T, et al. Acute pulmonary vasoconstriction and thromboxane release during protamine reversal of heparin anticoagulation in awake sheep: evidence for the role of reactive oxygen metabolites following nonimmunological complement activation. Circ Res 1988;62:905–15.*

Table 9.5 Drugs That Inhibit Complement Activation and Its Effects

Corticosteroids

Free radical scavengers

Heparin

Nonsteroidal antiinflammatory drugs

Prostaglandin E_1

Protease inhibitors: Aprotinin, ϵ-aminocaproic acid, tranexamic acid

Pulmonary vasodilators: β_2-adrenergic agents, phosphodiesterase inhibitors, calcium entry blockers

Thromboxane antagonists

Thromboxane synthetase inhibitors

---

itive antagonists may also play an important role in inhibiting the indirect effects of complement activation. These agents may be important in treating or preventing acute thromboxane-mediated pulmonary vasoconstriction and acute right ventricular dysfunction that can occur after protamine or transfusion reactions.

Investigators have evaluated different antiinflammatory drugs to prevent or treat experimentally induced pulmonary vasoconstriction. In heparin–protamin-induced animal models, dimethylthiourea, a hydrogen peroxide scavenger, prevented lipid peroxidation and arachidonic acid release, whereas UK 38-485 specifically inhibited thromboxane synthesis (Morel et al., 1988). Cyclooxygenase inhibition with indomethacin also blocked pulmonary hemodynamic and arterial blood gas changes secondary to protamine reversal of heparin (Hobbhahn et al., 1988). Similar effects were also achieved using specific thromboxane A_2 receptor antagonists (Conzen et al., 1989; Montalescot et al., 1990). These drugs have been used only to pretreat animals for pulmonary vasoconstriction, however. Nuttall and coworkers showed that instituting thromboxane A_2 receptor blockade with L-6705696 attenuated the degree and duration of complement-mediated pulmonary hypertension in pigs (Nuttal et al., 1991).

Lyew and Levy reported the first clinical use of an intravenous nonsteroidal antiinflammatory drug (ketorolac tromethanol), administered in an attempt to inhibit cyclooxygenase to block thromboxane synthesis and blunt protamine-induced pulmonary vasoconstriction and acute right ventricular failure after cardiopulmonary bypass (Figure 9.4) (Lyew and Levy, in press). Hemodynamic improvement occurred gradually and was attributed to residual cyclooxygenase activity. The patient was also receiving inotropic support, including catecholamines with β_2-adrenergic activity (epinephrine) and a phosphodiesterase fraction III inhibitor (amrinone), which may have also treated the pulmonary vasoconstriction and right ventricular dysfunction (see Figure 9.4).

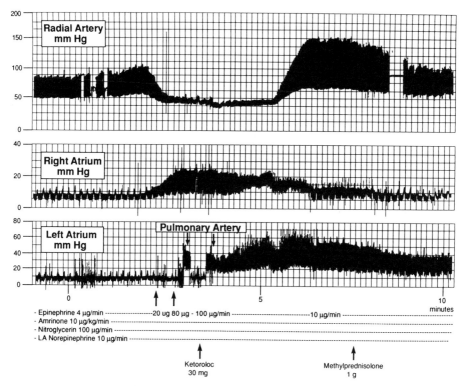

Figure 9.4 Acute systemic hypotension, and right ventricular failure after protamine administration in an NPH insulin-dependent diabetic patient after aortic valve replacement and coronary artery bypass grafting. The right atrial pressures increased acutely because of pulmonary vasoconstriction; the left atrial pressures were low. Epinephrine dose was increased and ketorolac, 30 mg, was administered intravenously. As the patient improved and right ventricular function improved, right atrial pressures decreased and systemic arterial pressures increased. LA = left atrial. *Reprinted with permission from Lyew MA, Levy JH. Treatment of protamine induced pulmonary hypertension following cardiopulmonary bypass with ketorolac. In press.*

Prostaglandin E₁ (Prostin VR)

Prostaglandin E_1 (PGE_1) is both a potent arterial vasodilator and an antiinflammatory drug (Table 9.6). PGE_1 has been used therapeutically in patients with refractory pulmonary hypertension and right heart failure after cardiopulmonary bypass (D'Ambra et al., 1985) because of its profound relaxation of arteriolar vascular smooth muscles, which decreases vascular resistance in the pulmonary and systemic circulation (Sczeklik et al., 1978). PGE_1 also exerts antiinflammatory effects, including a dose-dependent inhibition of IgE-dependent antigen-induced histamine release (Tauber et al., 1973) and inhibition of platelet

Table 9.6 Effects of Prostaglandin E_1

Pulmonary vasodilator

Bronchodilator

Coronary vasodilator

Antiinflammatory

aggregation (Sinha and Colman, 1978), and functions as a bronchodilator (Rosenthal et al., 1971). PGE_1 may also inhibit polymorphonuclear leukocyte-induced injury.

PGE_1 may have a role in the therapy of pulmonary vasoconstriction refractory to vasodilators, β_2-specific catecholamines, and cAMP specific phosphodiesterase inhibitors (e.g., amrinone). PGE_1 is taken up by the pulmonary endothelium, but uptake is decreased after cardiopulmonary bypass because of its inflammatory effects (Gillis and Pitt, 1982). PGE_1, which is normally infused into the right atrium, must be administered in combination with norepinephrine and infused into a left atrial cannula to prevent systemic vasodilation and avoid the vasoconstricting effects on the pulmonary vasculature. D'Ambra and coworkers reported 5 patients with refractory pulmonary hypertension who responded to right atrial PGE_1 infusion (30 to 150 ng/kg/min) in combination with left atrial norepinephrine infusion (up to 1 µg/kg/min) (D'Ambra et al., 1985). The reported simultaneous manipulation of pulmonary and systemic circulations provided excellent urine output, preservation of renal function, and cardiovascular improvement. PGE_1 has also been used to treat refractory pulmonary artery hypertension and noncardiogenic pulmonary edema after protamine and transfusion reactions (see Chapter 12).

Pharmacologic Approaches to Pulmonary Vasoconstriction

Vasodilation in the pulmonary arterial vasculature can be produced by any drug that 1) decreases calcium entry in vascular smooth muscle; 2) increases cAMP; and 3) increases cGMP, as illustrated in Figure 9.5. The dihydropyridine calcium entry blockers (e.g., isradipine, nicardipine, nifedipine) are specific for calcium channels in vascular smooth muscle, but their role in the therapy of acute pulmonary vasoconstriction is not established. cAMP can be increased by stimulating the β_2-adrenergic receptor in vascular smooth muscle or by inhibiting its breakdown by phosphodiesterase. Increasing cAMP in vascular smooth muscle facilitates calcium uptake by intracellular storage sites, thus decreasing calcium available for contraction. The net effect of increasing calcium uptake is to produce vascular smooth muscle relaxation and, therefore, vasodilation. Not all drugs that relax smooth muscle act through generation or accumulation of cAMP. This effect can also occur through the action of drugs that stimulate the formation

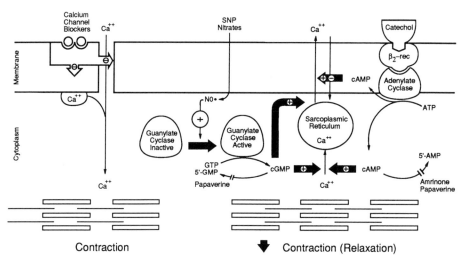

Figure 9.5 Pharmacologic reversal of pulmonary vasoconstriction. Pulmonary arterial vasodilation can be produced by increasing cyclic nucleotide formation, inhibiting its breakdown, or decreasing calcium entry. β_2-adrenergic receptor stimulation removes free cellular calcium ions by increasing uptake into the sarcoplasmic reticulum. The decrease in available calcium relaxes vascular smooth muscle and produces vasodilation. By inhibiting phosphodiesterase (PDE) metabolism of cAMP, drugs (i.e., amrinone and papaverine) also relax vascular smooth muscle and produce vasodilation. Nitrates and nitroprusside generate nitric oxide, which increases the formation of soluble cGMP, in turn increasing calcium uptake and extrusion. Drugs that are nonspecific phosphodiesterase inhibitors (i.e., papaverine) increase both cAMP and cGMP. Both cAMP and cGMP increase calcium uptake into the sarcoplasmic reticulum and extrusion from the cell. Calcium entry blockers inhibit calcium entry through calcium channels into vascular smooth muscle. PGE_1 also stimulates adenylate cyclase to increase cAMP by non-β_2-adrenergic receptors. When treating acute pulmonary vasoconstriction, the concomitant administration of nitroglycerin, β_2-adrenergic agents, and phosphodiesterase inhibitors may have additive effects to maximally stimulate cyclic nucleotide formation in the pulmonary vasculature.

of or inhibit the breakdown of cGMP. Drugs can stimulate the pulmonary vascular endothelium to release an endothelium-derived relaxing factor (EDRF or nitric oxide), which activates guanylate cyclase to generate cGMP. Nitrates and sodium nitroprusside generate nitric oxide independent of vascular endothelium. Drugs such as aminophylline, amrinone, and papaverine that are phosphodiesterase inhibitors also produce vascular smooth muscle dilation through augmentation of both cAMP and cGMP (Gain and Appleman, 1978; Kukovetz et al., 1981; Weishaar et al., 1986). PGE_1 stimulates vascular adenylate cyclase independent of the β_2-adrenergic receptor to increase cAMP in vascular smooth muscle (see Figure 3.3). The author uses these different pharmacologic pathways to generate cyclic nucleotides in pulmonary vasculature when treating pulmonary hypertension and right heart failure (see Chapter 10).

Pharmacologic Approaches to Increased Capillary Permeability

Increases in vascular permeability result from mediator-induced endothelial cell contraction and the formation of junctional gaps between adjacent endothelial cells (Hill, 1990). Because endothelial cells possess these contractile proteins, Hill raises the possibility of using drugs that produce relaxation of the endothelial contractile apparatus as antipermeability drugs (Hill, 1990). β_2-adrenergic agonists (isoproterenol and terbutaline), PGE_1, and phosphodiesterase inhibitors are all active antipermeability drugs in experimental models (Grega, 1986; Killackey et al., 1986; Svensjoe and Romempke, 1985). These agents effectively stimulate cAMP accumulation in endothelial cells from various vascular beds. cAMP may mediate relaxation of endothelial cells by interfering with the phosphorelaxation of myosin light chain kinase (Hill, 1990).

# 10

Management of Anaphylaxis

A plan for treating an anaphylactic or anaphylactoid reaction should be established well in advance of any possible occurrence. Retrospective studies of anaphylactic shock indicate a 3% to 4.3% mortality rate (Clarke et al., 1975; Fisher and More, 1981; Mantz et al., 1982). The longer initial therapy is delayed, the greater the likelihood of fatality (Barnard, 1973). If an anaphylactic reaction is considered a definite possibility and is planned for, adverse outcomes may be reduced substantially, as demonstrated by the decreased mortality from anaphylaxis associated with the use of chymopapain for chemonucleolysis (Agre et al., 1984).

Although various drugs are used to treat anaphylactic and anaphylactoid reactions, cessation of the offending drug, maintenance of the airway, administration of 100% oxygen, intravascular volume expansion, and administration of epinephrine are the mainstays of therapy (Table 10.1). These procedures are necessary to treat the sudden hypotension and hypoxia that result from vasodilation, increased capillary permeability, and bronchospasm that occur secondary to release of the different mediators described. Enough consistency exists throughout the literature and anecdotal case reports, along with experience obtained intraoperatively and postoperatively in managing cardiopulmonary dysfunction, to allow proposal of one treatment protocol.

Anaphylactic reactions may be protracted, with persistent hypotension, pulmonary hypertension and right ventricular dysfunction, noncardiogenic pulmonary edema, lower respiratory obstruction, or laryngeal obstruction persisting for 5 to 32 hours despite vigorous therapy. Additional hemodynamic monitoring, including radial and pulmonary artery catheterization, may be required when hypotension persists despite therapeutic interventions and resuscitation (see Chapter 11).

Although anaphylactic and anaphylactoid reactions are triggered by different mechanisms, the mediators released and the treatment for these life-threatening reactions are identical. Clinical judgement in applying principles of cardiopulmonary resuscitation and in titrating specific pharmacologic agents is important in treating anaphylactic reactions. A protocol with representative doses for a 70-kg patient is discussed.

Table 10.1 Management of Anaphylaxis

Initial Therapy
1. Stop administration of antigen
2. Maintain airway with 100% oxygen
3. Discontinue all anesthetic agents
4. Start intravascular volume expansion (2–4 L of crystalloid/colloid [25–50 mL/kg] with hypotension)
5. Give epinephrine (5–10 μg intravenously with hypotension, titrate as needed; 0.5–1.0 mg intravenously with cardiovascular collapse)*

Secondary Treatment
1. Catecholamine infusions (starting doses:
    epinephrine 4–8 μg/min [0.05–0.1 μg/kg/min]†
    norepinephrine 4–8 μg/min [0.05 – 0.1 μg/kg/min]†
    isoproterenol 0.05–1 μg/min†
2. Antihistamines (0.5–1.0 mg/kg diphenhydramine)
3. Corticosteroids (0.25–1.0 g hydrocortisone; alternately 1–2 g [25 mg/kg] methylprednisolone)‡
4. Bicarbonate (0.5–1.0 mEq/kg with persistent hypotension or acidosis)
5. Airway evaluation (before extubation)

* Higher doses may be required if the patient fails to respond or is receiving spinal or epidural anesthesia.
† Higher doses may be required.
‡ Methylprednisolone may be the drug of choice if the reaction is suspected to be complement mediated.

INITIAL THERAPY
Stop the Infusion of the Suspected Allergen

Steps should be taken to interrupt further drug administration and, when possible, to decrease absorption of the offending agent. This may prevent further recruitment of mast cells and basophils during a reaction, producing less mediator release. Intravenous infusions of suspected drugs or blood products should be stopped immediately.

Maintain the Airway and Administer 100% Oxygen

Severe mismatching of ventilation and perfusion may occur from bronchospasm, pulmonary vasoconstriction, and pulmonary capillary leakage. These changes can persist for several hours during anaphylactic reactions, producing both hypoxemia and hypercapnia. The airway should be initially maintained with 100% oxygen until oxygenation is adequate. Oxygenation can be monitored initially by using a pulse oximeter, and subsequently by measuring arterial blood gases. Increased peak inspiratory pressures may be required during positive pressure ventilation due to bronchospasm or interstitial pulmonary edema, producing decreased lung compliance. Increased airway pressure during mask ventilation may also be a sign of upper airway edema if the patient is not intubated.

If the patient is not already intubated and if there is any suggestion of airway compromise secondary to laryngeal edema or respiratory distress, or if the patient requires cardiopulmonary resuscitation, then intubation should be performed immediately. Endotracheal intubation allows for effective positive pressure ventilation and mechanical ventilation if respiratory distress ensues. Effective positive pressure ventilation with 100% oxygen should be performed before laryngoscopy or elective endotracheal tube placement. If cardiopulmonary resuscitation is required, time should not be wasted attempting a nasotracheal intubation; rather, oral intubation, the easiest and fastest route, should be performed using a stileted endotracheal tube. The potential for laryngeal edema, distorted airway structures, and technical difficulties should be anticipated when intubating patients after anaphylactic reactions. If laryngospasm or laryngeal edema does not respond to therapy, then a catheter cricothyrotomy or emergency surgical cricothyrotomy may be necessary to establish an adequate airway.

Discontinue All Anesthetic Agents

Anesthetic agents have negative inotropic properties and may interfere with the reflex compensatory response to hypotension; therefore, they should be discontinued during an acute event. Halothane, enflurane, and isoflurane are not the bronchodilators of choice for mediator-related bronchospasm during anaphylaxis. Furthermore, halothane sensitizes the heart to catecholamines, which must be administered in the event of severe reactions.

Start Intravascular Volume Expansion

Intravascular volume expansion is essential to successful treatment of hypotension. Using hemoconcentration to assess blood volume changes, Fisher suggests that 20% to 37% of the intravascular volume may be immediately lost from the intravascular space during anaphylactic and anaphylactoid reactions (Fisher, 1977). Precipitous decreases in pulmonary capillary wedge pressure and left ventricular end diastolic volumes have also been demonstrated during anaphylaxis, further illustrating the profound intravascular volume depletion that occurs (Beaupre et al., 1984; Levy, 1989a; Obeid et al., 1975).

Initial therapy consists of rapid intravascular replacement of 25 to 50 mL/kg (approximately 2 to 4 L in an adult) of lactated Ringer's solution, normal saline, or colloid solutions. Further volume expansion may be necessary if hypotension persists. Although there is no proven advantage to using colloid solutions over crystalloid solutions, colloid solutions (e.g., 5% albumin, hydroxyethel starch) may have a role in volume administration, since colloids provide greater intravascular volume expansion at equally infused volumes. Hydroxyethel starch (hetastarch) is supplied in plastic bags and can be administered rapidly using pressurized transfusion sets. In emergency situations, military antishock trousers (MAST suit) have been used to autotransfuse patients with hypotension during anaphylaxis (Oertel, 1984). The MAST suit may also be helpful in obtaining peripheral venous access in the upper extremities.

Fulminant noncardiogenic pulmonary edema with protein-containing secretions may occur after anaphylaxis and transfusion reactions (Carlson et al., 1981; Culliford et al., 1980; Dubois et al., 1980; Levy and Rockoff, 1982). In this setting, patients lose intravascular volume into the lung because of a sudden increase in capillary permeability. Lasix should not be administered in this form of pulmonary edema (noncardiogenic) because it may exacerbate hypotension. This scenario often requires volume expansion as well as careful hemodynamic monitoring of right and left ventricular function. Patients with noncardiogenic pulmonary edema secondary to transfusion-related acute lung injury may also have pulmonary hypertension with right heart failure occurring with elevated central venous pressures but low pulmonary capillary wedge and left atrial pressure. These patients require special therapy (see the next section).

Administer Epinephrine

Epinephrine is the mainstay of therapy in acute anaphylaxis. Its α_1-adrenergic effects make it useful for hypotension and provide constriction of the vascular capacitance and resistance bed during rapid intravascular volume expansion. Its β_1-adrenergic actions produce positive inotropic effects, and the β_2-adrenergic actions produce both bronchodilation and inhibition of mediator release from stimulated mast cells or basophils, all by stimulating intracellular $3'5'$cyclic adenosine monophosphate (cAMP). Furthermore, epinephrine administration is essential to aborting mast cell and basophil degranulation. Although different recommendations for intravenous epinephrine use have been reviewed (Table 10.2), current clinical use based on daily experiences in the management of cardiovascular dysfunction is as follows.

For hypotension, when using a premixed 1:10,000 epinephrine syringe (100 μg/mL), epinephrine can be given as a 5- to 10-μg intravenous bolus (0.05 to 0.1 mL), with repeated or incremental doses administered until hypotension is corrected (Figures 10.1, 10.2). Epinephrine should be given initially as an intravenous bolus, and incremental doses of $5 \rightarrow 10 \rightarrow 25 \rightarrow 50 \rightarrow 100 \rightarrow 200 \ldots$ μg of epinephrine can be titrated at 30- to 60-second intervals to restore baseline blood pressure. The author routinely mixes 2 mg of epinephrine in 250 mL of solution and maintains an 8 μg/mL syringe or infusion for cardiac surgery, administering incremental doses of $4 \rightarrow 8 \rightarrow 16 \rightarrow 32 \rightarrow 64 \ldots$ μg to treat cardiovascular dysfunction (see Figures 10.1, 10.2; see also Figures 6.3, 6.4). The initial dose may need to be higher depending on the clinical conditions and volume status of the patient. Although an epinephrine infusion has been suggested to be the ideal method of administration to correct hypotension, it is virtually impossible to maintain a simultaneous intravenous drug infusion when rapid volume expansion is required with limited vascular access (Barach et al.,

Table 10.2 Recommendations for Intravenous Epinephrine Use in Anaphylactic Shock

Author	Dosage (mg)	Dilution	Rate
Barbar and Budassi, 1975	1.0–2.0	None	Unspecified
Ford, 1977	1.0	1:10,000	Very slowly
Orange and Donsky, 1978	0.1–0.2	1:10,000	Unspecified
Caranasos, 1978	0.3–0.5	10 mL NS	Slowly
Lockey and Fox, 1979	0.1	1:100,000	Several minutes
Criep, 1980	0.3	None	Unspecified
Harvey, 1980	Rarely up to 0.25 in adults	None	Very slowly
AMA Dept of Drugs, 1980	0.005–0.025	1:10,000	Unspecified
Rosenblatt and Lawlor, 1981	Up to 0.25	10 mL NS	1–2 min
Gonzales and Lewis, 1981	0.05–0.2	200 times	Slowly
Lichtenstein, 1982	Unspecified	None	Unspecified
Eisenberg and Copass, 1982	0.5	None	Unspecified
Bickerman, 1982	0.3–0.4	None	Unspecified
Kravis, 1983	0.05–0.1 mg	1:10,000	Unspecified
Egglestone, 1983	0.01 mL/kg	1:10,000	Unspecified
Sterback, 1983	0.1–0.2	1:10,000	Unspecified
Austen, 1983	Unspecified	1:50,000	Unspecified
Chatton, 1983	0.1–0.2	10 mL NS	Very slowly
Stoelting, 1983	0.005 mg/kg	1:10,000	Unspecified
Barach et al., 1984	0.1	10 mL NS	5–10 min

NS = normal saline.
Modified from Barach EM, Nowak RM, Lee TG, Tomlanovich MC. Epinephrine for treatment of anaphylactic shock. JAMA 1984;251:2118–22.

1984). During general anesthesia, patients may also have altered sympathoadrenergic responses to acute anaphylactic shock. In addition, during spinal or epidural anesthesia, the patient may be partially sympathectomized, requiring earlier intervention with even larger doses of epinephrine and other catecholamines (Caplan et al., 1988).

If cardiac arrest or a total loss of blood pressure or pulse occurs, full intravenous cardiopulmonary resuscitative doses, 0.5 to 1.0 mg [7.5 to 15.0 μg/kg (5 to 10 mL of a 1:10,000 dilution)], of epinephrine should be given, along with rapid volume expansion (see Figure 10.2). Additional incremental doses may be required to resuscitate the patient, using doses of 1 to 5 mg. Recent

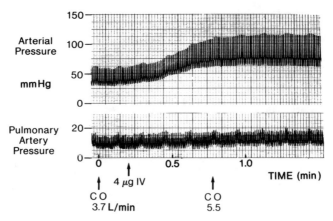

Figure 10.1 Effects of bolus epinephrine. After coronary artery bypass grafting, a patient manifested acute hypotension and hypovolemia after cardiopulmonary bypass. Epinephrine, 4 μg, was given through a central venous port, following by rapid volume expansion and hemodynamic improvement. Additional intravenous epinephrine would have been administered until the blood pressure returned to baseline.

studies in patients resuscitated after cardiac arrest suggest high-dose epinephrine may improve coronary perfusion pressure and rates of return of spontaneous circulation without increased complications from standard therapy (Callahan et al., 1991; Koscove and Paradis, 1988; Paradis et al., 1991).

Ventricular dysrhythmias and myocardial ischemia, previously reported with intravenous epinephrine administration, occurred only when full resuscitative doses (0.3 to 0.5 mg) were administered intravenously to patients with normal blood pressures (Horak et al., 1983; Sullivan, 1982). The use of carefully titrated doses is not associated with ventricular dysrhythmias in patients receiving intravenous epinephrine for cardiovascular dysfunction or anaphylactic/anaphylactoid reactions during cardiac surgery (Levy, 1989a).

If intravenous access is not available, epinephrine can be administered intratracheally using 0.5 to 1.0 mg (5 to 10 mL of 1:10,000 premixed syringes). Intramuscular or subcutaneous administration of epinephrine is unreliable in a patient in shock who requires immediate therapy to restore cerebral and coronary perfusion pressures. Absorption of epinephrine after subcutaneous injection is slow because of the drug's local vasoconstrictive effects. If a patient has minimal changes in his or her blood pressures, then common sense should prevail and intramuscular epinephrine or low doses of an epinephrine infusion should be considered. If laryngeal edema occurs with minimal hemodynamic changes, then epinephrine, either aerosolized (3 inhalations of 0.16 to 0.20 mg epinephrine per inhalation) or nebulized (8 to 15 drops of 2.25% epinephrine in 2 mL normal saline) should be administered. Intramuscular or subcutaneous routes of administration should be considered as possible alternatives.

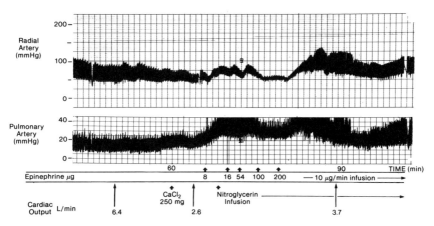

Figure 10.2 Use of intravenous epinephrine during anaphylactic shock. After a suspected anaphylactic reaction to protamine, incremental doses of epinephrine were administered until blood pressure returned to baseline values; then an epinephrine infusion was started. Pulmonary artery hypertension, a result of vasoactive mediators, calcium administration, epinephrine administration, or left ventricular failure, was treated with intravenous nitroglycerin.

SECONDARY TREATMENT
Antihistamines

Although histamine is only one of the mediators released in anaphylactic or anaphylactoid reactions, it may account for many of the initial adverse manifestations. No clinical evidence indicates that administration of antihistamines is effective in treating anaphylaxis once mediators have been released. Administration of antihistamines is therefore recommended only as an adjuvant therapy in acute anaphylactic and anaphylactoid reactions. The suggested dose of diphenhydramine is 1 mg/kg as an H_1 receptor antagonist. Although there is no evidence demonstrating the efficiency of H_2 antagonist administration during anaphylaxis, cimetidine or ranitidine may be considered for persistent hypotension, in combination with an H_1 receptor antagonist.

Catecholamine Infusions
Epinephrine

When hypotension or bronchospasm persist, an intravenous epinephrine infusion may be useful after intravascular volume expansion and boluses of epinephrine have been administered. Suggested starting doses of epinephrine are 0.05 to 0.10 µg/kg/min (4 to 8 µg/min); these should be titrated to raise or maintain arterial pressure after the initial resuscitation. Tachycardia may be a troublesome side effect and norepinephrine may be more effective in maintaining perfusion pressures. Persistent hypotension after the initial resuscitation in patients without preexisting cardiovascular disease suggests hypovolemia requiring additional intravascular volume expansion.

Treatment of anaphylaxis may also be complicated by increased use of β-adrenergic blocking agents (Jacobs et al., 1981). Patients who receive $β_1$-selective adrenergic blocking agents (metoprolol, atenolol) may demonstrate vasodilation after epinephrine administration in response to unopposed $β_2$-adrenergic stimulations, and norepinephrine may be more effective.

Norepinephrine (Levophed)

In persistent hypotension, norepinephrine may be useful in restoring blood pressure to preoperative values until adequate volume expansion has been achieved. Hypotension is deleterious to both cerebral and coronary perfusion and must be treated aggressively. Suggested starting doses of norepinephrine are 0.05 to 0.1 µg/kg/min (4 to 8 µg/min) and should be titrated to the desired effect.

Isoproterenol

If bronchospasm is refractory to previous therapies, isoproterenol may be useful as a pure β-adrenergic agonist and bronchodilator. The $β_2$-adrenergic effects of this drug cause pulmonary and systemic vasodilation and possibly hypotension, especially in patients already experiencing vasodilation or intravascular volume depletion. Tachyarrhythmias and ventricular ectopic beats are also possible $β_1$-adrenergic mediated side effects. Because isoproterenol dilates the pulmonary artery, it may be useful in treating the increased pulmonary vascular resistance of severe anaphylactic reactions when refractory bronchospasm or right ventricular dysfunction occurs (Figure 10.3). Starting doses for persistent bronchospasm are 0.01 µg/kg/min (0.5 to 1 µg/min).

Corticosteroids

Although corticosteroids should be administered in severe reactions such as shock or refractory bronchospasm/hypotension, no evidence delineates what constitutes an appropriate dose or preparation (Halevy et al., 1982). The administration of 1 g of hydrocortisone or its equivalent is appropriate for severe cardiopulmonary dysfunction. Corticosteroids may be useful in preventing potential late-phase reactions but may not have an immediate effect. Hydrocortisone, 5–10 mg/kg (up to 1 g initial dose) and then 2.5 mg/kg every 6 hours, or methylprednisolone, 1 mg/kg initially and every 6 hours for the first 24 hours, may be given. Large methylprednisone doses (35 mg/kg) have been shown to inhibit complement-induced polymorphonuclear cell aggregation and lysosomal enzyme release in vitro (Hammerschmidt et al., 1979). This may be the drug of choice if the reaction is suspected to be complement mediated (i.e., protamine or transfusion reactions) (Hammerschmidt et al., 1979; Sheagrin, 1981). In addition, very high doses of corticosteroids are a rational adjunct if used early in the therapy of leukoagglutinin-mediated, noncardiogenic pulmonary edema.

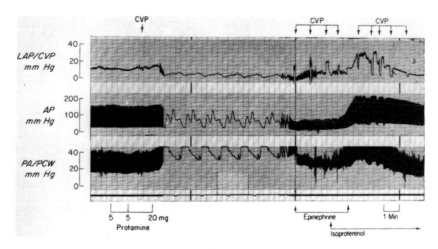

Figure 10.3 Pulmonary hypertension with left atrial and systemic hypotension during a suspected anaphylactic reaction to protamine after cardiopulmonary bypass. The patient had unstable angina pectoris and an intraaortic balloon pump was placed preoperatively. The patient was initially resuscitated with epinephrine but isoproterenol was substituted because of pulmonary hypertension and right ventricular failure. *Reprinted with permission from Lowenstein E, Johnston WE, Lappas DG, et al. Catastrophic pulmonary hypertension associated with protamine reversal of heparin. Anesthesiology 1983; 59:470–3.*

Sodium Bicarbonate

When hypotension does not respond to therapy, acidosis should be suspected and sodium bicarbonate, 0.5 to 1 mEq/kg, should be administered initially. Acid–base status must be monitored using arterial blood gases to guide rational therapeutic interventions. Persistent acidosis can be corrected by administering half the calculated milliequivalent dose according to the formula

$$\text{base excess} \times \text{body weight (kilograms)} \times 1/3.$$

Airway Evaluation

Laryngeal edema may occur in anaphylactic reactions and upper airway swelling can persist despite hemodynamic stability. Once intubated, patients should remain intubated until airway edema resolves. The presence of an air leak around the endotracheal tube after cuff deflation is a useful sign that laryngeal edema or swelling of other airway structures has subsided and that a trial of extubation is justified. Alternatively, laryngeal structures might be examined with direct laryngoscopy before the trachea is extubated. It may be advisable to extubate over a flexible endotracheal tube-changer that can deliver oxygen to maintain access to the airway. Equipment should be available for prompt reintubation and positive pressure ventilation with oxygen. Postextubation airway management is discussed in Chapter 11.

Intensive Care Unit Observation

Patients resuscitated after an anaphylactic reaction should be admitted to an intensive care unit for observation. Reports have demonstrated a recurrence of manifestations 8 to 12 hours after successful treatment of anaphylaxis (Stark and Sullivan, 1986). This form of relapse has also been called a late-phase reaction.

ADDITIONAL THERAPEUTIC CONSIDERATIONS

Despite all of the above measures, some patients may develop severe bronchospasm or pulmonary hypertension with right ventricular failure that requires additional therapeutic interventions. Because of the interdependence of the right heart and lung, air trapping due to severe bronchospasm can passively increase pulmonary vascular resistance and cause the right ventricle to fail (Figure 10.4). The right ventricle is accustomed to ejecting against a low resistance system;

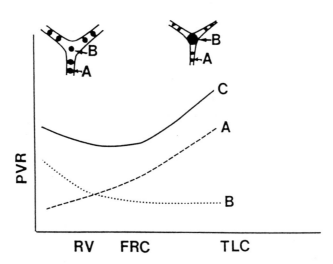

Figure 10.4 The effects of lung volume expansion on the caliber and resistance of the alveolar (A) and extraalveolar (B) pulmonary vessels. The net effect on total pulmonary vascular resistance (C) is the lowest at functional residual capacity (FRC). When the lung is over-distended during acute bronchospasm with air trapping, passive compression on pulmonary vessels increases pulmonary vascular resistance and produces acute right ventricular failure. *Reprinted with permission from Gal TJ. Respiratory Physiology in Anesthetic Practice. Baltimore, Williams and Wilkins, 1991.*

Table 10.3 Treatment of Anaphylaxis with Refractory Bronchospasm

Reassess ventilatory mode

β_2-specific drugs

Corticosteroids

Anticholinergic drugs

Aminophylline

Cardiopulmonary bypass (femoral)

---

normal pulmonary artery pressures are 25/10 mmHg. Acute increases in pulmonary artery pressures that can occur after bronchospasm, protamine, or leukoagglutinin reactions cause the right ventricle to dilate, shifting the intraventricular septum into the left ventricle and decreasing left ventricular end-diastolic compliance. The net effect is systemic hypotension. The inability to ventilate and eliminate carbon dioxide properly further increases pulmonary vascular resistance. Therefore, bronchospasm or right ventricular failure that is refractory to previous treatment must be aggressively treated (Table 10.3, 10.4).

Treatment of Anaphylaxis with Refractory Bronchospasm

Reassess Ventilatory Mode

Patients with severe bronchospasm and air trapping require longer expiratory times to prevent over-distention of the lung. Air trapping increases total lung capacity, passively increasing pulmonary vascular resistance. Longer inspiratory-to-expiratory (I:E) ratios of 1:3 are important to prevent air trapping. The use of an end-tidal CO_2 monitor is helpful in judging the relative degree of air trapping as well as response to bronchodilator therapy.

Administer β_2-Specific Drugs

β_2-specific adrenergic agents are the cornerstone of therapy for bronchospasm and can be aerosolized through an endotracheal tube. Albuterol or ter-

Table 10.4 Treatment of Anaphylaxis with Right Ventricular Failure

Reassess ventilation

Treat bronchospasm

Pulmonary vasodilators

β_2-specific catecholamines

Phosphodiesterase inhibitors

Intraaortic balloon pump

Prostaglandin E_1/norepinephrine infusions

Ventricular assist devices or cardiopulmonary bypass

butaline can be delivered by metered inhaler using a specific endotracheal tube adaptor (Figure 10.5). The β_2-specific agents should be administered using several puffs during forced inspiratory flow. Repeated doses can be administered and the desired improvement can be monitored by measuring pulmonary compliance, end-tidal CO_2 elimination, or the actual morphology of the end-tidal CO_2 curve.

Administer Corticosteroids

If corticosteroids have not been administered, they must be given as discussed previously.

Anticholinergic Drugs

Although anticholinergic drugs are not a primary therapeutic approach in this clinical situation, the use of ipratropium as a metered dose administered into the endotracheal tube may have some benefit, especially in patients with chronic obstructive pulmonary disease who develop bronchospasm. Alternatively, glycopyrolate administered as a nebulized mist may be helpful. Multiple pathways may stimulate parasympathetic–cholinergic-mediated pathways to increase bronchial tone during anaphylaxis.

Aminophylline

If bronchospasm persists, then aminophylline can be administered as an adjuvant to therapy. Aminophylline's other effects in treating right heart failure and increasing diaphragmatic contractility may be important, as discussed in Chapter 9. The initial loading dose is 5 to 6 mg/kg, which should be given over a 20-minute period, followed by a maintenance dose of 0.9 mg/kg/hr. In patients

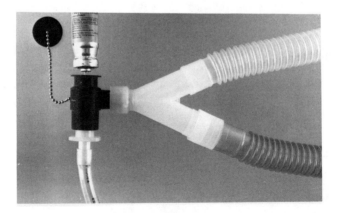

Figure 10.5 Adaptor for administering metered-dose inhalational therapy of β_2-specific adrenergic agents (albuterol, terbutaline) or anticholinergic agents (ipratropium) into the endotracheal tube during anesthesia or in the intensive care unit. The aerosol cannister is placed into the adaptor for administration.

with liver disease or congestive heart failure, the maintenance dose should be lowered to 0.25 to 0.5 mg/kg/hr.

Cardiopulmonary Bypass

Venovenous extracorporeal membrane oxygenation or cardiopulmonary bypass has been described as a last-ditch effort in the treatment of refractory hypoxemia (Pilato et al., 1988). The new portable cardiopulmonary bypass systems (BARD CPS) offer a unique approach but require significant time for femoral vascular access and are not routinely available.

Treatment of Anaphylaxis with Pulmonary Hypertension and Right Ventricular Failure

Reassess Ventilatory Mode and Treat Bronchospasm as Previously Described

Air trapping will passively increase pulmonary vascular resistance and must be avoided when patients develop right ventricular failure. As previously described, longer I:E ratios during mechanical ventilation, and aggressive pharmacologic therapy for bronchospasm, should be instituted to treat this reversible cause of increased pulmonary artery pressures.

Administer β_2-Specific Catecholamines and Pulmonary Vasodilators

Catecholamines with β_2-specific adrenergic effects and nitroglycerin are initial therapeutic approaches to pulmonary hypertension produced by active pulmonary vasoconstriction. Patients with pulmonary hypertension and right ventricular failure should be treated with intravenous β_2-specific catecholamines, drugs that include isoproteranol, epinephrine, and dobutamine. The β_2-specific effects provide pulmonary vasodilation. The α_1-adrenergic actions of a drug like epinephrine can have variable effects on the pulmonary vasculature but can also support perfusion pressure. Norepinephrine is actively taken up by the pulmonary vasculature (Pitt, 1984), and when infused through a central venous catheter, should be used cautiously in patients with pulmonary vasoconstriction. Left atrial administration, in cardiac surgical patients with right ventricular failure or pulmonary hypertension can be a preferred route (Coyle et al., 1990).

Phosphodiesterase Inhibitors

The administration of cAMP-specific (fraction III) phosphodiesterase inhibitors, including amrinone, milrinone, and enoximone, offers an important therapeutic approach to the treatment of right ventricular failure. These drugs produce pulmonary vasodilation independent of endothelium-derived relaxing factors, nitrates, or nitroprusside, and can act additively with β_2-specific agents to increase vascular cAMP more effectively (see Chapter 9). Furthermore, the fraction III phosphodiesterase inhibitors cause less tachycardia and other ventricular arrhythmias than aminophylline, offering distinct therapeutic advantages in patients who are already hemodynamically compromised (Levy et al., 1990).

To avoid systemic hypotension, intravenous loading doses of 1.5 to 2.0 mg/kg should be given over 5 to 10 minutes, followed by an infusion of 5 to 20 μg/kg/min (Levy et al., 1990).

Intraaortic Balloon Pump

Patients with acute right ventricular failure develop high intraventricular wall stress of the right ventricle. The right ventricle is perfused in both systole and diastole; therefore, perfusion pressure should be maintained. The use of an intraaortic balloon pump increases diastolic perfusion pressure, unloads the left ventricle, and allows for increased epicardial-to-endocardial flow of the right ventricle. Maintaining appropriate perfusion pressure is important when treating right ventricular failure and may necessitate the use of left atrial norepinephrine administration.

Prostaglandin E_1/Norepinephrine Infusion

In cardiac surgical patients with pulmonary hypertension refractory to the above therapeutic interventions, the use of a right atrial prostaglandin E_1 infusion at doses of 0.01 to 0.15 μg/kg/min infused into the right atrium in association with norepinephrine infused into a left atrial catheter at doses up to 1.0 μg/kg/min can help to unload the right ventricle pharmacologically, while at the same time maintaining perfusion pressures (D'Ambra et al., 1985). Prostaglandin E_1 is metabolized in the pulmonary endothelium whereas norepinephrine is metabolized in the periphery (Pitt, 1984). This therapy is usually reserved for patients who have had cardiac surgery where left atrial lines are in place or can be established to provide separate drug administration. In addition, the use of a right atrial and left atrial catheter to monitor right and left ventricular filling separately provides an important method of monitoring bi-ventricular function during reactions characterized by catastrophic pulmonary vasoconstriction. Low filling pressure of the left ventricle may be present in the place of pulmonary hypertension.

Ventricular Assist Devices or Cardiopulmonary Bypass

Ventricular assist devices and cardiopulmonary bypasses are also reserved for cardiac surgical patients and represent important therapeutic approaches after cardiopulmonary bypass and surgery. Patients developing acute right heart failure after protamine or blood product administration can be reheparinized with the reinstitution of cardiopulmonary bypass. In addition, reports have suggested that heparin administration alone can reverse acute cardiovascular dysfunction after some protamine reactions (Lock and Hessel, 1990).

11

Managing Sequelae in the Recovery Room and Intensive Care Unit

Following resuscitation after a major anaphylactic reaction, patients should be closely evaluated and monitored. Clinical observations of patients after anaphylaxis indicate that late-phase responses occur, with recurrent manifestations appearing 12 to 24 hours after the initial episode (Sheffer, 1985). Stark and Sullivan reported the clinical courses of 25 patients with life-threatening anaphylaxis who were observed for at least 12 hours (Stark and Sullivan, 1986). The agents responsible for the reactions included antibiotics (12 reactions), radiocontrast media (3 reactions), foods (3 reactions), and miscellaneous (7 reactions). Twelve patients (48%) manifested a single episode of anaphylaxis with no clinically detectable recurrence. Six patients (24%) experienced two distinct anaphylactic events separated by symptom-free intervals of 2 to 8 hours. Initial therapy included epinephrine, H_1 and H_2 antihistamines, and, in 5 of the 6 patients, 2 high doses of glucocorticoids—the initial dose within the first hour of therapy and the second dose 6 hours later. Three had recurrent laryngeal edema and 3 had recurrent hypotension. Five of the patients with recurrent episodes responded to conventional therapy for acute reactions, and 1 patient died of laryngeal edema. Seven patients (28%) suffered prolonged hypotension, bronchospasm, or laryngeal edema requiring intensive therapy and observation for 5 hours to 8 days. Two of these patients died.

These findings indicate that patients should be admitted to an intensive care unit or recovery room for observation after an anaphylactic reaction. If hypotension requires ongoing therapy, or if hypoxemia or hypercapnia persists, a careful assessment of the patient and underlying problems should be made, specific tests performed, and additional monitoring instituted as described. Guidelines to initial management in the recovery room and intensive care unit start with the following evaluation.

HISTORY, PHYSICAL EXAMINATION, LABORATORY DATA

Following initial resuscitation of the patient after an anaphylactic reaction, a complete history, physical examination, and laboratory evaluation must be performed. Specific problems pertinent to the patient following an anaphylactic reaction will be reviewed.

History

Information can be obtained from the patient, family, nurses, and old records. Specific information that should be obtained includes:

All Previous Medical Problems and Their Management
Problems that may be contributing to the shock state include a history of previous myocardial infarction or angina pectoris, endocrinologic abnormality, or infection.

Medications
Drugs that may contribute to the shock state include β-adrenergic blocking agents, digoxin, diuretics, vasodilators, nitrates, calcium entry blockers, or tricyclic antidepressants. Patients receiving β-adrenergic blocking agents may be refractory to the effects of epinephrine. This problem should be considered with refractory shock after adequate resuscitation. Further, patients receiving $β_1$-adrenergic selective blocking agents such as metoprolol (Lopressor) or atenolol (Tenormin) may develop further hypotension after the administration of epinephrine due to unopposed $β_2$-adrenergic effects on the peripheral vasculature. Instead of epinephrine, norepinephrine, a drug with primarily α- and $β_1$-adrenergic stimulation, or other pure alpha agonists should be considered.

Physical Examination

A complete physical examination should be performed after resuscitation, emphasizing important aspects of the initial assessment, to evaluate other causes or sequelae of shock.

Neurologic
The overall mental status after resuscitation should be noted. If the mental status is depressed, a coma score can be determined and followed. Seizures may also be present after anaphylaxis and should be treated with intravenous diazepam or barbiturates.

Cardiovascular
The heart should be auscultated, evaluating the quality of the heart tones, gallops, murmurs, or pericardial friction rubs. Neck veins and the quality of peripheral pulses should be noted.

Chest
Chest wall excursion should be observed for adequacy of ventilation. Labored ventilation and chest wall retractions during spontaneous ventilation can indicate upper airway obstruction or severe bronchospasm. Both lung fields should be auscultated, assessing for symmetry and quality of breath sounds, especially after intubation and during mechanical ventilation. Wheezing or other airway sounds should be noted.

Abdomen
The abdomen should be palpated for masses, tenderness, and rigidity and should be auscultated for bowel sounds and bruits. Diarrhea and abdominal pain are complications of anaphylaxis. Masive abdominal distension may occur after attempts at positive pressure mask ventilation before intubation.

Extremities
The extremities should be examined for pulses, color, and capillary refill. After anaphylactic reactions patients often have bounding pulses with warm extremities. For potential radial artery catheter insertion, the adequacy of collateral blood flow to the wrist should be noted by performing an Allen's test.

Laboratory Evaluation

The laboratory evaluation of a patient after an anaphylactic reaction should include the following.

Complete Blood Count with Differential and Serial Hematocrits
The hematocrit is a useful guide to intravascular blood volume expansion. Persistent hemoconcentration may suggest an ongoing capillary leak problem. Patients requiring intensive care admission should also have a baseline white blood cell count for future reference if long-term care is required, especially when an invasive hemodynamic monitor has been inserted or the patient requires intubation.

Serum Electrolytes
After massive volume resuscitation, serum potassium and other electrolytes should be evaluated. Patients will mobilize their third space fluid losses after capillary permeability alterations as they improve clinically. As a result, profound diuresis may occur, requiring continuous potassium replacement. If the diuresis is vigorous, requiring frequent potassium supplementations, a urine sample for potassium concentration is useful in calculating replacement requirements.

Chest Radiograph
Following resuscitation after anaphylaxis, a chest radiograph is important to evaluate the presence of interstitial edema due to increased capillary perme-

ability or hyperinflation from bronchospasm and air trapping. Furthermore, after intubation or central venous cannulation, proper endotracheal tube and catheter placement should be confirmed. The chest radiograph should also be carefully observed for the presence of pneumothorax after internal jugular and subclavian needle insertion.

Electrocardiogram

Persistent hypotension or potential coronary vasoconstrictive effects of mediators released during anaphylaxis may produce myocardial injury. Therefore, an electrocardiogram should be evaluated for ST–T wave changes or other evidence of myocardial ischemia after resuscitation. Serial tracings should be obtained if evidence of myocardial ischemia or injury exists along with serum for creatine phosphokinase-MB levels.

Clotting Parameters

Platelet count, prothrombin time (PT), and partial thromboplastin time (PTT) may be altered, producing values consistent with disseminated intravascular coagulation (i.e., decreased platelet count and elevated PT, PTT) after anaphylaxis. Baseline values should be obtained and followed until they normalize. Fresh frozen plasma may be necessary to replace clotting factors if bleeding occurs or if central venous cannulation using internal jugular or subclavian access is required.

Blood Urea Nitrogen, Creatinine

Baseline renal function tests should be evaluated after persistent hypotension, because transient renal dysfunction may occur.

MONITORS

If hypotension does not quickly reverse after resuscitation, or if persistent hypotension during anaphylaxis produces myocardial ischemia, injury, or even cardiogenic shock, additional hemodynamic monitoring is indicated to evaluate the cause and the response to therapy.

Electrocardiographic Monitoring

Electrocardiographic monitors should be placed in all patients after anaphylactic reactions, especially to diagnose and treat arrhythmias if patients require ongoing vasoactive drug administration. In addition, in the monitor mode with proper calibration, leads II and V_5 can be used to evaluate myocardial ischemia.

Pulse Oximetry

Pulse oximetry should also be used in all patients after anaphylactic reactions. Cardiopulmonary dysfunction commonly occurs with ventilation–perfusion mismatching to produce hypoxemia. During the initial clinical presentations of the reaction, during therapy, or as a consequence of late phase reactions, careful monitoring using pulse oximetry should be used to diagnose and treat these problems when they occur.

End-Tidal CO_2

End-tidal CO_2 monitoring can be useful to diagnose and treat cardiopulmonary dysfunction in patients requiring intubation and mechanical ventilation after anaphylaxis. The exhaled CO_2 waveform can be used to determine if persistent small airway obstruction and air trapping is occurring or used as a guide to therapy. In addition, end-tidal CO_2 is an immediate measure of the adequacy of mechanical ventilation, especially in contrast to the process of analyzing arterial blood gases. In the patient with pulmonary hypertension and right ventricular failure, elevations of $PaCO_2$ can exacerbate pulmonary vasoconstriction, and should be rapidly normalized.

Automated Blood Pressure Monitoring

If the patient does not have an intraarterial catheter, then an automated blood pressure monitor should be placed. Frequent and rapid assessment of blood pressure is essential to diagnose and treat the cardiovascular dysfunction that can occur in the recovery room and the intensive care unit.

Central Venous Cannula

A central venous cannula is useful for vasoactive drug administration and for central venous monitoring as a guide to fluid replacement in patients with normal ventricular function. A low central venous pressure (less than 2 to 3 mmHg) suggests intravascular volume depletion. A high central venous pressure (greater than 10 to 12 mmHg) suggests increased intravascular volume or ventricular dysfunction. Central venous pressure may not adequately reflect left ventricular preload in the presence of left ventricular dysfunction, mechanical ventilation, right ventricular dysfunction, or pulmonary hypertension (e.g., after transfusion or protamine reactions).

Pulmonary Artery Catheter

A pulmonary artery (Swan-Ganz) catheter can be inserted to assess both left and right ventricular preload, cardiac output, and pulmonary artery pressure to guide rational therapeutic interventions. In addition, the newer pulmonary artery catheters (Multipurpose pacing and continuous $S\bar{v}O_2$ oximetry) provide the ability for atrial or ventricular pacing in patients manifesting atrioventricular conduction defects, asystolic episodes, or tachydysrhythmias, or continuous measurements of oxygen saturation of the mixed venous blood in patients with persistent cardiopulmonary dysfunction. Measurements useful in managing hemodynamic instability after anaphylaxis include the following.

Pulmonary Capillary Wedge Pressure approximates left ventricular end-diastolic pressure by measuring distal pulmonary venous pressure. The goal of intravascular volume administration is to provide adequate left ventricular end-diastolic volume, a major determinant of cardiac output. After anaphylaxis, optimal intravascular volume expansion can be achieved at a pulmonary capillary wedge pressure of 12 to 15 mmHg in patients without preexisting ventricular dysfunction.

Cardiac Output may be increased initially in anaphylactic shock states; however, persistent hypotension in patients with ischemic heart disease can produce myocardial dysfunction. Cardiac output determinations also allow calculation of systemic and pulmonary vascular resistance. Persistent hypotension after anaphylactic shock may be due to either increased or decreased systemic vascular resistance.

Pulmonary Artery Pressure is an important monitor of right ventricular and pulmonary function. Pulmonary hypertension due to increased pulmonary vascular resistance occurs after leukoagglutinin reactions, protamine reactions, or sepsis. In patients without pulmonary artery catheters, later clinical manifestations include hypoxemia or findings consistent with the adult respiratory distress syndrome. Pulmonary artery pressure also increases with left ventricular failure or fluid overload, but often without an increased pulmonary vascular resistance. If pulmonary capillary wedge pressure approximates or is slightly lower than pulmonary artery diastolic pressure (less than 5 mmHg), increased pulmonary vascular resistance is not likely. Conversely, if pulmonary catheter wedge pressure is much lower than pulmonary artery diastolic pressure, pulmonary vascular resistance is increased (see Figure 6.2) (Latson et al., 1986). Pulmonary vascular resistance is normally 80 to 160 dynes $\times$ second $\times$ centimeter^{-5} and can be calculated as follows

$$\frac{\text{mean pulmonary artery pressure} - \text{pulmonary capillary wedge pressure}}{\text{cardiac output}} \times 80$$

Foley Catheter

A Foley catheter is essential to assess renal function, providing an indicator of adequate intravascular volume replacement and cardiac output. As adult patients improve following anaphylaxis, they may mobilize third space fluid losses of 10 to 12 L (Royston and Wilkes, 1978).

Intraarterial Cannula

An intraarterial cannula facilitates continuous assessment of cardiovascular changes as well as allowing frequent arterial blood gas sampling. Blood pressure cuff measurements can be unreliable during anaphylaxis, especially with epinephrine or norepinephrine administration. In addition, careful observations of the quality of the arterial tracing on the oscilloscope provide useful information regarding cardiovascular status. Large fluctuations of systolic and diastolic arterial pressure during positive pressure ventilation can be seen with hypovolemia (Figure 11.1). Percutaneous radial artery cannulation of the nondominant hand is frequently used; however, femoral or axillary artery access may be necessary if radial artery pulses are not palpable.

RENAL FUNCTION

Urine output should be maintained at 0.5 to 1.0 mL/kg/hr after resuscitation after anaphylactic shock. Oliguria in patients without previous renal dysfunction suggests persistent hypovolemia and inadequate intravascular volume expansion. If oliguria persists despite adequate intravascular volume administration as determined by hemodynamic monitoring, then diuretics or low-dose dopamine (1 to 2 µg/kg/min) should be administered intravenously.

METABOLIC STATUS

Metabolic status should be assessed from the laboratory evaluation discussed previously and abnormalities corrected as needed. Anaphylactic or other shock syndromes may be associated with metabolic acidosis (secondary to elevated lactic acid), hyperglycemia, and renal failure. In addition, blood glucose levels should be measured during epinephrine infusions since they may cause glycogenolysis and gluconeogenesis.

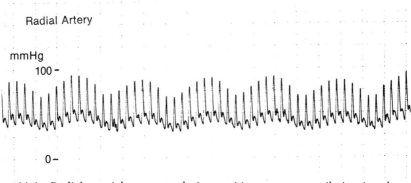

Figure 11.1 Radial arterial pressures during positive-pressure ventilation in a hypovolemic patient. Note the fluctuations in both systolic and diastolic arterial pressures. The pulmonary capillary wedge pressure was 3 mmHg.

RESPIRATORY MANAGEMENT AFTER ANAPHYLAXIS

Once a severe anaphylactic or anaphylactoid reaction has occurred and the patient has been successfully treated, the lung may suffer consequences of the physiologic insult, producing an acute adult respiratory distress syndrome. This is characterized by

1. Decreased pulmonary compliance
2. Increased alveolar–arterial oxygen gradient
3. Increased intrapulmonary shunt
4. Bilateral infiltrates on the chest radiograph
5. Pulmonary hypertension (Zapol and Falker, 1985).

Consequences of the adult respiratory distress syndrome have a final common pathway through the liberation of inflammatory mediators producing endothelial damage with increased capillary permeability and resultant perivascular edema (see Chapter 4). In addition to leukoagglutinins and complement activation, experimentally induced anaphylaxis from immunoglobulin-G (IgG) reactions has produced aggregates of white blood cells and platelets in the pulmonary vasculature, leading to microvascular occlusion and inflammation (Smedegärd et al., 1980). Acute noncardiogenic pulmonary edema can also occur after immunoglobulin-E (IgE)-mediated reactions, producing acute lung injury (Levy and Rockoff, 1982). Postmortem examination of the lungs of a patient after a fatal anaphylactoid reaction from radiocontrast media (Diatrizoate) revealed numerous pure granulocyte aggregates impacted in the microscopic pulmonary arteries and capillaries (Schneiderman et al., 1983). The lungs were markedly edematous and free of pneumonia or thromboemboli.

Mechanical ventilation is often required after a severe anaphylactic reaction when the lung is a major shock organ. Often, 24 to 72 hours of mechanical ventilation may be necessary to support the patient until the lung resolves the inflammatory insult. Some patients may require longer periods of mechanical ventilation, however. Unfortunately, there is no way to predict the clinical course. Rather, therapy should be directed at providing respiratory support until the patient improves.

Postextubation Stridor

Postextubation stridor can be caused by residual laryngeal edema after an anaphylactic reaction or may be due to the effects of prolonged intubation. Stridor should be differentiated from bronchospasm, because both can produce inspiratory as well as expiratory wheezing. The acute onset of wheezing after extubation is consistent with laryngeal edema and should be managed as follows.

1. Place airway equipment at the bedside for prompt reintubation.
2. Continue to administer 100% oxygen by face mask with a cool humidified mist.

3. Sit the patient up at an angle of 45 degrees or greater to decrease laryngeal venous congestion, especially in view of laryngeal injury and potentially altered capillary permeability.
4. Administer inhaled racemic epinephrine by nebulizer with oxygen (0.5 mL of 2.25% solution in 2 to 2.5 mL normal saline) every 1 to 4 hours.
5. Administer dexamethasone, 0.1 mg/kg intravenously every 6 hours, if corticosteroids have not already been given.
6. Continue close monitoring in the recovery room or intensive care unit even when the patient responds to therapy.
7. Additional therapy can include
    a. Helium–oxygen mixture (Heliox) administration may temporarily improve ventilation because of its decreased viscosity if there is upper airway edema.
    b. With acute respiratory compromise in a stridorous patient, positive-pressure assisted ventilation applied during inspiration using a 100% oxygen ambu-bag with a mask can help the patient until an artificial airway is reestablished.
8. Reasons to reintubate the patient with stridor include
    a. Fatigue
    b. Hypercapnia
    c. Mental status changes (i.e., obtundation)
    d. Inadequate tidal volume.

IRREVERSIBLE SHOCK

When anaphylactic shock does not respond to treatment, *reconsider* the causes. Additional monitoring and evaluation are essential in sorting out the problems. The following potentially reversible contributing factors should be evaluated and corrected

1. Hypoxemia or inadequate ventilation
2. Vasopressors not infusing
3. Inadequate intravascular volume expansion
4. Pneumothorax
5. Myocardial ischemia or infarction

12

Human Physiologic Responses During Anaphylactic or Anaphylactoid Reactions

The following cases illustrate the physiologic responses during anaphylactic and anaphylactoid reactions as well as individualized responses to therapy. The purpose of this section is to emphasize the variability of clinical responses and the importance of using an established therapeutic plan.

ANAPHYLACTOID REACTION TO VANCOMYCIN

A 60-year-old, 65-kg man with 3-vessel coronary disease was scheduled for coronary artery bypass grafting. Radial artery and pulmonary artery catheters were inserted preoperatively in the operating room before anesthetic induction. Baseline hemodynamic data were obtained as shown in Figure 12.1. Vancomycin, 100 mg, administered for wound prophylaxis, was accidentally given as a rapid intravenous bolus. Arterial pressure decreased precipitously to 75/30 mmHg and was associated with an increased cardiac output. The patient was noted to have diffuse cutaneous flushing and complained of a "warm feeling." Ephedrine, 5 mg, was administered intravenously with a rapid return of baseline blood pressure (Figure 12.2). The electrocardiogram was unchanged in leads II and V_5 and despite the transient hypotension, the patient underwent an otherwise uneventful operation.

Although vancomycin has been suggested to produce myocardial depression, the author has shown nonimmunologic histamine release as the mechanism responsible for both hypotension and flushing (Levy et al., 1987). For these reasons, vancomycin must be administered as a slow dilute infusion over a *minimum* of 30 minutes. The rapid administration of vancomycin produces a self-limiting reaction consistent with a bolus dose of morphine or *d*-tubocurarine, or an infusion of histamine.

Pulmonary artery or central venous pressures did not change, but systemic vascular resistance decreased. Histamine infused in volunteers produces similar

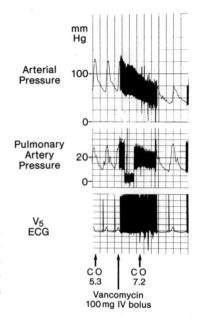

Figure 12.1 Cardiovascular changes during an anaphylactoid reaction to vancomycin after rapid administration. Central venous pressure was measured as shown in the pulmonary artery tracing. The hypotension was associated with a sudden reduction in systemic vascular resistance.

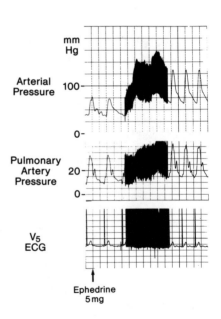

Figure 12.2 Cardiovascular changes after ephedrine administration to treat the hypotension. Blood pressure returned to baseline values and lead V_5 of the electrocardiogram was unchanged.

effects (Vigorito et al., 1983). The duration of the reaction is short, because histamine is rapidly cleared by tissues. The hypotension responds to vasoconstrictors, volume administration, or Trendelenburg positioning.

SUSPECTED ANAPHYLAXIS TO CEFAZOLIN

A 20-year-old, 70-kg man was scheduled for an elective rhinoplasty for recurrent nasal bleeding. There was no history of allergy to prior anesthetics, and the patient had received penicillin in the past without a reaction. Induction and intubation were uneventful after 500 mg thiamylal and 100 mg succinylcholine, and anesthesia was maintained with 1.5% enflurane and 70% nitrous oxide (Figure 12.3, arrow 1). Lidocaine, 9 mL of a 1% solution with 1:100,000 epinephrine, was administered submucosally in the nares, and cocaine packs containing 4 mL of 4% solution were placed (arrow 2). To prevent postoperative swelling, 500 mg sodium methylprednisolone was given intravenously, and the patient was prepared and draped (arrow 3). One gram of cefazolin was then administered intravenously over 4 minutes (arrow 4).

Within 8 minutes after the initial administration of cefazolin, the sudden onset of bronchospasm was noted and was treated with 0.25 mg terbutaline subcutaneously and controlled ventilation with 100% oxygen (arrow 5). Acute hypotension ensued, enflurane was discontinued, and phenylephrine, 200 µg, was initially administered intravenously followed by a rapid 1 L Ringer's lactate infusion over 10 minutes for blood pressure support (arrow 6). Epinephrine, 0.3 mg, was then given subcutaneously (arrow 7). The initial arterial blood gas tensions during controlled ventilation with 100% oxygen after epinephrine were pH 7.28, $PaCO_2$ 45 mmHg, and PaO_2 394 mmHg (arrow 8). Sodium bicarbonate, 50 mEq, was administered intravenously for metabolic acidosis (arrow 9).

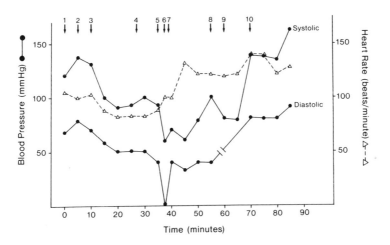

Figure 12.3 Cardiovascular changes during an anaphylactic reaction to cefazolin. The arrows refer to events described in the text.

The surgery was rapidly completed while anesthesia was maintained with 1% enflurane and 50% nitrous oxide (arrow 10). In the recovery room 1 hour after the administration of cefazolin, the patient was awake and alert although facial swelling persisted. A chest radiograph taken before extubation was normal. The patient was extubated uneventfully after cuff deflation demonstrated a large air leak.

The manifestations of bronchospasm, hypotension, and facial edema are classic for an anaphylactic reaction. Although a variety of drugs was administered, the temporal sequence of cefazolin administration and the incidence of allergic reactions to penicillin and its derivatives in the general population suggest this agent as the allergen responsible. Although most anaphylactic reactions have an immediate onset, clinical manifestations may occur as late as 15 minutes after the parenteral injection of an antigen. Furthermore, a prior history of penicillin or other drug allergy is not required for a life-threatening anaphylactic reaction to penicillin.

Incidental pretreatment for the patient's reaction potentially occurred with 90 μg epinephrine (from the lidocaine) and 0.5 g methylprednisolone 25 to 30 minutes before the onset of acute anaphylaxis. Although the dose of epinephrine was too small to inhibit mediator release effectively, the use of cocaine may theoretically have potentiated its effcts. Despite corticosteroid pretreatment in this patient, a life-threatening anaphylactic reaction occurred.

Terbutaline, a β_2-specific adrenergic agonist, was administered before the decrease in blood pressure and may have precipitated hypotension by acting as a vasodilator. Pure α-adrenergic agonists are not the drugs of choice and were initially administered in this case before the recognition of a true anaphylactic reaction. Epinephrine, administered subcutaneously in this patient with moderate hypotension, along with rapid intravascular volume expansion, restored blood pressure to baseline values. Subcutaneous epinephrine is not the preferred route of administration with life-threatening hypotension. Airway evaluation to assess laryngeal edema in this patient with facial swelling was important before extubation. The air leak around the endotracheal tube after deflating the cuff is a useful sign of a patent airway.

ANAPHYLAXIS TO MEPERIDINE*

A 2.5-year-old, 12-kg girl was scheduled for sigmoidoscopy to evaluate rectal bleeding. She was in excellent health with no known allergies, no previous history of asthma, and a normal physical examination.

An intravenous infusion was started in the examining room and meperidine, 25 mg, was given intravenously. Within 1 minute, facial urticaria developed and coughing was noted. Diphenhydramine 25 mg, was given, but the child suddenly began to wheeze and cyanosis was noted. Oxygen was administered by facemask

---

*Reprinted with permission from Levy JH, Rockoff MR. Anaphylaxis to meperidine. Anesth Analg 1982;61:301–3.

Table 12.1 Arterial Blood Gases, pH, and Alveolar-Arterial Gradients After Anaphylaxis to Meperidine

Hours Postarrest	FiO₂ (%)	Ventilation	Medications Given	PaO₂ (mmHg)	PaCO₂ (mmHg)	pH	A-aO₂ Gradient
0	100	Ambu-bag	Epinephrine	80	50	7.25	571
1	100	IMV	Dexamethasone Aminophylline	98	56	7.21	546
3	100	IMV	Isoproterenol	106	38	7.31	560
4	100	IMV	Isoproterenol	410	25	7.47	272
6	50	IMV	Isoproterenol	221	27	7.46	102
10	35	CPAP		175	37	7.40	27
20	30	CPAP		157	34	7.42	15
28	21	Extubated		98	37	7.41	6

IMV = intermittent mandatory ventilation; CPAP = continuous positive airway pressure.

but cyanosis persisted, pulses become unobtainable, and cardiopulmonary resuscitation was instituted immediately. An endotracheal tube was inserted and profuse frothy proteinaceous secretions were suctioned from the trachea. Epinephrine was administered intravenously in 50 to 100 µg/repeated doses along with a rapid 500 mL infusion of normal saline until systolic blood pressure increased to 90 mmHg. The initial arterial blood gas tensions during hand ventilation with 100% oxygen were pH 7.25, $PaCO_2$ 50 mmHg, and PaO_2 80 mmHg (Table 12.1).

The patient was admitted to the pediatric intensive care unit where the initial chest radiograph showed pulmonary edema, an electrocardiogram demonstrated sinus tachycardia, and physical examination revealed bilateral inspiratory and expiratory wheezing (Figure 12.4). Mechanical ventilation with positive end-expiratory pressure at 8 cm water was instituted and aminophylline, 5 mg/kg, was infused over 30 minutes followed by an infusion of 0.9 mg/kg/hr (see Table 12.1). Despite these interventions, wheezing and respiratory failure persisted. Therefore, dexamethasone, 0.75 mg/kg, was given and an infusion of

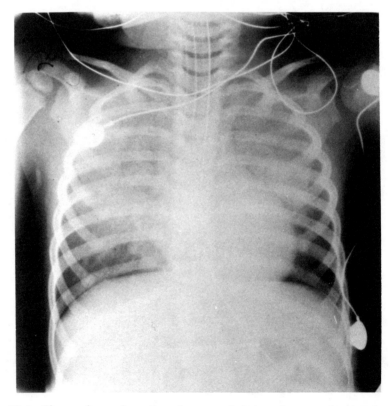

Figure 12.4 Chest radiograph on intensive care admission after resuscitation after anaphylaxis to meperidine. Note the diffuse bilateral infiltrates.

isoproterenol at 0.15 µg/kg/min was begun for persistent wheezing. Within 6 hours, mechanical ventilation and the isoproterenol were discontinued and spontaneous ventilation with an inspired oxygen content of 35% showed arterial pH 7.4, $PaCO_2$ 37 mmHg, and PaO_2 176 mmHg.

Twenty-four hours later the patient appeared alert, the chest radiograph revealed resolution of the pulmonary edema, and extubation was accomplished uneventfully (Figure 12.5). She was discharged and given a MedAlert bracelet. Six weeks later, serum revealed the presence of immunoglobulin-E (IgE) antibodies specific for meperidine by RAST testing.

The rapid onset of urticaria, bronchospasm, cyanosis, and shock is consistent with the diagnosis of anaphylaxis. The demonstration of IgE antibodies immunospecific for meperidine confirmed the diagnosis. The use of intravenous resuscitative epinephrine doses along with rapid volume expansion promptly restored blood pressure. Pulmonary edema after the anaphylactic reaction, before intravascular volume administration, was likely due to increased capillary permeability. Positive end-expiratory pressure was administered because interstitial

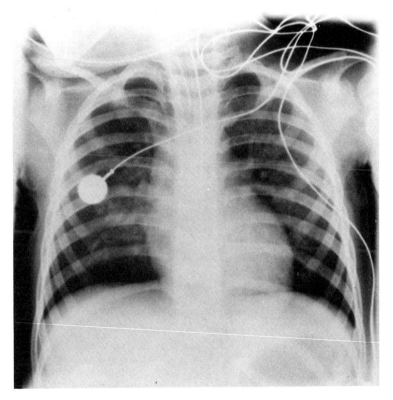

Figure 12.5 Chest radiograph 24 hours after the onset of anaphylaxis. Note the marked resolution of pulmonary edema that corresponded to arterial blood gas improvement.

edema was thought to be contributing to her respiratory failure. Bronchospasm, refractory to aminophylline and corticosteroids, was treated with the β-adrenergic agonist isoproterenol, with marked clinical improvement. For this child, the dose was 0.15 μg/kg/min; when using isoproterenol in adults, the starting dose should be smaller (i.e., 0.01 μg/kg/min). Finally, after resuscitation and stabilization, the patient was readily weaned from mechanical ventilation and extubated.

ANAPHYLAXIS TO PROTAMINE

A 61-year-old, 72-kg man with a history of coronary artery disease and NPH insulin use underwent four-vessel coronary artery bypass grafting. After a stable anesthetic induction and cardiopulmonary bypass run, termination of extracorporeal circulation was uneventful. Before protamine administration, the arterial pressure was 110/60 mmHg, mean pulmonary artery pressure was 12 mmHg, and the cardiac output was 4.8 L/min (Figure 12.6). Arterial blood gases obtained immediately after cardiopulmonary bypass were normal.

After aortic decannulation, a protamine infusion was started. Within 2 minutes after the infusion of approximately 80 mg protamine, there was a precipitous decrease in radial artery pressure to approximately 60/40 mmHg, the cardiac output had increased to 8.4 L/min, and the systemic vascular resistance was profoundly reduced to approximately 400 dynes/sec/cm^{-5}. The patient was resuscitated with incremental bolus doses of 4 μg epinephrine followed by 8 μg, and an epinephrine infusion was started at 10 μg/min. Additional volume

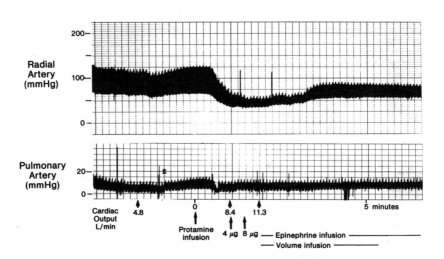

Figure 12.6 Cardiovascular changes during anaphylaxis to protamine. The patient was initially resuscitated with intravenous epinephrine boluses followed by an infusion of 10 μg/min, along with rapid volume infusion.

was infused and within 3 minutes after a rapid infusion of 2 L of lactated Ringer's, the blood pressure had returned to approximately 90/60 mmHg. At an epinephrine infusion of 8 to 10 μg/min, the patient began to manifest an increased heart rate of 120 to 130 beats/min and continued moderate hypotension. Therefore, additional volume was administered and a norepinephrine infusion was started at 6 μg/min while the epinephrine was tapered off (Figure 12.7). By 10 minutes after the initial protamine administration, the blood pressure had returned to baseline values and the patient was hemodynamically stable. The norepinephrine infusion was continued postoperatively and discontinued in the intensive care unit.

This is an example of an IgE-mediated anaphylactic reaction to protamine. The patient was an NPH diabetic and evidence suggests that some of these patients may be sensitized to protamine (Weiss et al., 1989). Further, the precipitous and persistent hypotension after the administration of low protamine doses is characteristic of anaphylaxis. During IgE-mediated anaphylaxis to protamine, histamine, prostacyclin (PGI$_2$), and other vasoactive mediators are released that produce vasodilation without changes in pulmonary artery pressure (see Figure 6.3). During complement activation by immunoglobulin-G (IgG) anaphylaxis to protamine or direct heparin–protamine-mediated effects, however, thromboxane A$_2$ is liberated, producing acute pulmonary vasoconstriction, right ventricular failure, and hypotension (see Figure 6.4).

The intravenous administration of incremental epinephrine doses followed by an epinephrine infusion in conjunction with rapid volume administration allowed prompt increase of arterial blood pressure. When an epinephrine infusion

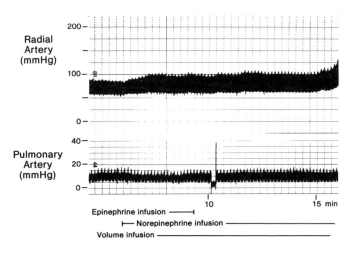

Figure 12.7 During epinephrine and volume administration after protamine anaphylaxis, the patient had persistent hypotension and tachycardia. Therefore, a norepinephrine infusion was started at 6 μg/min with restoration of blood pressure.

194 | MANAGEMENT OF ANAPHYLAXIS

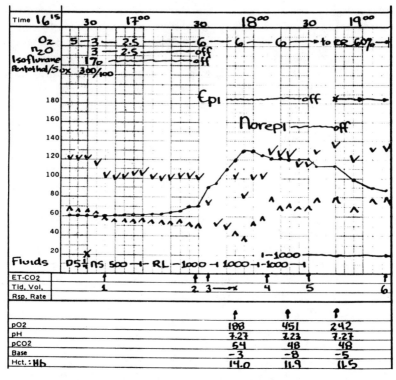

1: Diphenhydramine 50 mg
Cimetidine 300 mg
Dexamethasone 20 mg

2: Chymopapain test dose

3: Epinephrine IV boluses

    10 μg
    50 μg
    100 μg
      0.5 mg ×2
      1.0 mg ×2

4: arterial line #16 g IV

5: to RR 18^{35}
132/80
112 reg
20 spont

6: extubated in RR awake, alert no evidence of airway edema

Figure 12.8 Anesthetic record during anaphylactic reaction to chymopapain injected for chemonucleolysis.

was not restoring the blood pressure to baseline value or when additional side effects resulted (i.e., tachycardia), the noreinephrine infusion was begun. The prompt restoration of blood pressure emphasizes the importance of rapid recognition and appropriate therapy.

ANAPHYLAXIS TO CHYMOPAPAIN DESPITE PRETREATMENT

A 37-year-old woman with a history of extravasated nucleus pulposus underwent chemonucleolysis under general anesthesia. The patient had an uneventful anesthetic induction with thiopental and succinylcholine and was easily intubated. Anesthesia was maintained using a 1% inspired concentration of isoflurane (Figure 12.8).

After the anesthetic induction, the patient received pretreatment for a potential anaphylactic reaction which consisted of 50 mg diphenhydramine, 300 mg cimetidine, and 20 mg dexamethasone (Figure 12.8, arrow 1). The patient was turned to a left lateral decubitus position and a chymopapain test dose of 0.3 mg was administered into the disc. Within 2 minutes there was a precipitous decrease in systolic arterial pressure to 70 mmHg followed by 50 mmHg systolic. The isoflurane was discontinued, 100% oxygen was administered, volume was rapidly infused, and the patient received incremental doses of intravenous epinephrine using a 1:10,000 dilution. The patient received 10 µg, 50 µg, and 100 µg, 0.5 mg, and then 1 mg doses as intravenous boluses followed by an epinephrine infusion. A total of 3 L of lactated Ringer's was rapidly infused into the patient and a norepinephrine infusion was started because of persistent hypotension. Because of the hemodynamic instability, an additional 16-gauge intravenous catheter was placed for additional volume administration. A radial artery catheter was also inserted for frequent blood gas determination as well as intraarterial pressure monitoring.

After resuscitation, the patient was rapidly weaned off epinephrine while the norepinephrine infusion was continued. In the recovery room, the blood pressure was 132/80 mmHg, the spontaneous respiratory rate was 20 per minute, and the patient's heart rate was 112 beats/min. Because of improved hemodynamic stability but persistent bronchospasm, an epinephrine infusion was started at 1 to 2 µg/min and the norepinephrine infusion was stopped. The patient showed continued improvement in the recovery room and was awake and alert. There was no evidence of facial edema and the patient was extubated without any upper airway problem. The epinephrine infusion was discontinued within the first hour. After subsequent recovery room monitoring the patient continued her improvement and was discharged to the intensive care unit for overnight observation.

This case illustrates the profound hypotension that can occur after anaphylaxis. Despite the absence of invasive hemodynamic monitoring, the patient received incremental doses of epinephrine in addition to rapid intravascular volume administration to restore baseline blood pressures rapidly. When the epinephrine infusion was ineffective despite acceptable arterial blood gas levels, a norepinephrine infusion was started. Because of persistent bronchospasm in the recovery room, the epinephrine infusion was restarted at low doses. This case demonstrates the importance of rapid volume administration along with titrating appropriate doses of intravenous epinephrine to a desired endpoint, i.e., restoration of blood pressure. Once blood pressure returned to baseline values, specific catecholamine infusions were used effectively to fine-tune the restored cardiopulmonary function. Rapid recognition and appropriate, carefully titrated drug therapy saved this patient's life.

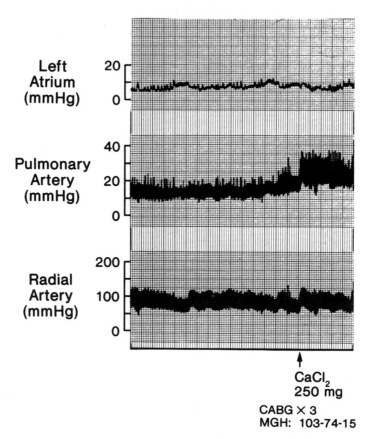

Figure 12.9 Hemodynamic changes during transfusion-related acute lung injury. After coronary artery bypass grafting (CABG), a patient was hypovolemic with a left atrial pressure of 5 mmHg, and 1 unit of whole blood was rapidly transfused. After the transfusion, the pulmonary artery pressure gradually began to increase, but systolic blood pressure was less than 100 mmHg, and $CaCl_2$, 250 mg, was given as a bolus. The radial artery pressure increased acutely, but pulmonary artery pressure also increased and stayed persistently elevated.

TRANSFUSION-RELATED ACUTE LUNG INJURY, A SUSPECTED LEUKOAGGLUTININ REACTION

A patient was hypovolemic after coronary artery bypass grafting, with a left atrial pressure of 5 mmHg, and normal pulmonary artery pressures after chest closure (Figure 12.9). One unit of whole blood was rapidly administered, but despite the volume infusion, the patient was still hypotensive. Calcium, 250 mg, was administered because of the rapid transfusion, and mean pulmonary artery pressure increased acutely to 25 mmHg, without changes in left atrial pressure (see Figure 12.9). Cardiac output was 3.3 L/min and several repeated doses of calcium were then administered to treat the persistent hypotension; however, pulmonary artery pressures continued to increase in association with calcium administration, as shown in Figure 12.10. There were no changes in the heart rate or rhythm as the patient was atrioventricularly paced (Figure 12.11). The pulmonary artery pressure had increased to a mean of 35 mmHg, the cardiac output was still decreased, and ongoing hypotension required that the chest be reopened to exclude a mechanical cause for the hemodynamic instability. The right ventricle was noted to be dilated, and the patient developed acute frothing pulmonary edema with a left atrial pressure of 5 mmHg. The protein content of the tracheal fluid was 2.8%. The acute increase in capillary permeability was manifested by fulminant pulmonary edema and sudden hemoconcentration to a hematocrit of 55%, as illustrated in Table 12.2. Hemoconcentration and intra-

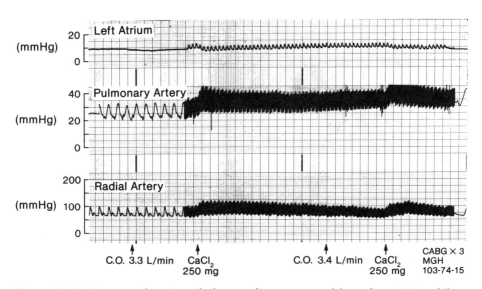

Figure 12.10 Because of persistently low cardiac output and hemodynamic instability after rapid infusion of 1 unit of whole blood, additional bolus doses of $CaCl_2$ were administered. Pulmonary artery pressures continued to increase and the patient developed acute frothing pulmonary edema.

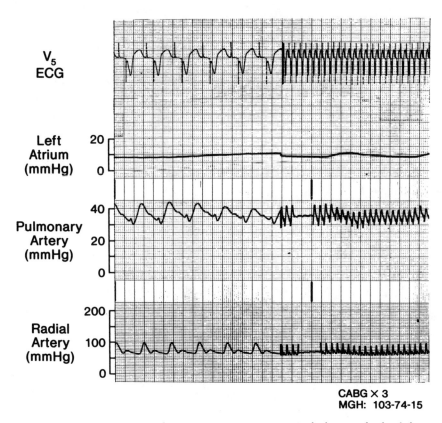

Figure 12.11 At 25 mm/sec the patient was atrioventricularly paced, the left atrial pressure was 7 mmHg, the mean pulmonary artery pressure was 35 mmHg, and the blood pressure was 100/60 mmHg.

vascular hypovolemia persisted despite the administration of 4 L of intravenous fluid, including both lactated Ringer's and 5% albumin, because of ongoing volume loss into the lung from increased capillary permeability. Methylprednisolone, 2 g; diphenhydramine, 50 mg; cimetidine, 300 mg; and various catecholamines, including isoproterenol, epinephrine, and norepinephrine, were in-

Table 12.2 Serial Hematocrits and Arterial Blood Gases During a Transfusion-Related Acute Lung Injury Reaction to Blood After Cardiopulmonary Bypass

Time	FIO_2	PaO_2	$PaCO_2$	pH	Hct
0	1.0	326	40	7.37	28
15 min	1.0	157	70	7.10	55
1.5 hr	1.0	290	62	7.23	56
3.0 hr	1.0	229	55	7.25	50

fused in an attempt to maintain hemodynamic stability. Oxygenation and ventilation were inadequate despite hand ventilation, as shown in Table 12.2. Persistent acidosis was treated with repeated doses of sodium bicarbonate. Because of the persistent systemic arterial hypotension, pulmonary hypertension, and right ventricular failure despite low left atrial pressures, norepinephrine and isoproterenol were given to increase perfusion pressure and dilate the pulmonary vasculature (Figure 12.12). Phentolamine, an α-adrenergic antagonist, was administered to decrease pulmonary artery pressures, but it decreased systemic arterial pressure as well (Figure 12.12). Despite infusions of isoproterenol, the right ventricle was still failing due to persistently elevated pulmonary artery pressures; therefore right atrial prostaglandin E_1 (PGE_1) was administered in combination with left atrial norepinephrine. As the PGE_1 infusion was increased, norepinephrine was also increased to maintain systemic perfusion pressure (Fig-

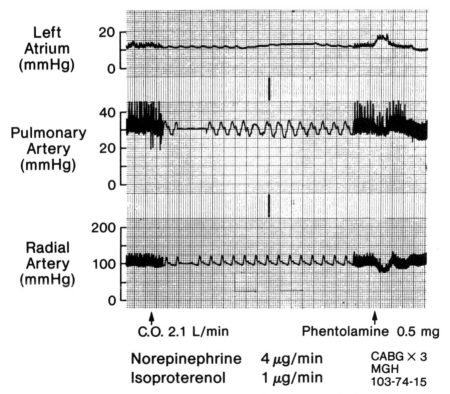

Figure 12.12 The patient had persistent low cardiac output with elevated pulmonary artery pressures and right ventricular failure due to pulmonary vasoconstriction. Norepinephrine was administered to increase perfusion pressure, and isoproterenol was infused to dilate the pulmonary artery. Phentolamine was subsequently given in an attempt to dilate the pulmonary artery; however, both systemic and pulmonary artery pressures decreased.

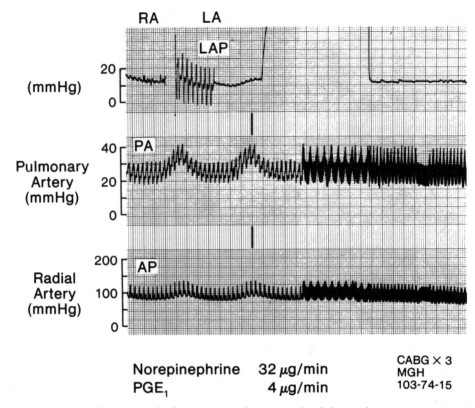

Figure 12.13 The patient had persistent right ventricular failure refractory to standard therapeutic interventions, therefore PGE_1 was infused into the right atrium to reverse the pulmonary vasoconstriction, and norepinephrine was infused into the left atrium to maintain systemic perfusion pressures. After approximately 2 hours of resuscitation, pulmonary artery pressures had decreased, right atrial and left atrial pressures had equalized, and right ventricular function had improved.

ure 12.13). The right ventricular function improved as pulmonary artery pressures decreased, and right and left atrial pressures equalized (Figure 12.13). After 5 hours of resuscitation in the operating room, the patient was taken to the intensive care unit, where the chest radiograph, when compared with the preoperative one (Figure 12.14), demonstrated bilateral pulmonary edema despite low left atrial pressures (Figure 12.15). Mechanical ventilation and positive end expiratory pressure (PEEP) were required for an additional 4 days until the interstitial edema resolved and the patient was weaned from the ventilator, as shown in Table 12.3.

This case illustrates the acute pulmonary vasoconstriction and right heart failure that can occur after transfusion reactions. Antibodies (IgG) in the donor blood, called leukoagglutinins, aggregate neutrophils to produce vascular injury,

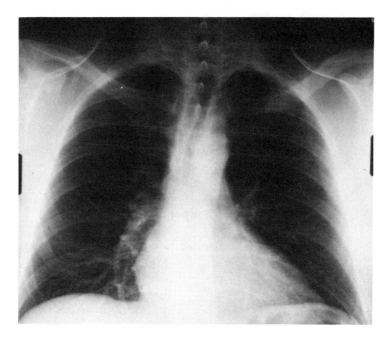

Figure 12.14 Preoperative chest radiograph in the patient before coronary artery bypass grafting.

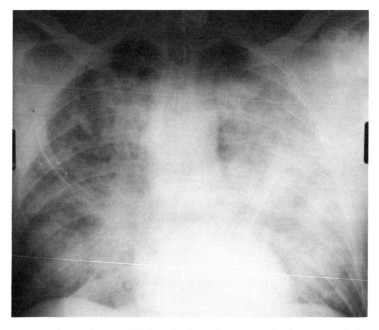

Figure 12.15 Radiograph on arrival to the intensive care unit after a transfusion-related acute lung injury. Note the bilateral pulmonary edema and changes from the preoperative film. The pulmonary artery catheter has been pulled back into the superior vena cava.

Table 12.3 Serial Arterial Blood Gases and Hematocrits in the Intensive Care Unit Following a Transfusion-Related Acute Lung Injury Reaction After Cardiac Surgery

Time (hr)	PIP	PEEP	IMV	FiO_2	PaO_2	$PaCO_2$	pH	Hct
5	50	5	9	1.0	84	61	7.21	49
6	53	5	15	1.0	73	38	7.33	49
8	50	10	12	1.0	81	34	7.29	50
9	50	12	12	1.0	126	33	7.27	50
10	52	15	12	1.0	153	29	7.33	43
12	52	15	12	1.0	209	32	7.35	45
14	46	15	12	0.8	108	30	7.45	42
15	46	15	12	0.7	163	30	7.45	43
20	42	15	12	0.7	146	35	7.43	41
24	40	10	12	0.7	115	35	7.47	40
30	36	10	8	0.6	151	37	7.48	40
36	38	10	8	0.5	112	38	7.48	39
48	38	10	7	0.4	124	38	7.47	35
60	34	10	7	0.4	117	43	7.46	37
72	38	10	8/12	0.4	127	42	7.48	33
84	36	10	8/14	0.4	153	37	7.52	32
96	–	5	CPAP	0.4	107	47	7.45	34
108	–	–	extub	1.0	142	46	7.46	34

PIP = peak inspiratory pressure (cm H_2O); PEEP = positive end expiratory pressure (cm H_2O); IMV = intermittent mandatory ventilation (breaths/min); Hct = hematocrit; CPAP = continuous positive airway pressure; extub = extubated.

thromboxane A_2-mediated pulmonary vasoconstriction, and transfusion-related acute lung injury characterized by pulmonary edema despite low left ventricular filling pressures (noncardiogenic). The patient was refractory to standard pharmacologic therapy, so PGE_1 was infused into the right atrium. Norepinephrine was administered into the left atrium to avoid first-pass effects on the pulmonary vasculature, and to support perfusion pressure. The technique of left-sided norepinephrine infusion can be used only when a left atrial catheter is present. This reaction occurred in 1982, but now a cyclic adenosine monophosphate specific phosphodiesterase inhibitor like amrinone, milrinone, or enoximone could be administered in combination with a catecholamine with β_2-adrenergic activity to treat the pulmonary vasoconstriction (see Chapters 9 and 10). PGE_1 has potent antiinflammatory effects and may be an ideal agent for treating pulmonary hypertension and right ventricular failure after transfusion-related acute lung injury refractory to other therapeutic interventions. Also notable is the persistent respiratory failure requiring mechanical ventilation and PEEP. As the alterations in capillary permeability resolved, peak inspiratory pressures decreased, PEEP was weaned, oxygenation improved, and the hematocrit decreased. Measuring the hematocrit for resolution of the hemoconcentration is another way of monitoring the patient for the degree of increased capillary permeability.

The patient also developed acute increases in pulmonary artery pressure after intravenous calcium administration. Calcium is essential to inflammatory cell activation and mediator synthesis. The use of calcium entry blockers decreases mediator release and removal of calcium prevents mast cell activation (see Chapter 9). Tanz and coworkers demonstrated exacerbations of cardiovascular dysfunction when calcium was given in experimental anaphylaxis (Tanz et al., 1985). This explains the increased pulmonary vasoconstriction seen with bolus calcium administration, which suggests that calcium should not be administered when treating anaphylaxis or other episodes of thromboxane-mediated pulmonary vasoconstriction.

SUMMARY

Preventing Anaphylactic Reactions

It would be ideal if physicians could prevent anaphylactic or anaphylactoid reactions. Certain patients may be at an increased risk and certain procedures or agents are more often implicated in producing reactions than others. Patients with a history of allergy, atopy, or asthma have been suggested to be at an increased risk. In addition, blood products, antibiotics, and chymopapain may be associated with an inordinately high incidence of reactions. Identifying high-risk patients and the development of specific tests aids in preventing anaphylactic or anaphylactoid reactions. Suggestions for specific prevention of these reactions include the following approaches (Sheffer, 1984).

1. Careful medical histories including drug or latex allergy should always be obtained preoperatively before drug or blood product administration. Patients at high risk for latex allergy (i.e., spina bifida) should be carefully questioned for adverse reactions to latex or previous intraoperative cardiovascular collapse. In patients with a known history of latex allergy, latex should be strictly avoided. Latex is ubiquitous in the operating room environment and materials to which the patient will be exposed must be carefully checked for their latex content.
2. Blood and blood product administration should be carefully considered before transfusions. Blood products pose the risk of infectious disease transmission as well as allergic reactions. If blood is to be administered for anemia, then packed red blood cells should be administered instead of whole blood. After the transfusion of 19,126 units of whole blood and 42,648 units of red blood cells, Milner reported the reaction rate to whole blood was substantially greater than that to packed red blood cells (Table 1) (Milner and Butcher, 1978).
3. Drugs known to release histamine (e.g., morphine, meperidine, d-tubocurarine, metocurine, atracurium, mivacurium, vancomycin) should be injected slowly as dilute solutions, or avoided when possible in patients with preexisting cardiopulmonary dysfunction.
4. Evaluate patients preoperatively for chymopapain allergy either by skin testing or enzyme-linked immunosorbent assay testing (Chymo-Fast). Patients with positive skin tests or Chymodiactin immunoglobu-

Table 1 Reported Transfusion Reactions to Packed Red Blood Cells (PRBC) and Whole Blood (WB)

	42,678 Units PRBC Transfused		19,126 Units WB Transfused	
Reaction	No.	Percent	No.	Percent
Allergic	34	0.0796	57	0.298
WBC antibodies	12	0.0023	14	0.073

Data from Milner LV, Butcher K. Transfusion reactions reported after transfusion of red blood cells and of whole blood. Transfusion 1978;18:493–5.

lin-E concentrations of 0.06 IU/mL should not undergo chymopapain injections.
5. Always administer intraoperative antibiotics slowly after dilutions into 100, 150, or 250 mL bags. Vital signs should be carefully noted after the initial drug administration.
6. Patients with a prior history of anaphylactic reaction to an anesthetic drug or during surgery should be evaluated when 1) multiple anesthetic drugs have been administered, 2) the agent in question is unclear, 3) a muscle relaxant or latex is implicated, and 4) the patient is to undergo repeated anesthesia in the future. Patients with known reactions to anesthetic drugs should be given a letter or bracelet with their medical history.
7. Consider pretreating patients at risk for potential anaphylactic reactions (i.e., latex allergy). Although pretreatment for anaphylaxis does not prevent reactions, drugs such as H_1 and H_2 receptor antagonists, corticosteroids, and ephedrine may attentuate the physiologic responses. Antihistamines may initially modify hypotensive responses during anaphylaxis. Therefore, blood pressure should be carefully monitored whenever antihistamines have been administered as pretreatment. One must not be lulled into a false sense of security after pretreatment for potential anaphylactic reactions.
8. Physicians must be alert to the early signs and symptoms of anaphylaxis. Patients should be carefully observed for 15 to 30 minutes after parenteral injections. Resuscitation equipment should always be available whenever parenteral drugs are administered. Anaphylaxis is an acute, potentially fatal reaction. However, with anticipation, prompt recognition, and appropriate therapy, a disastrous outcome can be avoided.

References

Abada RP, Owens WD. Hereditary angioneurotic edema, an anesthetic dilemma. Anesthesiology 1977; 46:428–30.
Abraham GN, Petz LD, Fudenberg HH. Cephalothin hypersensitivity associated with anti-cephalothin antibodies. Int Arch Allergy 1968; 34:65–74.
Abraham GN, Petz LD, Fudenberg HH. Immunohaematological cross-allergenicity between penicillin and cephalothin in humans. Clin Exp Immunol 1968; 3:343–57.
Adkinson NF, Newball HH, Findlay S, Adams K, Lichtenstein LM. Anaphylactic release of prostaglandins from human lungs in vitro. Am Rev Respir Dis 1980; 121:911–20.
Adkinson NF Jr, Wheeler B. Risk factors for IgE-dependent reactions to penicillin. In: Kerr JW, Ganderton MA, eds. XI International Congress of Allergology and Clinical Immunology. London, MacMillan Press, 1983; 55–9.
Adkinson NF Jr, Swabb EA, Sugerman AA. Immunology of the monobactam aztreonam. Antimicrob Agents and Chemother 1984; 25:93–7.
Adkinson NF. Risk factors for drug allergy. J Allergy Clin Immunol 1984; 74:567–72.
Adkinson NF. Tests for immunological drug reactions. In: Rose NR, Friedman H, Fahey JL, eds. Manual of Clinical Laboratory Immunology, 3rd ed. Baltimore, American Society for Microbiology 1986; 692–7.
Agre K, McDermott DJ, Wilson RR. Anaphylaxis from chymopapain. JAMA 1984; 251, 1953.
Aguilera L, Martinez-Bourio R, Cid C, Arino JJ, Saez de Eguilaz JL, Arizaga A. Anaphylactic reaction after atropine. Anaesthesia 1988; 43:955–7.
Albin MS, Carroll RG, Maroon JC. Clinical considerations concerning detection of venous air embolism. Neurosurgery 1978; 3:380–91.
Aldrete JA, Johnson DA. Allergy to local anesthetics. JAMA 1969; 207:356–7.
Alexopoulos D, Raine AEG, Cobbe SM. Serum sickness complicating intravenous streptokinase therapy in acute myocardial infarction. Eur Heart J 1984; 5:1010–2.
Alexsson JG, Johansson SG, Wrangsjö K. IgE-mediated anaphylactoid reactions to rubber. Allergy 1987; 42:46–50.
Alving BM. Hypotension associated with prekallikrein activator (Hageman-factor fragments) in plasma protein fraction. N Engl J Med 1978; 299:66–8.
AMA Department of Drugs. Drugs used to treat shock. In AMA Drug Evaluations. Chicago, American Medical Association, 1980: 552.
American Thoracic Society, Medical Section of American Lung Association. Standards for the diagnosis and care of patients with chronic obstructive pulmonary disease (COPD) and asthma. New York, American Lung Association, 1987.
Ammann AJ, Hong R. Selective IgA deficiency: presentation of 30 cases and a review of the literature. Medicine 1971; 50:223–36.

Andrews AT, Zmijewski CM, Bowman HS, Rehart JK. Transfusion reaction with pulmonary infiltration associated with HL-A-specific leukocyte antibodies. Am J Clin Pathol 1976; 66:483–7.

Ansell G, Tweedie MCK, West CR, Evans P, Cough L. The current status of reactions to intravascular contrast media. Invest Radiol 1980; 15:532–9.

Antohe F, Heltianu C, Simionescu N. Further evidence for the distribution and nature of histamine receptors on microvascular endothelium. Microcirc Endothelium Lymphatics 1986; 3:163–85.

Anuras J, Cheng FHF, Richerson HB. Experimental leukocyte-induced pulmonary vasculitis with inquiry into mechanism. Chest 1977; 71:383–7.

Armstrong B, Dinan B, Jick H. Fatal drug reactions in patients admitted to surgical services. Am J Surg 1976; 132:643.

Assem ESK, Ling YB. Fatal anaphylactic reaction to suxamethonium: new screening test suggests possible prevention. Anaesthesia 1988; 43:958–61.

Assem ESK. Anaphylactic reactions affecting the human heart. Agents Actions 1989; 27:142–5.

Atkins PC, Wasserman SI. Chemotactic mediators. Clin Rev Allergy 1983; 1:385–95.

Atkinson JP, Frank MM. Role of complement in the pathophysiology of hematologic disease. Prog Hematol 1977; 10:211–45.

Austen KF. Tissue mast cells in immediate hypersensitivity. Hosp Pract 1972; 17:98–108.

Austen KF. Systemic anaphylaxis in the human being. N Engl J Med 1974; 291:661–4.

Austen KF. Diseases of the immediate hypersensitivity type. In: Peterdorf RG, Adams RD, Braunwald E, eds. Harrison's Principles of Internal Medicine. New York, McGraw-Hill, 1983:374.

Baenziger NL, Force LE, Becherer PR. Histamine stimulates prostacyclin synthesis in cultured human umbilical vein endothelial cells. Biochem Biophys Res Commun 1980; 92:1435–40.

Baenziger NL, Fogerty FJ, Mertz LF, Chernuta LF. Regulation of histamine-mediated prostacyclin synthesis in cultured human vascular endothelial cells. Cell 1981; 24:915–23.

Baldo BA, Fisher MM. Detection of serum IgE antibodies that react with alcuronium and tubocurarine after life threatening reactions to muscle-relaxant drugs. Anaesth Intensive Care 1983a; 11:194–7.

Baldo BA, Fisher MM. Anaphylaxis to muscle relaxant drugs: cross-reactivity and molecular basis of binding of IgE antibodies detected by radioimmunoassay. Mol Immunol 1983b; 20:1393–1400.

Baldo BA, Fisher MM. Substituted ammonium ions as allergenic determinants in drug allergy (letter). Nature 1983c; 306:262–4.

Baldo BA, Harle DG, Fisher MM. In vitro diagnosis and studies on the mechanism(s) of anaphylactoid reactions to muscle relaxant drugs. Ann Fr Anesth Réanim 1985; 4:139–45.

Barach EM, Nowak RM, Lee TG, Tomlanovich MC. Epinephrine for treatment of anaphylactic shock. JAMA 1984; 251:2118–22.

Barandun S, Kistler P, Jeunet F, Isliker H. Intravenous administration of human γ-globulin. Vox Sang 1962; 7:157–74.

Barbar JM, Budassi SA. Mosby's Manual of Emergency Care: Practices and Procedures. St. Louis, CV Mosby, 1975: 352–4.

Barcroft H, Star I. Comparison of the actions of adrenaline and noradrenaline on the cardiac output in man. Clin Sci 1951; 10:295–303.

Barnard JH. Studies of 400 Hymenoptera sting deaths in the United States. J Allergy Clin Immunol 1973; 52:259–63.

Barnes PJ. New concepts in the pathogenesis of bronchial hyperresponsiveness and asthma. J Allergy Clin Immunol 1989a; 83:1013–26.

Barnes PJ. A new approach to the treatment of asthma. N Engl J Med 1989b; 321:1517–27.

Barnes PK, de Renzy-Martin N, Thomas VJE, Watkins J. Plasma histamine levels following atracurium. Anaesthesia 1986; 41:821–4.
Barton JC. Nonhemolytic, noninfectious transfusion reactions. Semin Hematol 1981; 18:95–121.
Bashir H. Adverse reactions due to leucocyte and platelet antibodies. Anaesth Intens Care 1980; 8:132–8.
Basta SJ, Savarese JJ, Ali HH, Moss J, Gionfriddo M. Histamine-releasing potencies of atracurium, dimethyl tubocurarine and tubocurarine. Br J Anaesth 1983; 55:105S–6S.
Beamish D, Brown DT. Adverse responses to I.V. anesthetics. Br J Anaesth 1981; 53:55–8.
Beaupre PN, Roizen MF, Cahalan MK, Alpert RA, Cassorla L, Schiller NB. Hemodynamic and two-dimensional transesophageal echocardiographic analysis of an anaphylactic reaction in man. Anesthesiology 1984; 60:482–4.
Beaven MA. Histamine. N Engl J Med 1976; 294:30–6; 320–5.
Beaven MA, Robinson-White A, Roderick NB, Kauffman GL. The demonstration of histamine release in clinical conditions: a review of past and present assay procedures. Klin Wochenschr 1982; 60:873–81.
Bedard RM, Busse WW. Nifedipine inhibition of human basophil histamine release. J Allergy Clin Immunol 1983; 71:104.
Beemer GH, Dennis WL, Platt PR, Bjorksten AR, Carr AB. Adverse reactions to atracurium and alcuronium; a prospective surveillance study. Br J Anaesth 1988; 61:680–4.
Beladinelli L, Linden J, Berne RM. The cardiac effects of adenosine. Prog Cardiovasc Dis 1989; 32:73–97.
Bennet MJ, Anderson LK, McMillan JC, Ebertz JM, Hirshman CA. Anaphylactic reaction during anesthesia associated with positive intradermal skin test to fentanyl. Can Anaesth Soc J 1986; 33:75–8.
Berg TLO, Johansson SGO. Allergy diagnosis with the radioallergosorbent test: a comparison with the results of skin and provocation tests in an unselected group of children with asthma and hay fever. J Allergy Clin Immunol 1974; 54:209–21.
Best N, Sinosich MJ, Teisner B, Grudzinskas JG, Fisher M McD. Complement activation during cardiopulmonary bypass by heparin-protamine interaction. Br J Anaesth 1984; 56:339–43.
Best N, Teisner B, Grudzinskas JG, Fisher MM. Classical pathway activation during an adverse response to protamine sulphate. Br J Anaesth 1983; 55:1149–53.
Bevan JA, Brayden JE. Nonadrenergic neural vasodilator mechanisms. Circ Res 1987; 60:309–26.
Bickerman HA. Antiallergic drugs. In: Model LW, ed. Drugs of Choice 1982–1983. St. Louis, CV Mosby, 1982; 573.
Bidstrup BP, Royston D, Sapsfort RN, Taylor KM. Reduction in blood loss and blood use after cardiopulmonary bypass with high dose aprotinin (Trasylol). J Thorac Cardiovasc Surg 1989; 97:364–72.
Bienenstock J, Tomioka M, Matsuda H, et al. The role of mast cells in inflammatory processes: evidence for nerve/mast cell interactions. Int Arch Allergy Appl Immunol 1987; 82:238–43.
Björk J, Smedegard G. The microvasculature of the hamster cheek pouch as a model for studying acute immune-complex induced inflammatory reactions. Int Arch Allergy Appl Immun 1984; 74:178–85.
Blanca M, Fernandez J, Miranda A, et al. Cross-reactivity between penicillins and cephalosporins: clinical and immunologic studies. J Allergy Clin Immunol 1989; 83:381–5.
Bland JHL, Laver BM, Lowenstein E. Vasodilator effect of commercial 5% plasma protein fractin solutions. JAMA 1973; 224:1721–4.
Bochner BS, Lichtenstein LM. Anaphylaxis. N Engl J Med 1991; 324:1785–90.
Boe J. Hypoxic and embolic pulmonary vasoconstriction. Gen Pharmacol 1983; 14:149–51.

Boileau S, Hummer-Sigiel M, Moeller R, Drouet N. Reevaluation des risques respectifs d'anaphylaxie et d'histaminoliberation avec les substances anesthesiologiques. Ann Fr Anesth Reanim 1985; 4:195–204.

Booij LHD, Krieg N, Crul JF. Intradermal histamine releasing effect caused by Org-NC 45: a comparison with pancuronium, metocurine and d-tubocurarine. Acta Anaesth Scand 1980; 24:393–4.

Booth BH, Patterson R. Electrocardiographic changes during human anaphylaxis. JAMA 1970; 211:627–31.

Borchard U, Hafner D, Hirth C. Electrophysiological actions of histamine and H_1-, H_2-receptor antagonists in cardiac tissue. Agents Actions 1986; 18:186–90.

Borda T, Slone D, Jick H. Assessment of adverse drug reactions within drug surveillance program. JAMA 1986; 205:645.

Borgeat P, Laclos BF, Maclove J. New concepts in the modulation of leukotriene synthesis. Br J Pharmacol 1983; 32:381–7.

Bork K, Witzke G. Long-term prophylaxis with C1-inhibitor (C1 INH) concentrate in patients with recurrent angioedema caused by hereditary and acquired C1-inhibitor deficiency. J Allergy Clin Immunol 1989; 83:677–82.

Bouma BN, Miles LA, Beretta G, Griffin JH. Human plasma prekallikrein: studies of its activation by activated Factor XII and of its inactivation by diisopropylphosphofluoridate. Biochemistry 1980; 19:1151–60.

Bouma BN, Griffin JH. Human blood coagulation factor XI: purification properties and mechanisms of activation by activated Factor XII. J Biol Chem 1977; 252:6432–40.

Bove J. Delayed complications of transfusion. Conn Med 1968; 32:36–9.

Boyce MJ. Pharmacological characterization of cardiovascular histamine receptors in man in vivo. Klin Wochenschr 1982; 60:978–82.

Branch DR, Houghton MT. Allergic reaction to transfused cephalothin antibody. JAMA 1979; 241:495–6.

Brasch RC. Allergic reactions to contrast media: accumulated evidence. Am J Roentgenol 1980a; 134:797–801.

Brasch RC. Evidence supporting an antibody mediation of contrast media reactions. Invest Radiol 1980b; 15:S29–31.

Briggs LP, Clarke RSJ, Watkins J. An adverse reaction to the administration of disoprofol (Diprivan). Anesthesia 1982; 37:1099–101.

Brittingham TE, Chaplin H. Febrile transfusion reactions caused by sensitivity to donor leukocytes and platelets. JAMA 1957; 161:819–25.

Bristow MR, Ginsburg R, Harrison DC. Histamine and the human heart: the other receptor system (editorial). Am J Cardiol 1982; 49:249–51.

Brocklehurt WE, Lahiri SC. The production of bradykinin in anaphylaxis. J Physiol (Lond) 1952; 160:15P–16P.

Brown DT, Beamish D, Wildsmith JAW. Allergic reaction to an amide local anaesthetic. Br J Anaesth 1981; 53:435–7.

Bruno LA, Smith DS, Bloom MJ. Sudden hypotension with a test dose of chymopapain. Anesth Analg 1984; 63:533–5.

Burke JA, Levi R, Guo ZG, Corey EJ. Leukotrienes C_4, D_4, and E_4: effects on human and guinea-pig cardiac preparations in vitro. J Pharmacol Exp Ther 1982; 211:235–42.

Burks AW, Sampson HA, Buckley RH. Anaphylactic reactions after gamma globulin administration in patients with hypogammaglobulinemia. Detection of IgE antibodies to IgA. N Engl J Med 1986; 314:560–4.

Burman D, Hodson AK, Wood CBS, Brueton NFW. Acute anaphylaxis, pulmonary oedema, and intravascular haemolysis due to crypoprecipitate. Arch Dis Child 1973; 48:483–5.

Busse WW, Reed CE. Asthma: definition and pathogenesis. In: Middleton E, et al., eds. Allergy Principles and Practice, 3rd ed. St. Louis, CV Mosby, 1988; 969–98.

Busse WW. The role of inflammation in asthma: a new focus. J Resp Dis 1989; 10:72–80.
Butchers PR, Skidmore IF, Vardey CJ, Wheeldon A: Characterization of the receptor mediating the antianaphylactic effects of beta-adrenoceptor agonists in human lung tissue in vitro. Br J Pharmacol 1980; 71:663–7.
Butler VP Jr, Beiser SM. Antibodies to small molecules: biologic and clinical applications. Adv Immunol 1973; 17:255–310.
Byrne JP, Dixon JA. Pulmonary edema following blood transfusion reaction. Arch Surg 1971; 102:91–4.
Callahan M, Barton CW, Kayser S. Potential complications of high-dose epinephrine therapy in patients. JAMA 1991; 265:1117–22.
Campbell FW, Tabak C. Management of the patient with a history of protamine hypersensitivity for cardiac surgery. Anesthesiology 1984; 61:761–4.
Caplan RA, Su JY. Differences in threshold for protamine toxicity in isolated atrial and ventricular tissue. Anesth Analg 1984; 63:1111–5.
Caplan RA, Ward RJ, Posner K, Cheney FW. Unexpected cardiac arrest during spinal anesthesia: a closed claims analysis of predisposing factors. Anesthesiology 1988; 68:5–11.
Caplan SN, Berkman EM. Protamine sulfate and fish allergy. N Engl J Med 1976; 295:172.
Caranasos GJ. Drug reactions. In: Schwartz GR, Safar P, Stone JH, eds. The Principles and Practice of Emergency Medicine. Philadelphia, WB Saunders, 1978: 1310.
Carilli AD, Ramanamurty MV, Chang YS, Shin D, Sethi V. Noncardiogenic pulmonary edema following blood transfusion. Chest 1978; 74:310–12.
Carlson RW, Schaeffer RC Jr, Puri VK, Brennan AP, Weil MH. Hypovolemia and permeability pulmonary edema associated with anaphylaxis. Crit Care Med 1981; 9:883–5.
Carstairs JR, Nimmo AJ, Barnes PJ. Autoradiographic visualization of beta-adrenoceptor subtypes in human lung. Am Rev Resp Dis 1985; 132:541–7.
Carrington DM, Earl HS, Sullivan TJ. Studies of human IgE to a sulfonamide determinant. J Allergy Clin Immunol 1987; 79:442–7.
Casale TB, Bowman S, Kaliner M. Induction of human cutaneous mast cell degranulation by opiates and endogenous opioid peptides: evidence for opiate and nonopiate receptor participation. J Allergy Clin Immunol 1984; 73:775–81.
Casey L, Clarke J, Fletcher J, Ramwell P. Cardiovascular, respiratory, and hematologic effects of leukotriene D_4 in primates. In: Samuelsson B, Paoletti R, eds. Leukotrienes and Other Lipoxygenase Products. New York, Raven, 1982; 201–10.
Cassidy JT, Burt A, Petty R. Selective IgA deficiency in connective tissue disease. N Engl J Med 1969; 80:275.
Castaneda AB. Must heparin be neutralized following open-heart operations? J Thorac Cardiovasc Surg 1966; 52:716–24.
Caulfield JP, El-Lati S, Thomas G, Church MK. Dissociated human foreskin mast cells degranulate in response to anti-IgE and substance P. Lab Invest 1990; 63:502–10.
Cavarocchi NG, Schaff HV, Orszulak TA, Homburger HA, Schnell WA, Pluth JR. Evidence for complement activation by protamine–heparin interaction after cardiopulmonary bypass. Surgery 1985; 98:525.
Chand N, Perhach JL, Diamantis W, Sofia RD. Heterogeneity of calcium channels in mast cells and basophils and the possible relevance to pathophysiology of lung diseases: a review. Agents Actions 1985; 17:407–17.
Chapuis B, Helg C, Jeannet M, Zulian G, Huber P, Gumovski P. Anaphylactic reaction to intravenous cyclosporin. N Engl J Med 1985; 312:1259.
Chatton MJ. Anaphylactic reactions. In: Krupp MA, Chatton MJ, eds. Current Medical Diagnosis and Treatment. Los Altos, Lange Medical Publications, 1983:15.
Chenoweth DE, Cooper SW, Hugli TE, Stewart RW, Blackstone EH, Kirklin JW. Com-

plement activation during cardiopulmonary bypass. N Engl J Med 1981; 304:497–503.
Chiu RCJ, Samson R. Complement (C3,C4) consumption in cardiopulmonary bypass, cardioplegia, and protamine administration. Ann Thorac Surg 1984; 37:339–42.
Chung F, Miles J. Cardiac arrest following protamine administration. Can Anaesth Soc J 1984; 31:314–8.
Church MK, Lowman MA, Robinson C, Holgate ST, Benyon RC. Interaction of neuropeptides with human mast cells. Int Arch Allergy Appl Immunol 1989a; 88:70–8.
Church MK, Lowman MA, Reese PH, Benyon RC. Mast cells, neuropeptides and inflammation. Agents Actions 1989b; 27:8–16.
Clarke RSJ. Adverse effects of intravenously administered drugs used in anaesthetic practice. Drugs 1981; 22:26–41.
Clarke RSJ. Epidemiology of adverse reactions in anaesthesia in the United Kingdom. Klin Wochenschr 1982; 60:1003–5.
Clarke RSJ, Dundee JW, Garrett RT, McArdle GK, Suddon JA. Adverse reactions to intravenous anaesthetics: a survey of 100 reports. Br J Anaesth 1975; 47:575–85.
Cobb CA, Fung DL. Shock due to protamine hypersensitivity. Surg Neurol 1982; 17:245–6.
Cochrane CG, Revak SD, Aikin BS, Wuepper KD. The structural characteristics and activation of Hageman factor. In: Lepow IH, Ward PA, eds. Inflammation: Mechanisms and Control. New York, Academic Press, 1972:119–31.
Cochrane CG, Revak SD, Wuepper KD. Activation of Hageman factor in solid and fluid phases; a critical role of kallikrein. J Exp Med 1973; 138:1564–83.
Cochrane CG, Griffin JH. The biochemistry and pathophysiology of the contact system of plasma. Adv Immunol 1982; 33:241–306.
Cogen FC, Norman ME, Dunsky E, Hirschfeld J, Zweiman B. Histamine release and complement changes following injection of contrast media in humans. J Allergy Clin Immunol 1979; 64:299–303.
Cohen C, Smith T. The intraoperative hazard of acrylic bone cement. Anesthesiology 1971; 35:547–9.
Cohen LS, Wechsler AS, Mitchell JH, Glick G. Depression of cardiac function by streptomycin and other antimicrobial agents. Am J Cardiol 1970; 26:505–11.
Collett B, Alhag A, Abdullah NB. Pathways to complement activation during cardiopulmonary bypass. Br Med J 1984; 289:1251–8.
Colman RW. Activation of plasminogen by human plasma kallikrein. Biochem Biophys Res Commun 1969; 35:273–9.
Colman RW. Surface-mediated defense reactions: the plasma contact activation system. J Clin Invest 1984; 73:1249–53.
Colman RW, Schmaier AH. The contact activation system: biochemistry and interactions of these surface-mediated defense reactions. CRC Crit Rev Oncol Hematol 1986; 5:57–85.
Conahan TJ, Andrews RW, NacVaygh H. Cardiovascular effects of protamine sulfate in man. Anesth Analg 1981; 60:33–6.
Conroy MC, Adkinson NF, Lichtenstein LM. Measurement of IgE on human basophils: relation to serum IgE and anti-IgE-induced histamine release. J Immunol 1977a; 118:1317–21.
Conroy MC, Adkinson NF, Sobotka AK, Lichenstein LM. Releasibility of histamine from human basophils. Fed Proc 1977b; 36:1216.
Conzen PF, Habazettl H, Guttmann R, et al. Thromboxane mediation of pulmonary hemodynamic responses after neutralization of heparin by protamine in pigs. Anesth Analg 1989; 68:25–31.
Cook FV, Farrar WE. Vancomycin revisited. Ann Intern Med 1978; 88:813–8.
Council on Scientific Affairs. In vitro testing for allergy: report II of the Allergy Panel. JAMA 1987; 258:1639.

Cox JV, Steane E, Cunningham G, Frenkel EP. Risk of alloimmunization and delayed hemolytic transfusion reactions in patients with sickle cell disease. Arch Intern Med 1988; 148:2485–9.

Coyle JP, Carlin HM, Lake CR, Lee CK, Chernow B. Left atrial infusion of norepinephrine in the management of right ventricular failure. J Cardiothorac Anesth 1990; 4:80–3.

Craddock PR, Fehr J, Brigham KL, Kronenberg RS, Jacob HS. Complement and leukocyte-mediated pulmonary dysfunction in hemodialysis. N Engl J Med 1977; 296:769–74.

Criep LH. Guarding against, guides to anaphylaxis, and emergency treatment. Mod Med 1980; 48:54–63.

Culliford AT, Thomas S, Spencer FC. Fulminating noncardiogenic pulmonary edema: a newly recognized hazard during cardiac operations. J Thorac Cardiovasc Surg 1980; 80:868–75.

Curling PE, Duke PG, Levy JH, Finlayson DC. Management of the postoperative cardiac patient. In: Hurst J, ed. Clinical Essays on the Heart, Vol. III. New York, McGraw-Hill, 1984: 257–86.

D'Ambra MN, LaRaia PJ, Philbin DM, Watkins WD, Hilgenberg AD, Buckley MJ. Prostaglandin E_1: a new therapy for refractory right heart failure and pulmonary hypertension after mitral valve replacement. J Thorac Cardiovasc Surg 1985; 89:567–72.

Dahlén SE, Bjök J, Hedqvist P, et al. Leukotrienes promote plasma leakage and leukocyte adhesion in postcapillary venules: in vivo effects of relevance to acute inflammatory response. Proc Natl Acad Sci 1981; 78:3887–91.

Dajee H, Laks H, Miller J, Oren R. Profound hypotension from rapid vancomycin administration during cardiac operation. J Thorac Cardiovasc Surg 1984; 87:145–6.

Degges RD, Foster ME, Dang AQ, Read RC. Pulmonary hypertensive effect of heparin and protamine interaction: evidence for thromboxane B2 release from the lung. Am J Surg 1987; 154:696–9.

Delage C, Irey NS. Anaphylactic deaths: a clinicopathologic study of 43 cases. J Forensic Sci 1972; 17:525–40.

Delage C, Mullick FG, Irey NS. Myocardial lesions in anaphylaxis. Arch Pathol 1973; 95:185–9.

Descotes J, Laschi A, Tachon P, Evreux JC. Propriétés anti-anaphylactiques du verapamil. J Pharmacol (Paris) 1982; 13:573–8.

deShazo RD, Nelson HS. An approach to the patient with a history of local anesthetic hypersensitivity: experience with 90 patients. J Allergy Clin Immunol 1989; 63:387–94.

DeSwarte RD. Drug allergy: an overview. Clin Rev Allergy 1986; 5:143–69.

DeSwarte RD. Drug allergy. In: Patterson R, ed. Allergic Diseases: Diagnosis and Management, 3rd ed. Philadelphia, JB Lippincott, 1989; 505–661.

Didier A, Cador D, Bongrand P, et al. Role of the quaternary ammonium ion determinants in allergy to muscle relaxants. J Allergy Clin Immunol 1987a; 79:578–84.

Didier A, Benzarti M, Senft M, et al. Allergy to suxamethonium: persisting abnormalities in skin tests, specific IgE antibodies and leukocyte histamine release. Clin Allergy 1987b; 17:385–92.

Dietrich W, Hahnel C, Richter JA. Routine application of high-dose aprotinin in open heart surgery: a study on 1,784 patients. Anesthesiology, 1990; 73:A146.

Doenicke A, Lorenz W. Histamine release in anaesthesia and surgery. Premedication with H_1- and H_2-receptor antagonists: indications, benefits and possible problems. Klin Wochenschr 1982; 60:1039–45.

Doolan L, McKenzie I, Krafchek J, Barsons B, Buxton B. Protamine sulfate hypersensitivity. Anaesth Intens Care 1981; 9:147.

Dorn R, Page G, Giroud M. Choc anaphylactique apres injection locale de Zymofren. Lyon Medical 1976; 236:177.

Dubois M, Lotze MT, Diamond WJ, Kim YD, Flye MW, Macnamara TE. Pulmonary shunting during leukoagglutinin-induced noncardiac pulmonary edema. JAMA 1980; 244:2186–9.

Dueck R, O'Connor RD. Thiopental: false positive RAST in patient with elevated serum IgE. Anethesiology 1984; 61:337–8.

Dundee JW, Fee JPH, McDonald JR, Clarke RSJ. Frequency of atopy and allergy in an anaesthetic patient population. Br J Anaesth 1978; 50:793–8.

Dutcher JP, Aisner J, Hogge DE, Schiffer CA. Donor reaction to hydroxyethyl starch during granulocytapheresis. Transfusion 1984; 24:66–7.

Dvorak AM. Mast cell degranulation in human hearts. N Engl J Med 1986; 315:969–70.

Dye D, Watkins J. Suspected anaphylactic reaction to Cremophor EL. Br Med J 1980; 280:1353.

Dykewicz MS, McGrath KG, Davison R, Kaplan KJ, Patterson R. Identification of patients at risk for anaphylaxis due to streptokinase. Arch Int Med 1986; 146:305–7.

Ebertz JM, Hermens JM, McMillan JC, Uno H, Hirshman C, Hanifin JM. Functional differences between human cutaneous mast cells and basophils: a comparison of morphine-induced histamine release. Agents Actions 1986; 18:455–62.

Eggleston PA. Anaphylaxis and serum sickness. In: Conn HF, ed. Current Therapy. Philadelphia, WB Saunders, 1983; 573.

Eggleston PA, Kagey-Sobotka A, Schleimer RP, Lichtenstein LM. Interaction between hyperosmolar and IgE-mediated histamine release from basophils and mast cells. Am Rev Respir Dis 1984; 130:86–91.

Eisen HN. Hypersensitivity to simple chemicals. In: Lawrence HS, ed. Cellular and Humoral Aspects of the Hypersensitive States. New York, PB Hoeber, 1959; 111–26.

Eisenberg MS, Copass MK. Emergency Medical Therapy. Philadelphia, WB Saunders, 1982; 563.

Ellison N, Behar M, MacVaugh H, Marshall BE. Bradykinin, plasma protein fraction, and hypotension. Ann Thorac Surg 1978; 29:15–9.

Erdos EG. Kinases in bradykinin, kallidin and kallikrein. In: Erdos, EG, ed. Handbook of Experimental Pharmacology, Vol 25(S). Heidelberg, Springer-Verlag, 1979.

Etter MS, Helrich M, Mackenzie CF. Immunoglobulin E fluctuation in thiopental anaphylaxis. Anesthesiology 1980; 52:181–3.

Ettlin R, Hougne R, Bruppacher R, Muller V, Stocker F. Atopy and adverse drug reactions. Int Arch Allergy 1981; 66:93–5.

Eyre P, Lewis AJ. Production of kinins in bovine anaphylactic shock. Br J Pharmacol 1972; 44:311–3.

Ezra D, Boyd LM, Feuerstein G, Goldstein RE. Coronary constriction by leukotriene C_4, D_4, and E_4 in the intact pig heart. Am J Cardiol 1983; 51:1451–4.

Fabian I, Aronson M. Polycations as possible substitutes for protamine in heparin neutralization. Thrombosis Res 1980; 37:237–9.

Fadali MA, Papacostas CA, Duke JJ, Ledbetter M, Osbakken M. Cardiovascular depressant effect of protamine sulphate: experimental study and clinical implications. Thorax 1976; 31:320–3.

Fahmy NR, Sunder N, Soter NA. Role of histamine in the hemodynamic and plasma catecholamine responses to morphine. Clin Pharmacol Ther 1983; 33:615–20.

Fairman RP, Morrow C, Glauser FL. Methylmethacrylate induces pulmonary hypertension and increases lung vascular permeability in sheep. Am Rev Respir Dis 1984; 130:92–5.

Falk RH. Allergy to diazepam. Br Med J 1977; 2:287.

Faraj BA, Gottlieb GR, Camp VM, Kutner M, Lolies P. Development of a sensitive radioassay of histamine for in vitro allergy testing. J Nucl Med 1983; 25:56–63.

Fazackerley EJ, Martin AJ, Tolhurst-Cleaver CL, Watkins J. Anaphylactoid reaction following the use of etomidate. Anaesthesia 1988; 43:953–4.

Fearon DT, Ruddy S, Schur PH, McCabe WR. Activation of the properdin pathway of

complement in patients with gram-negative bacteremia. N Engl J Med 1975; 292:937–40.
Fee JPH, McDonald JR, Clarke RSJ, Dundee JW, Pal PK. The incidence of atopy and allergy in 10,000 preanaesthetic patients. Br J Anaesth 1978; 50:74–8.
Fehr J, Rohr H. In vivo complement activation by polyanion–polycation complexes: evidence that C_{5a} is generated intravascularly during heparin-protamine interaction. Clin Immunol Immunopathol 1983; 29:7–14.
Felbo M, Jensen KG. Death in childbirth following transfusion of leukocyte incompatible blood. Acta Haematol 1962; 27:113–9.
Feldberg W, Paton WD. Release of histamine from skin and muscle in the cat by opium alkaloids and other histamine liberators. J Physiol 1951; 114:490–509.
Fiedel A, Rent R, Myhrman R, Gewurz H. Complement activation by interaction of polyanions and polycations. Immunology 1976; 30:161–9.
Findlay SR, Dvorak AM, Kagey-Sobotkg A, Lichtenstein LM. Hyperosmolar triggering of histamine release from human basophils. J Clin Invest 1981; 67:1604–13.
Fiser WP, Fewell JE, Hill DE, Barnes RW, Read RC. Cardiovascular effects of protamine sulfate are dependent on the presence and type of circulating heparin. J Thorac Cardiovasc Surg 1985; 89:63–70.
Fisher MM. Severe histamine mediated reactions in althesin. Anaesth Inten Care 1976; 4:33–5.
Fisher MM. Blood volume replacement in acute anaphylactic cardiovascular collapse related to anaesthesia. Br J Anaesth 1977; 49:1023–6.
Fisher MM. Intradermal testing in the diagnosis of acute anaphylaxis during anesthesia–results of five years experience. Anaesth Inten Care 1979; 7:58–61.
Fisher MM. Reaginic antibodies to drugs used in anesthesia. Anesthesiology 1980; 52:318–20.
Fisher MM. The diagnosis of acute anaphylactoid reactions to anaesthetic drugs. Anaesth Inten Care 1981; 9:235–41.
Fisher MM, More DG. The epidemiology and clinical features of anaphylactic reactions in anaesthesia. Anaesth Inten Care 1981; 9:226–34.
Fisher MM. The epidemiology of anaesthetic anaphylactoid reactions in Australasia. Klin Wochenschr 1982; 60:1017–20.
Fisher MM, Munro I. Life threatening, anaphylactoid reactions to muscle relaxants. Anesth Analg 1983; 62:559–64.
Fisher MM. Intradermal testing after anaphylactoid reaction to anaesthetic drugs: practical aspects of performance and interpretation. Anaesth Intensive Care 1984; 12:115–20.
Fisher MM, Roffe DJ. Allergy, atopy and IgE. Anaesthesia 1984; 39:213–7.
Fisher MM, Teisnner B, Charlesworth J. Significance of sequestial changes in serum complement levels during acute anaphylactoid reactions. Crit Care Med 1984; 12:351–3.
Fisher M McD. Clinical observations on the pathophysiology and treatment of anaphylactic cardiovascular collapse. Anaesth Intensive Care 1986; 14:17–21.
Forbes CG, Pensky J, Ratnoff OD. Inhibition of activated Hageman factor and activated thromboplastin antecedent by purified C1 inactivator. J Lab Clin Med 1970; 76:809–15.
Ford RM. Management of acute allergic disease including anaphylaxis. Med J Aust 1977; 1:222–3.
Foreman JC, Piotrowski W. Peptides and histamine release. J Allergy Clin Immunol 1984; 74:127–31.
Forman MB, Oates JA, Robertson D, Robertson RM, Roberts LJ, Virmani R. Increased adventitial mast cells in a patient with coronary spasm. N Engl J Med 1985; 313:1138–41.
Frank MM, Gelfand JA, Atkinson JP. Hereditary angioedema: the clinical syndrome and its management. Ann Intern Med 1976; 84:580–93.

Frank MM. Complement: a brief review. J Allergy Clin Immunol 1988; 84:411–20.
Freedman MD, Schocket AL, Chapel N, Gerber JG. Anaphylaxis after intravenous methylprednisolone administration. JAMA 1981; 245:607–8.
Freeman JG, Turner GA, Vernables GA, Latner AL. Serial use of aprotinin and incidence of allergic reactions. Curr Med Res Opin 1983; 8:559–561.
Frick OL. Immediate hypersensitivity. In: Stites DP, Stobo JD, Fudenberg HH, Wells JV, eds. Basic and Clinical Immunology, 14th ed. Los Angeles, Lange Medical Publications, 1982.
Fuerstein G, Siren AL. The opioid system in cardiac and vascular regulation of normal and hypertensive states. Circulation 1987; 75(Suppl 1):125–9.
Furchgott RF, Vanhoutte PM. Endothelium-derived relaxing and contracting factors. FASEB J 1989; 3:2007–18.
Furhoff AK. Anaphylactoid reactions to dextran: a report of 133 cases. Acta Anaesthesiol Scand 1977; 21:161–7.
Futo J, Kupferberg JP, Moss J. Inhibition of histamine N-methyltransferase (HNMT) in vitro by neuromuscular relaxants. Biochem Pharmacol 1990; 39:415–20.
Gain KR, Appleman MM. Distribution and regulation of the phosphodiesterases of muscle tissues. In: George WJ, Ignarro LJ, eds. Advances in Cyclic Nucleotide Research. New York, Raven Press, 1978:221–31.
Gal TJ. Respiratory Physiology in Anesthetic Practice. Baltimore, Williams and Wilkins, 1991.
Gallo JA, Cork RC, Puchi P. Comparison of effects of atracurium and vecuronium in cardiac surgical patients. Anesth Analg 1988; 67:161–5.
Galpin JE, Chow AW, Yoshikawa TT, Guze LB. "Pseudoanaphylactic" reactions from inadvertent infusion of procaine penicillin G. Ann Intern Med 1974; 81:358.
Geha RS. Human IgE. J Allergy Clin Immunol 1984; 74:109–20.
Gell PGH, Coombs RRA, Lachmann PJ, eds. Clinical Aspects of Immunology, 3rd ed. Oxford, Blackwell Scientific Publications, 1975.
Gerber AC, Jorg W, Zbinden S, Seger RA, Dangel PH. Severe intraoperative anaphylaxis to surgical gloves: Latex allergy, an unfamiliar condition. Anesthesiology 1989; 71:800–2.
Ghebrehiwit B, Silverberg M, Kaplan AP. Activation of the classical complement pathway by Hageman factor fragments. J Exp Med 1981; 153:665–76.
Ghosh JS. Allergy to diazepam and other benzodiazepines. Br Med J 1977; 1:902–3.
Gibbs PS, LoSasso AM, Moorthy SS, Hutton CE. The anesthetic and perioperative management of a patient with documented hereditary angioneurotic edema. Anesth Analg 1977; 56:571–3.
Gill C, Michaelides PL. Dental drugs and anaphylactoid reactions: report of a case. Oral Surg 1980; 50:30–2.
Gill DS, Barradas MA, Fonseca VA, Dandona P. Plasma histamine concentrations are elevated in patients with diabetes mellitus and peripheral vascular disease. Metabolism 1989; 38:243–7.
Gillis DN, Pitt BR. The fate of circulating amines within the pulmonary circulation. Ann Rev Physiol 1982; 44:1503–7.
Ginsburg R, Bristow MR, Stinson EB, Harrison DC. Histamine receptors in the human heart. Life Sci 1980; 26:2245–9.
Ginsburg R, Bristow MR, Kantrowitz N, Baim FS, Harrison DC. Histamine provocation of clinical coronary artery spasm: implications concerning pathogenesis of variant angina pectoris. Am Heart J 1981; 102:819–22.
Gleich GJ, Flavahan NA, Fujisawa T, Vanhoutte PM. The eosinophil as a mediator of damage to respiratory epithelium: a model for bronchial hyperreactivity. J Allergy Clin Immunol 1988; 81:776–80.
Gleichmann H, Breininger J. Over 95% sensitization against allogeneic leukocytes following single massive blood transfusion. Vox Sang 1975; 28:66–73.
Glovsky MM, Hugli TE, Ishizaka T, Lichtenstein LM, Erickson BW. Anaphylatoxin-

induced histamine release with human leukocytes: studies of C3a leukocyte binding and histamine release. J Clin Invest 1979; 64:804–11.
Goetzl EJ. Mediators of immediate hypersensitivity derived from arachidonic acid. N Engl J Med 1980; 303:822–925.
Goetzl EJ. Asthma: new mediators and old problems. N Engl J Med 1984; 311:252–3.
Gold M, Swartz JS, Braude BM, Dolovich J, Shandling B, Gilmour RF. Intraoperative anaphylaxis: an association with latex sensitivity. J Allergy Clin Immunol 1991; 87:662–6.
Goldberg M. Systemic reactions to intravascular contrast media. Anesthesiology 1984; 60:46–56.
Goldenberg M, Pines KL, Baldwin EF. The hemodynamic response of man to norepinephrine and epinephrine and its relation to the problem of hypertension. Am J Med 1948; 5:792–806.
Goldfinger D, Lowe C. Prevention of adverse reactions to blood transfusion by administration of saline-washed red blood cells. Transfusion 1981; 21:277–80.
Gomez E, Corrado OJ, Baldwin DL, Swanston AR, Davies RJ. Direct in vivo evidence for mast cell degranulation during allergen-induced reactions in man. J Allergy Clin Immunol 1986; 78:637–45.
Gonzales GD, Lewis AJ, eds. Modern Drug Encyclopedia and Therapeutic Index. New York, Yorke Medical Books, 1981: 339.
Gorden FM, Simon GL, Wofsy CB. Adverse reactions to trimethoprin-sulfamethoxazole in patients with the acquired immunodeficiency syndrome. Ann Intern Med 1984; 100:495.
Gottschlich GM, Gravlee GP, Georgitis JW. Adverse reactions to protamine sulfate during cardiac surgery in diabetic and non-diabetic patients. Ann Allergy 1988; 61:277–81.
Gould L, Reddy CV, Zen B, Singh BK. Life-threatening reaction to thiazides. NY State J Med 1980; 80:1975–6.
Grammer LC, Patterson R. Proteins: chymopapain and insulin. J Allergy Clin Immunol 1984; 74:635–40.
Grammer LC, Metzger BE, Patterson R. Cutaneous allergy to human (recombinant DNA) insulin. JAMA 1984a; 251:1459–60.
Grammer LC, Roberts M, Nicholls AJ, Platts MM, Patterson R. IgE against ethylene oxide-altered human serum albumin in patients who have had acute dialysis reactions. J Allergy Clin Immunol 1984b; 74:544–6.
Grant JA, Dupree E, Goldman AS, Schultz DR, Jackson AL. Complement-mediated release of histamine from human leukocytes. J Immunol 1975; 114:1101–6.
Grant JA, Settle L, Whorton WB, Dupree E. Complement-mediated release of histamine from human basophils. J Immunol 1976; 117:450–6.
Grant JA, Cooper JR, Arens JF, et al. Anaphylactic reactions to protamine in insulin-dependent diabetics during cardiovascular surgery. Anesthesiology 1983; 59:A74.
Green GR, Rosenblum A. Report of the penicillin study group, American Academy of Allergy. J Allergy Clin Immunol 1971; 48:331–43.
Greenberger P, Patterson R, Kelly J, Stevenson DD, Simon R, Lieberman P. Administration of radiographic contrast media in high risk patients. Invest Radiol 1980; 15:540–3.
Greenberger P, Patterson R, Simon R. Pretreatment of high-risk patients requiring radiographic contrast media studies. J Allergy Clin Immunol 1981; 67:185–7.
Greenberger PA. Contrast media reactions. J Allergy Clin Immunol 1984; 74:600–5.
Greenberger PA, Patterson R, Tapio CM. Prophylaxis against repeated radiocontrast media reactions in 857 cases: adverse experience with cimetidine and safety of β-adrenergic antagonists. Arch Intern Med 1985; 145:2197–200.
Greenblatt EP, Chen L. Urticaria pigmentosa: an anesthetic challenge. J Clin Anesth 1990; 2:108–15.
Greer IA, Fellows K. Anaphylactoid reaction to ranitidine in labour. Br J Clin Pract 1990; 44:78.

Grega GA. Contractile elements in endothelial cells as potential targets for drug action. Trends Pharmacol Sci 1986; 7:452–7.

Gregori P. Allergischer schock nach behandlung mit protease-inhibitoren. Med Klin 1967; 62:1868–9.

Grieco MH. Cross-allergenicity of the penicillins and the cephalosporins. Arch Intern Med 1967; 119:141–6.

Griffin JH, Cochrane CG. Mechanisms of involvement of high molecular weight kininogen in surface-dependent reactions of Hageman factor (coagulation Factor XII). Proc Natl Acad Sci USA 1976; 73:2554–8.

Gross NJ. Ipratropium bromide. N Engl J Med 1988; 319:486–94.

Guo Z-G, Levi R, Graver M, Robertson DA, Gay WA. Inotropic effects of histamine in human myocardium: differentiation between positive and negative components. J Cardiovasc Pharmacol 1984; 6:1210–5.

Habazettl H, Conzen PF, Volmar B, et al. Pulmonary hypertension after heparin-protamine: role of left sided infusion, histamine, platelet-activating factor. Anesth Analg 1990; 71:637–44.

Hagedorn HC, Jensen BN, Krarup NB, et al. Protamine insulinate. JAMA 1936; 106:177–80.

Halevy S, Altura BM. H_1- and H_2-histamine receptor antagonists and protection against traumatic shock. Proc Soc Exp Biol Med 1977; 154:453–6.

Halevy S, Altura BT, Altura BM. Pathophysiological basis for the use of steroids in the treatment of shock and trauma. Klin Wochenschr 1982; 60:1021–30.

Halpern GM. Nonreaginic anaphylactic and/or blocking antibodies: introduction. Clin Rev Allergy 1983; 1:179–81.

Hamilton RG, Rendellin, Adkinson NF. Serological analysis of human IgG and IgE anti-insulin antibodies by solid-phase radioimmunoassays. J Lab Clin Med 1980; 96:1022–36.

Hammerschmidt DE, White JG, Craddock PR, Jacob HS. Corticosteroids inhibit complement-induced granulocyte aggregation: a possible mechanism for their efficacy in shock states. J Clin Invest 1979; 63:798–803.

Hammerschmidt DE. Of lungs and leukocytes (editorial). JAMA 1980; 244:2199–2200.

Hammerschmidt DE, Weaver LJ, Hudson LD, Craddock PR, Jacob HS. Association of complement activation and elevated plasma-C_{5a} with adult respiratory distress syndrome. Lancet 1980; 1:947–9.

Hammerschmidt DE, Harris PD, Wayland JH, Craddock PR, Jacob HS. Complement-induced granulocyte aggregation in vivo. Am J Pathol 1981; 102:146–50.

Hammerschmidt DE, Jacob HS. Adverse pulmonary reactions to transfusion. In: Stollerman GH, ed. Advances in Internal Medicine. Chicago, Year Book Medical Publishers, 1982:511–30.

Hanashiro PK, Weil MH. Anaphylactic shock in man. Arch Intern Med 1967; 119:129–40.

Hanko JH, Hardebo JE. Enkephalin-induced dilatation of pial arteries in vitro probably mediated by opiate receptors. Eur J Pharmacol 1978; 51:295–7.

Hanna CJ, Bach MK, Pare PD, Schellenberg RR. Slow-reacting substances (leukotrienes) contract human airway and pulmonary vascular smooth muscle in vitro. Nature 1981; 290:343–4.

Hansbrough JR, Wedner JH, Chaplin DD. Anaphylaxis to intravenous furosemide. J Allergy Clin Immunol 1987; 80:538–41.

Hardy CC, Robinson C, Tattersfield AE, Holgate ST. The bronchoconstriction effect of inhaled prostaglandin D_2 in normal and asthmatic men. N Engl J Med 1984; 311:209–13.

Harle DG, Baldo BA, Fisher MM. Detection of IgE antibodies to suxamethonium after anaphylactoid reactions during anaesthesia. Lancet 1984; 1:930–2.

Harle DG, Baldo BA, Fisher MM. Assays for, and cross-reactivities of, IgE antibodies to the muscle relaxants gallamine, decamethonium and succinylcholine (suxamethonium). J Immunol Methods 1985a; 78:293–305.

Harle DG, Baldo BA, Fisher MM. Cross-reactivity of metocurine, atracurium, vecuronium and fazadinium with IgE antibodies from patients unexposed to these drugs but allergic to other myoneural blocking drugs. Br J Anaesth 1985b; 57:1073–6.

Harle DG, Baldo BA, Smal MA, Wagon P, Fisher MM. Detection of thiopentone-reactive IgE antibodies following anaphylactoid reactions during anaesthesia. Clin Allergy 1986; 16:493–8.

Harle DG, Baldo BA. Atracurium and anaphylaxis (letter). Med J Aust 1986; 144:220.

Harle DG, Baldo BA, Smal MA, Fisher MM. Drugs as allergens: the molecular basis of IgE binding to thiopentone. Int Arch Allergy Appl Immunol 1987; 84:277–83.

Harle DG, Baldo BA, Coroneos NJ, Fisher MM. Anaphylaxis following administration of papaveretum: case report, implication of IgE antibodies that react with morphine and codeine and identification of an allergenic determinant. Anesthesiology 1989; 71:489–94.

Hashim SW, Ray HR, Hammond GL, Kopf GS, Geha AS. Noncardiogenic pulmonary edema from cardiopulmonary bypass: an anaphylactic reaction to fresh frozen plasma. Am J Surg 1984; 147:560–4.

Haslam PL, Townsend PJ, Branthwaite MA. Complement activation during cardiopulmonary bypass. Anaesthesia 1980; 35:22–6.

Harvey SC. Sympathomimetic drugs. In: Osol A, ed. Remington's Pharmaceutical Sciences. Easton, Mack Publishing, 1980; 815–24.

Hatano Y, Arai T, Noda J, et al. Contribution of prostacyclin to d-tubocurarine-induced hypotension in humans. Anesthesiology 1990; 72:28–32.

Hatton F, Tiert L, Maujol L, et al. Enquête épidémiologique sur les anesthésies. Ann Fr Anesth Réanim 1983; 2:333–5.

Hauptmann G, Goetz J, Steib A, Otteni JC. Médicaments inhibant l'activation du complément. Ann Fr Anesth Réanim 1985; 4:210–3.

Heinrich D, Eckhardt CM, Stier W. The specificity of leukocyte and platelet alloantibodies in sera of patients with nonhemolytic transfusion reactions. Vox Sang 1973; 25:442–6.

Hellema HWJ, Rumke P. Sperm autoantibodies as a consequence of vasectomy: I. Within one year postoperation. Clin Exp Immuol 1978; 31:18–29.

Hermens JM, Ebertz JM, Hanifin JM, Hirshman CA. Comparison of histamine release in human skin mast cells by morphine, fentanyl, and oxymorphone. Anesthesiology 1985; 62:124–9.

Hill SJ. Distribution, properties, and functional characteristics of three classes of histamine receptor. Pharmacol Rev 1990; 42:45–74.

Hines RL, Barash PG. Protamine: does it alter right ventricular performance? Anesth Analg 1986; 65:1271–4.

Hirshman CA, Downes H, Butler J. Relevance of plasma histamine levels to hypotension. Anesthesiology 1982; 57:424–5.

Hirshman CA, Peters J, Cartwright-Lee I. Leukocyte histamine release to thiopental. Anethesiology 1983; 56:64–7.

Hirshman CA, Edelstein RA, Eastman CL. Histamine release by barbiturates in human mast cells. Anesthesiology 1985; 63:353–6.

Hobbhahn J, Conzen PF, Zenker B, Goetz AE, Peter K, Brendel W. Beneficial effect of cyclogenase inhibition on adverse hemodynamic response after protamine. Anesth Analg 1988; 67:253–60.

Hoffman BB, Lefkowitz RJ. Catecholamines and sympathomimetic drug. In: Gilman AG, Rall TW, Nies AS, Taylor P, eds. The Pharmacologic Basis of Therapeutics. New York, Pergamon Press, 1990: 187–220.

Holland CL, Singh AK, McMaster PRB, Fang W. Adverse reactions to protamine sulfate following cardiac surgery. Clin Cardiol 1984; 7:157–62.

Hong SL, Levine L. Inhibition of arachidonic acid release from cells as the biochemical action of anti-inflammatory corticosteroids. Proc Natl Acad Sci 1976; 73: 1730–4.

Hook WA, Siraganian RP. Influence of anions, cations and osmolarity on IgE-mediated histamine release from human basophils. Immunology 1981; 43:723–31.

Horak A, Raine R, Opie LH, Lloyd EA. Severe myocardial ischemia induced by intravenous adrenaline. Br Med J 1983; 286:519.

Horrow JC. Protamine: a review of its toxicity. Anesth Analg 1985; 64:348–61.

Horrow J, Hlavacek J, Strong MD, et al. Prophylactic tranexamic acid decreases bleeding after cardiac operations. J Thorac Cardiovasc Surg 1990; 99:70–4.

Hudson JC, Wurm WH, O'Donnell TF, et al. Ibuprofen pretreatment inhibits prostacyclin release during abdominal exploration in aortic surgery. Anesthesiology 1990; 72:443–9.

Huestis DW. Anti-IgA in blood donors. Transfusion 1976; 16:289–90.

Hurst JW, ed. The Heart, 5th ed. New York, McGraw-Hill, 1982.

Huttel MS, Schou Olesen A, Stoffersen M. Complement mediated solvent reactions to diazepam with cremophor as solvent (Stesolid MR). Br Anaesth J 1980; 52:77–9.

Idsoe O, Guthe T, Willcox RR, DeWeck AL. Nature and extent of penicillin side-reactions with particular reference to fatalities from anaphylactic shock. Bull WHO 1968; 38:159–88.

Immunology: A Scope publication. The Upjohn Company, Kalamazoo, MI, 1981.

Incaudo G, Schatz M, Patterson R, Rosenberg M, Yamamato F, Hamburger RN. Administration of local anesthetics to patients with a history of prior adverse reaction. J Allergy Clin Immunol 1978; 61:339–45.

Ind PW, Brown MJ, Lhoste FJM, Macquin J, Dollery CT. Concentration effect relationships of infused histamine in normal volunteers. Agents Actions 1982; 12:12–6.

Ishikawa S, Sperelakis N. A novel class (H_3) of histamine receptors on perivascular nerve terminals. Nature 1987; 327:158–60.

Ishizaka T. Analysis of triggering events in mast cells for immunoglobulin E-mediated histamine release. J Allergy Clin Immunol 1981; 67:90–6.

Isles AF, McLeod SM, Levison H. Thiophylline: new thoughts about an old drug. Chest 1982; 82:495–54S.

Jacob HS, Craddock PR, Hammerschmidt DE, Moldow CF. Complement-induced granulocyte aggregation: an unsuspected mechanism of disease. N Engl J Med 1980; 302:789–94.

Jacobs RL, Geoffrey WR Jr, Fournier DC, Chilton RJ, Culver WG, Beckmann CH. Potentiated anaphylaxis in patients with drug-induced beta-adrenergic blockade. J Allergy Clin Immunol 1981; 68:125–7.

James LP, Austen KF. Fatal systemic anaphylaxis in man. N Engl J Med 1964; 270:597–603.

Jancelowica A, Sussman G, Tarlo S, Dolovich J. Clinical presentation of five patients allergic to latex. J Allergy Clin Immunol 1989; 83:267.

Jaques LB. A study of the toxicity of the protamine, salmine. Br J Pharmacol 1949; 4:135–44.

Jasani B, Kreil G, Mackler BF, Stanworth DF. Further studies on the structural requirements for polypeptide-mediated histamine release from rat mast cells. Biochem J 1979; 181:623–32.

Jick H. Adverse reactions to trimethoprim-sulfamethoxazole in hospitalized patients. Rev Infect Dis 1982; 4:326.

Jick H. Adverse drug reactions: the magnitude of the problem. J Allergy Clin Immunol 1984; 74:555–7.

Johansson SGO. In vitro diagnosis of reagin-mediated allergic diseases. Allergy 1978; 33:292–8.

Johnson AR, Erdös EG. Release of histamine from mast cells by vasoactive peptides. Proc Soc Exp Biol Med 1973; 142:1252–6.

Jones HM, Matthews N, Vaughan RS, Stark JM. Cardiopulmonary bypass and complement activation. Involvement of classical and alternate pathways. Anaesthesia 1982; 37:629–33.

Just-Viera JO, Fischer CR, Gago O, Morris JD. Acute reaction to protamine. Am Surg 1984; 50:52–60.

Kahan BD, Wideman CA, Flechner S, Van Buren CT. Anaphylactic reaction to intravenous cyclosporine. Lancet 1984; 1:52.

Kaliner M, Sigler R, Summers R, Shelhamer JH. Effects of infused histamine: analysis of the effects of H-1 and H-2 histamine receptor antagonists on cardiovascular and pulmonary responses. J Allergy Clin Immunol 1981; 68:365–71.

Kaliner M, Shelhamer JH, Ottesen EA. Effects of infused histamine: correlation of plasma histamine levels and symptoms. J Allergy Clin Immunol 1982; 69:283–9.

Kallos T. Impaired arterial oxygenation associated with use of bone cement in the femoral shaft. Anesthesiology 1975; 42:210–16.

Kalsner S, Richards R. Coronary arteries of cardiac patients are hyperreactive and contain stores of amines: a mechanism for coronary spasm. Science 1984; 223:1435–8.

Kaplan AP, Austen KF. Activation and control mechanisms of Hageman factor-dependent pathways of coagulation, fibrinolysis, and kinin generation and their contribution to the inflammatory process. J Allergy Clin Immunol 1975; 56:491–506.

Katz NM, Kim YD, Siegelman R, Ved SA, Ahmed SW, Wallace RB. Hemodynamics of protamine administration: comparison of right atrial, left atrial, and aortic injections. J Thorac Cardiovasc Surg 1987; 94:881–6.

Kazimierczak W, Diamant B. Mechanisms of histamine release in anaphylactic and anaphylactoid reactions. Prog Allergy 1978; 4:295–365.

Kay AB. Asthma and inflammation. J Allergy Clin Immunol 1991; 87:893–910.

Keitolu M, Okayama H, Satoh Y, Maruyama Y, Takishima T. Does diffuse intimal thickening in human coronary artery act as a diffusion barrier to endothelium-derived relaxing factor? Tohuko J Exp Med 1988; 154:413–4.

Kelly JF, Patterson R. Anaphylaxis: course, mechanisms and treatment. JAMA 1974; 227:1431–6.

Kelly JF, Patterson R, Lieberman P, Mathison DA, Stevenson DD. Radiographic contrast media studies in high risk patients. J Allergy Clin Immunol 1978; 62:181–4.

Kern RA, Langner PH Jr: Protamine and allergy. JAMA 1938; 113:198–200.

Kernoff PBA, Durrant IJ, Rizza CR, Wright FW. Severe allergic pulmonary oedema after plasma transfusion. Br J Haematol 1972; 23:777–81.

Khandelwal JK, Hough LB, Green JP. Histamine and some of its metabolites in human body fluids. Klin Wochenschr 1982; 60:914–18.

Killackey JJF, Johnston MG, Movat HZ. Increased permeability of microcarrier-cultured endothelial monolayers in response to histamine and thrombin. Am J Pathol 1986; 122:50–61.

Kilzer P, Chang K, Marvel J, Kilo C, Williamson JR. Tissue differences in vascular permeability changes induced by histamine. Microvasc Res 1985; 30:270–85.

Klarkowski DB. The serological investigation of red cell incompatible transfusion reactions. Anaesth Intensive Care 1980; 8:120–4.

Klausner JM, Paterson IS, Mannick JA, Valeri CR, Shepro D, Hechtman HB. Reperfusion pulmonary edema. JAMA 1989; 261:1030–40.

Knape JTA, Schuller JL, deHaan P, DeJong AP, Bovill JG. An anaphylactic reaction to protamine in a patient allergic to fish. Anesthesiology 1981; 55:324–5.

Knapp AB, Grimshaw RS Jr, Goldfarb JP, Farkas PS, Rubin M, Rosenstreich DL. Cimetidine-induced anaphylaxis. Ann Intern Med 1982; 97:374–5.

Kofke WA, Levy JH, eds. Postoperative Critical Care Procedures of the Massachusetts General Hospital. Boston, Little, Brown, 1986.

Kolstinen J. Selective IgA deficiency in blood donors. Vox Sang 1975; 29:192–202.

Kolstinen J, Sarna A. Immunologic abnormalities in the sera of IgA deficient blood donors. Vox Sang 1975; 29:203–13.

Konstam MA, Cohen SR, Weiland DS, et al. Relative contribution of inotropic and vasodilator effects to amrinone-induced hemodynamic improvement in congestive heart failure. Am J Cardiol 1986; 57:242–8.

Koscove EM, Paradis NA. Successful resuscitation from cardiac arrest using high-dose epinephrine therapy. JAMA 1988; 259:3031–4.

Kraenzler EJ, Starr NJ. Heparin-associated thrombocytopenia: management of patients for open heart surgery. Case reports describing the use of iloprost. Anesthesiology 1988; 69:964–7.

Kraft D. Other Antibiotics. de Weck AL, Bundgaard H, eds. In Allergic Reactions to Drugs. Berlin, Springer-Verlag, 1983: 483–520.

Kravis TC. Obstructive lung diseases. In: Kravis TC, Warner CG, eds. Emergency Medicine: A Comprehensive Review. Rockville, MD, Aspen Systems Corp., 1983: 838.

Kreil E, Montalescot G, Green E, et al. Nafamstat mesilate attenuates pulmonary hypertension in heparin-protamine reactions. J Appl Physiol 1989; 67:1463–71.

Kronenfeld MA, Garguilo R, Weinberg P, Grant G, Thomas SJ, Turndorf H. Left atrial injection of protamine does not reliably prevent pulmonary hypertension. Anesthesiology 1987; 67:578–80.

Kukovetz WR, Pöch G, Holzmann S. Cyclic nucleotides and relaxation of vascular smooth muscle. In: Vanhoutte PM, Leusen I, eds. Vasodilatation. New York, Raven Press, 1981: 331–53.

Kurachi K, Davie EW: Activation of human factor XI (plasma thromboplastin antecedent) by factor XIIa (activated Hageman factor). Biochemistry 1977; 16:5831–9.

Labatut A, Sorbette F, Virenque C. Shock states during injection of vitamin K_1. Therapie 1988; 43:58.

LaForest M, More D, Fisher M. Predisposing factors in anaphylactoid reactions to anaesthetic drugs in an Australian population: the role of allergy, atopy and previous anaesthesia. Anaesth Intensive Care 1980; 8:454–9.

Lagunoff D, Martin TW, Read G. Agents that release histamine from mast cells. Ann Rev Pharmacol 1983; 23:331–51.

Lakin JD, Blocker TJ, Strong DM, Yocum MW. Anaphylaxis to protamine sulfate mediated by a complement-dependent IgG antibody. J Allergy Clin Immunol 1978; 61:102–7.

Lalli AF. Contrast media reactions: data, analysis and hypothesis. Radiology 1980; 134:1–12.

Langer R, Linhardt RJ, Hoffberg S, et al. An enzymatic system for removing heparin in extracorporeal therapy. Science 1982; 217:261–3.

Langrehr D, Newton D, Agoston S. Epidemiology of adverse reactions in anaesthesia in Germany and The Netherlands. Klin Wochenschr 1982; 60:1010–6.

Laroche D, Vergnaud MC, Sillard B, Soufarapis H, Bricard H. Biochemical markers of anaphylactoid reactions to drugs: comparison of plasma histamine and tryptase. Anesthesiology 1991; 75:945–9.

Laser EC, Lang J, Sovak M, Kolb W, Lyon S, Hamlin AE. Steroids: theoretical and experimental basis for utilization in prevention of contrast media reactions. Radiology 1977; 125:1–12.

Laser EC, Lang JH, Lyon SG, Hamblin AE. Complement and contrast material reactors. J Allergy Clin Immunol 1979; 64:105–12.

Laser EC, Lang JH, Lyon SG, Hamblin AE. Changes in complement and coagulation factors in a patient suffering a severe anaphylactoid reaction to injected contrast media: some considerations of pathogenesis. Invest Radiol 1980a; 15:(suppl)S6–12.

Laser EC, Lang JH, Hamblin AE, et al. Activation systems in contrast idiosyncrasy. Invest Radiol 1980b; 15(suppl):S2–S5.

Lasser EC, Berry CC, Talner LB, et al. Pretreatment with corticosteroids to alleviate reactions to intravenous contrast material. N Engl J Med 1987; 317:845–9.

Latson TW, Kickler TS, Baumgartner WA. Pulmonary hypertension and noncardiogenic pulmonary edema following cardiopulmonary bypass associated with an antigranulocyte antibody. Anesthesiology 1986; 64:106–11.
Lawrence ID, Warner JA, Cohan VL, Hubbard WC, Kagey-Sobotka A, Lichtenstein LM. Purification and characterization of human skin mast cells: evidence for human mast cell heterogeneity. J Immunol 1987; 139:3062–9.
Laxenaire MC, Gueant JL, Bermejo E, Mouton C, Navez MT. Anaphylactic shock due to propofol. Lancet 1988; ii:739–40.
Laxenaire MC, Mata-Bermejo E, Moneret-Vautrin DA, Gueant JL. Life threatening anaphylactoid reactions to propofol (Diprivan). In press.
Laxenaire MC, Moneret-Vautrin DA, Boileau S, Moeller R. Adverse reactions to intravenous agents in anaesthesia in France. Klin Wochenschr 1982; 60:1006–9.
Laxenaire MC, Moneret-Vautrin DA, Boileau S, Borce J. Facteurs de risque d'histaminoliberation en anesthesie generale. Therapie 1983a; 38:529–34.
Laxenaire MC, Moneret-Vautrin DA, Watkins J. Diagnosis of the causes of anaphylactoid anesthetic reactions. Anaesthesia 1983b; 38:147–8.
Laxenaire MC, Moneret-Vautrin DA, Vervloet D. The French experience of anaphylactoid reactions. Int Anesthesiol Clin 1985; 23:145–60.
Laxenaire MC, Moneret-Vautrin DA, eds. Le Risque Allergique en Anesthésie-Réanimation. Paris, Masson, 1990.
Lebowitz PW, Newberg LA, Gillette MT. Clinical Anesthesia Procedures of the Massachusetts General Hospital. Boston, Little, Brown, 1982.
Lefrère JJ, Girot R. Acute cardiovascular collapse during intravenous vitamin K_1 injection. Thromb Haemost 1987; 58:790.
Leikola J, Koistinen J, Lehtinen M, Virolainen M. IgA-induced anaphylactic transfusion reactions: a report of four cases. Blood 1973; 42:111–9.
Leusen I, Van de Voorde J. Endothelium-dependent responses to histamine. In: Vanhoutte PM, ed. Vasodilatation: Vascular Smooth Muscle, Peptides, Autonomic Nerves, and Endothelium. New York, Raven Press, 1988: 469–74.
Levi R. Cardiac anaphylaxis: models, mediators, mechanisms, and clinical considerations. In: Marone G, Lichtenstein LM, Condorelli M, Fauci AS, eds. Human Inflammatory Disease, vol 1, Clinical Immunology. Toronto, Decker Inc, 1988.
Levi R, Rubin LE, Gross SS. Histamine in cardiovascular function and dysfunction: recent developments. In: Uvnäs B, ed. Handbook of Experimental Pharmacology, vol 97, Histamine and Histamine Antagonists. Berlin, Springer-Verlag, 1991.
Levine BB. Immunochemical mechanisms involved in penicillin hypersensitivity in experimental animals and in human beings. Fed Proc 1965; 24:45–50.
Levine BB. Immunologic mechanisms of penicillin allergy: a haptenic model system for the study of allergic diseases of man. N Engl J Med 1966; 275:1115–25.
Levine BB, Redmond AP, Fellner MJ, Voss HE, Levytska V. Penicillin allergy and the heterogeneous immune responses of man to benzylpenicillin. J Clin Invest 1966; 45:1895–906.
Levine BB, Redmond AP. Minor haptenic determinant-specific reagins of penicillin hypersensitivity in man. Int Arch Allergy 1969; 35:445–55.
Levy JH. Unusual reaction to Trasylol. Can Med Assoc J 1974; 111:1304.
Levy JH, Rockoff MR. Anaphylaxis to meperidine. Anesth Analg 1982; 61:301–3.
Levy JH. Intravenous epinephrine therapy in anaphylaxis. JAMA 1983; 249:3173.
Levy JH. Identification and treatment of anaphylaxis. In: Roizen M, ed. Chemonucleolysis Anaphylaxis: Mechanisms of Action and Strategies for Treatment under General Anesthesia, 21–34. Chicago, Smith Laboratories, 1983.
Levy JH. Anaphylaxis to chymopapain following antihistamine pretreatment. Anesth Analg 1985; 64:190.
Levy JH. Allergic reactions and the intraoperative use of foreign substances. In: Barash P, ed. Refresher Course in Anesthesiology, vol. 13, 1985; 129–41.

Levy JH, Zaidan JR, Faraj B. Prospective evaluation of risk of protamine reactions in NPH insulin dependent diabetics. Anesth Analg 1986a; 65:739–42.
Levy JH, Roizen MF, Morris JM. Anaphylactic and anaphylactoid reactions. Spine 1986b; 11:282–91.
Levy JH, Kettlekamp N, Goertz P, Hermens J, Hirshman CA. Histamine release by vancomycin: a mechanism for hypotension in man. Anesthesiology 1987; 67:122–5.
Levy JH, Hug CC. Cardiopulmonary bypass as a method of assessing the effects of anesthetics on myocardial function. Br J Anaesth 1988; 60:35S–37S.
Levy JH. Anaphylactic/anaphylactoid reactions during cardiac surgery. J Clin Anesth 1989a; 1:426–30.
Levy JH. Life-threatening reactions to intravenous protamine. N Engl J Med 1989b; 321:1684–5.
Levy JH, Brister NW, Shearin A, et al. Wheal and flare responses to opioids in humans. Anesthesiology 1989c; 70:756–60.
Levy JH, Schwieger IM, Zaidan JR, Faraj BA, Weintraub WS. Evaluation of patients at risk for protamine reactions. J Thorac Cardiovasc Surg 1989d; 98:200–4.
Levy JH, Faraj BA, Zaidan JR, Camp VM. Effects of protamine on histamine release from human lung. Agents Actions, 1989a; 28:70–72.
Levy JH, Ramsay JM, Bailey JM. Pharmacokinetics and pharmcodynamics of phosphodiesterase III inhibitors. J Cardiothorac Anesth 1990; 4(S):7–16.
Levy JH, Salmenpera MT. Aprotinin and its heparin-sparing effect. J Thorac Cardiovasc Surg 1991; 102:802.
Levy JH, Adelson DM, Walker BF. Wheal and flare responses to muscle relaxants in humans. Agents Actions 1991; 34:302–8.
Levy JH, Adelson DM. Effects of vecuronium induced histamine N-methyltransferase inhibition on cutaneous responses in humans. Agent Actions, in press.
Levy JH, Bailey JM. Perioperative experience with amrinone. Eur J Anaesth, in press.
Lewis RA, Austen KF. The biologically active leukotrienes: biosyntheses, metabolism, receptors, functions, and pharmacology. J Clin Invest 1984; 73:889–902.
Lewis RA, Austen KF, Soberman RJ. Leukotrienes and other products of the 5-lipoxygenase pathways. N Engl J Med 1990; 323:645–55.
Liberman P, Siegle RL, Taylor WW Jr. Anaphylactoid reactions to iodinated contrast media. J Allergy Clin Immunol 1978; 62:174–80.
Lichtenstein LM. Anaphylaxis. In: Wyngarden JB, Smith LH, eds. Cecil: Textbook of Medicine. Philadelphia, WB Saunders, 1982: 1805.
Ljungstroem KG, Renck H, Hedin H, Richter W, Rosenberg B. Prevention of dextran induced anaphylactic reactions by hapten inhibition. Acta Chir Scand 1983; 149:341–8.
Lock R, Hessel EA. Probable reversal of protamine reactions by heparin administration. J Cardiothorac Anesth 1990; 4:604–8.
Lockey RF, Fox RW. Allergic emergencies. Hosp Med 1979; 16:64–8.
Lörenz W, Doenicke A, Schoning B, Neugebauer E. The role of histamine in adverse reactions to intravenous agents. In: Thornton JA, ed. Adverse Reactions of Anaesthetic Drugs. Amsterdam, Elsevier/North Holland Biomedical Press, 1981: 169–238.
Lörenz W, Ennis M, Dick W, Doenicke A. Perioperative uses of histamine antagonists. J Clin Anesth 1990; 2:345–360.
Lowenstein E, Hallowell P, Levine FH, Daggett WM, Austen WG, Laver MB. Cardiovascular response to large doses of morphine in man. N Engl J Med 1969; 281:1389–94.
Lowenstein E, Johnston WE, Lappas DG, et al. Catastrophic pulmonary hypertension associated with protamine reversal of heparin. Anesthesiology 1983; 59:470–3.
Lowman MA, Rees PH, Benyon RC, Church MK. Human mast cell heterogeneity: histamine release from mast cells dispersed from skin, lung, adenoids, tonsils, and colon in response to IgE-dependent and nonimmunologic stimuli. J Allergy Clin Immunol 1988; 81:590–7.

Lloyd JE, Newman JH, Brigham KL. Permeability pulmonary edema: diagnosis and management. Arch Intern Med 1984; 144:143–7.
Lucchesi BR. Role of calcium on excitation contraction in cardiac and vascular smooth muscle. Circulation 1989; 80:IV-1–IV-13.
Lyew MA, Levy JH. Treatment of protamine induced pulmonary hypertension following cardiopulmonary bypass with ketorolac. In press.
Maggart M, Stewart S. The mechanisms and management of noncardiogenic pulmonary edema following cardiopulmonary bypass. Ann Thorac Surg 1987; 43:231–6.
Majno G, Palade GE. Studies on inflammation. I. The effect of histamine and serotonin on vascular permeability: an electron microscopic study. J Biophys Biochem Cytol 1961; 11:571–672.
Majno G, Gilmore V, Leventhal M. The effect of histamine and serotonin on the mechanism of vascular leakage caused by histamine-type mediators: a microscopic study in vivo. Circ Res 1967; 21:833–55.
Majno G, Shea SM, Leventhal M. Endothelial contraction induced by histamine-type mediators. J Cell Biol 1969; 42:647–72.
Malbran A, Hammer CH, Frank MM, Fries LF. Acquired angioedema: observations on the mechanisms of action of autoantibodies directed against C1 esterase inhibitor. J Allergy Clin Immunol 1988; 81:1199–1204.
Mansfield LE, Ting S, Haverly RW. Anaphylaxis caused by the sodium succinate ester of hydrocortisone and methylprednisolone. J Asthma 1986; 23:81–3.
Mantz JM, Gauli G, Meyer P, et al. Le choc anaphylactique. Rev Med Interne (Fr) 1982; 3:331–8.
Marshall I. Characterization and distribution of histamine H_1- and H_2-receptors in precapillary vessels. J Cardiovasc Pharmacol 1984; 6:S587–S597.
Mason JW, Kleeburg U, Dolan P, Colman RW. Plasma kallikrein and Hageman factor in gram-negative bacteremia. Ann Intern Med 1970; 73:545–51.
Mathé AA, Hedqvist P, Strandberg K, Leslie CA. Aspects of prostaglandin function in the lung. N Engl J Med 1977; 296:850–5; 910–4.
Mathews KP. Urticaria and angioedema. J Allergy Clin Immunol 1983; 72:1–16.
Mathieu A, Goudsouzian N, Snider MT. Reaction to ketamine: anaphylactoid or anaphylactic. Br J Anaesth 1975; 47:624.
Matsson P, Enander I, Andersson A-S, Nystrand J, Schwartz L, Watkins J. Evaluation of mast cell activation (tryptase) in two patients suffering from drug-induced hypotensive reactions. Agents Actions 1991; 33:218–20.
Matthay RA, Berger HJ, Loke J, Gottschalk A, Zoret BL. Effects of aminophylline upon right and left ventricular performance in chronic obstructive pulmonary disease. Am J Med 1978; 65:903–10.
May CD. The ancestry of allergy: being an account of the original experimental induction of hypersensitivity recognizing the contribution of Paul Portier. J Allergy Clin Immunol 1985; 75:485–95.
McBride P, Bradley D, Kaliner M. Evaluation of a radioimmunoassay for histamine measurement in biologic fluids. J Allergy Clin Immunol 1988; 82:638–46.
McGrath KG, Zeffren B, Alexander J, Kaplan K, Patterson R. Allergic reactions to streptokinase consistent with anaphylactic or antigen-antibody complex-mediated damage. J Allergy Clin Immunol 1985; 76:453–7.
McIntosh FC, Paton WDM. The liberation of histamine by certain organic bases. J Physiol 1949; 109:190–219.
McIntyre RW, Flezzani P, Knopes KD, Reves JG, Watkins WD. Pulmonary hypertension and prostaglandins after protamine. Am J Cardiol 1986a; 58:857–8.
McIntyre TN, Zimmerman GA, Prescott SM. Leukotrienes C_4 and D_4 stimulate human endothelial cells to synthesize platelet-activating factor and bind neutrophils. Proc Natl Acad Sci USA 1986b; 83:2204–8.
Meier HL, Pierce JV, Colman RW, Kaplan AP. Activation and function of human Hageman

factor: the role of high molecular weight kininogen and prekallikrein. J Clin Invest 1977; 60:18–31.

Meier HL, Kaplan AP, Lichtenstein LM, Revak S, Cochrane CG, Newball HH. Anaphylactic release of a prekallikrein activator from human lung in vitro. J Clin Invest 1983; 72:574–81.

Mendelson LM, Meltzer EO, Hamburger RN. Anaphylaxis-like reactions to corticosteroid therapy. J Allergy Clin Immunol 1974; 54:125–31.

Metcalf DD. Effector cell heterogeneity in immediate hypersensitivity reactions. Clin Rev Allergy 1982; 1:311–25.

Metzger H, Alcaraz G, Hohman R, Kinet JP, Pribluda V, Quarto R. The receptor with high affinity for immunoglobulin E. Ann Rev Immunol 1986; 4:419–70.

Michaels JA, Barash PG. Hemodynamic changes during protamine administration. Anesth Analg 1983; 62:831–5.

Michelassi F, Castorena G, Hill ED, et al. Leukotriene D_4: a potent coronary artery vasoconstrictor associated with impaired ventricular contraction. Science 1982; 217:841–3.

Michelassi F, Castorena G, Hill ED, et al. Effects of leukotrienes B_4 and C_4 on coronary circulation and myocardial contractility. Surgery 1983; 94:267–75.

Mikhail GR, Miller-Milinska A. Mast cell population in human skin. J Invest Dermatol 1964; 43:249–54.

Mikkelsen E, Sakr AM, Jespersen LT. Studies on the effect of histamine in isolated pulmonary arteries and veins. Acta Pharmacol Toxicol 1984; 54: 86–93.

Miller R, Tausk HC. Anaphylactoid reaction to vancomycin during anesthesia; a case report. Anesth Analg 1977; 56:870–2.

Milne B, Rogers K, Cervenko F. The haemodynamic effects of intraaortic versus intravenous administration of protamine for reversal of heparin in man. Can Anaesth Soc J 1983; 30:347–51.

Milner LV, Butcher K. Transfusion reactions reported after transfusion of red blood cells and of whole blood. Transfusion 1978; 18:493–5.

Mitchell EB, Askenase PW. Basophils in human disease. Clin Rev Allergy 1983; 1:427–48.

Moneret-Vautrin DA, Laxenaire MC, Mouton C. Anaphylaxie croisee avec le vecuronium. Ann Fr Anesth Réanim 1984; 3:467–70.

Moneret-Vautrin DA, Laxenaire MC, Bavoux F. Allergic shock to latex and ethylene oxide during surgery for spina bifida. Anesthesiology 1990; 73:556–8.

Moneret-Vautrin DA, Mouton C. Anaphylaxie aux myorelaxants: valeur prédictive des intradermoreactions et Recherche de l'anaphylaxie croisee. Ann Fr Anesth Réanim 1985; 4:186–91.

Moneret-Vautrin DA, Widmer S, Laxenaire MC, Maday T. Deux chocs anaphylactiques par sensibilisation probable au solvant du flunitrazepam. Ann Fr Anesth Réanim 1986; 5:556–7.

Moneret-Vautrin DA, Guéant JL, Kamel L, Laxenaire MC, Kholty SE, Nicolas JP. Anaphylaxis to muscle relaxants: cross-sensitivity studied by radioimmunoassays compared to intradermal tests in 34 cases. J Allergy Clin Immunol 1988; 82:745–52.

Montalescot G, Lowenstein E, Ogletree ML, et al. Thromboxane receptor blockade prevents pulmonary hypertension induced by heparin-protamine reactions in awake sheep. Circulation 1990; 82:1765–77.

Moorthy SS, Pond W, Rowland RG. Severe circulatory shock following protamine (an anaphylactic reaction). Anesth Analg 1980; 59:77–8.

Morel DR, Kitain E, Purcell MH, Thomas SJ, Zapol WM, Lowenstein E. Acute pulmonary sequestration of white blood cells produced by I.V. bolus of protamine after cardiopulmonary bypass. Anesthesiology 1984; 61:A49.

Morel DR, Zapol WM, Thomas SJ, et al. C5a and thromboxane generation association with pulmonary vaso- and bronchoconstriction during protamine reversal of heparin. Anesthesiology 1987; 66:597–604.

Morel DR, Lowenstein E, Nguyenduy T, et al. Acute pulmonary vasoconstriction and thromboxane release during protamine reversal of heparin anticoagulation in awake sheep: evidence for the role of reactive oxygen metabolites following nonimmunological complement activation. Circ Res 1988; 62:905–15.

Morrison DC, Roser JF, Cochrane CG, Henson PM. Two distinct mechanisms for the initiation of mast cell degranulation. Int Arch Allergy Appl Immunol 1975; 49:172–8.

Moscicki RA, Sockin SM, Corsello BF, Ostro MG, Bloch KJ. Anaphylaxis during induction of general anesthesia: subsequent evaluation and management. J Allergy Clin Immunol 1990; 86:325–32.

Moss J, Fahmy NR, Sunder N, Beaven MA. Hormonal and hemodynamic profile of an anaphylactic reaction in man. Circulation 1981; 63:210–13.

Moss J, Rosow CW, Savarese JJ, Philbin DM, Kniffen KJ. Role of histamine in the hypotensive action of d-tubocurarine in humans. Anesthesiology 1981; 55:19–25.

Moss J, Philbin DM, Rosow CE, Basta SJ, Gelb C, Savarese JJ. Histamine release by neuromuscular blocking agents in man. Klin Wochenschr 1982; 60:891–5.

Movat HZ. The role of histamine and other mediators in microvascular changes in acute inflammation. Can J Physiol Pharmacol 1987; 65:451–7.

Murano G. The "Hageman" connection: interrelationships of blood coagulation, fibro (geno)ysis, kinin generation, and complement activation. Am J Hematol 1978; 4:409–17.

Murray N, Lyons J, Chappell M. Crescentic glomerulonephritis: a possible complication of streptokinase treatment for myocardial infarction. Br Heart J 1986; 56:483–5.

Nagle JE, Fuscaldo JT, Fireman D. Paraben allergy. JAMA 1977; 237:1594–5.

Newfield P, Roizen MF. Hazards of rapid administration of vancomycin. Ann Intern Med 1979; 91:581.

Nicolas F, Villers D, Blanloeil Y. Hemodynamic pattern in anaphylactic shock with cardiac arrest. Crit Care Med 1984; 12:144–5.

Noel J, Rosenbaum LH, Gangadharan V, Stewart J, Galens G. Serum sickness-like illness and leukocytoclastic vasculitis following intracoronary arterial streptokinase. Am Heart J 1987; 113:395–7.

Nordström L, Fletcher R, Pavek K. Shock of anaphylactoid type induced by protamine: a continuous cardiorespiratory record. Acta Anaesthesiol Scand 1978; 22:195–201.

Norman PS, Lichtenstein LM, Ishizaka K. Diagnostic tests in ragweed hay fever. A comparison of direct skin tests, IgE antibody measurements, and basophil histamine release. J Allergy Clin Immunol 1973; 52:210–24.

North FC, Kettelkamp N, Hirshman CA. Comparison of cutaneous and in vitro histamine release by muscle relaxants. Anesthesiology 1987; 66:543–6.

Nossal GJV. The basic components of the immune system. N Engl J Med 1987; 316:1320–1325.

Nuttall GA, Murray MJ, Bowie EJW. Protamine-heparin-induced pulmonary hypertension in pigs: effects of treatment with a thromboxane receptor antagonist on hemodynamics and coagulation. Anesthesiology 1991; 74:138–45.

Oates JA, FitzGerald GA, Branch RA, Jackson EK, Knapp HR, Roberts LJ. Clinical implications of prostaglandin and thromboxane A_2 formation. N Engl J Med 1988; 319:689–98; 761–9.

Obeid AI, Johnson L, Potts J, Mookherjee S, Eich RH. Fluid therapy in severe systemic reaction to radiopaque dye. Ann Intern Med 1975; 83:317–20.

Ocelli G, Saban Y, Pruneta RM, Pourcher N, Michel AM, Maestracci P. Anaphylaxis to droperidol: two cases. Ann Fr Anesth Réanim 1984; 3:440–2.

O'Connor PC, Erskine JG, Pringle TH. Pulmonary oedema after transfusion with fresh frozen plasma. Br Med J 1981; 282:379–80.

Oertel T. Bee-sting anaphylaxis: the use of military antishock trousers. Ann Emerg Med 1984; 13:6:459–61.
O'Flaherty JT, Wykle RL. Biology and biochemistry of platelet-activating factor. Clin Rev Allergy 1983; 1:353–67.
O'Keefe J, Domalik-Wawrzynski L, Guerrero JL, Rosow CE, Lowenstein E, Powell WJ Jr. Local and neurally mediated effects of sufentanil on canine skeletal muscle vascular resistance. J Pharmacol Exp Ther 1987; 242:699–706.
Okuno T. Anti-penicillin antibodies in transfused blood. JAMA 1971; 218:95.
Olinger GN, Becker RM, Bonchek LI. Noncardiac pulmonary edema and peripheral vascular collapse following cardiopulmonary bypass; rare protamine reaction? Ann Thorac Surg 1980; 19:20–5.
Olridge A, Hollis TM. Aortic endothelial and smooth muscle histamine metabolism in experimental diabetes. Arteriosclerosis 1982; 2:142–50.
Olsson P, Hammarlund A, Pipkorn U. Wheal-and-flare reactions induced by allergen and histamine: evaluation of blood flow with laser doppler flowmetry. J Allergy Clin Immunol 1988; 82:291–6.
Ong R, Sullivan T. Detection and characterization of human IgE to cephalosporin determinants. J Allergy Clin Immunol 1988; 81:222.
Orange RP, Austen WG, Austen KF. Immunological release of histamine and slow-reacting substance of anaphylaxis from human lung. J Exp Med 1971; 134:136s–148s.
Orange RP, Donsky GJ. Anaphylaxis. In: Middleton E, Reed CE, Ellis EF, eds. Allergy: Principles and Practice. St. Louis, CV Mosby, 1978:563.
Orfan N, Patterson R, Dykewicz R. Severe angioedema related to ACE inhibitors in patients with a history of idiopathic angioedema. JAMA 1990; 264:1287–9.
Oswalt CE, Gales GA, Holmstrom FM. Pulmonary edema as a complication of acute airway obstruction. JAMA 1977; 238:1833–5.
Ottensmeyer EP, Whiting RF, Korn AP. Three-dimensional structure of herring sperm protamine Y-I with the aid of dark field electron microscopy. Proc Natl Acad Sci 1975; 72:4953–5.
Owen DAA, Harvey CA, Boyce MJ. Effects of histamine on the circulatory system. Klin Wochenschr 1982; 60:972–7.
Padfield A, Watkins J. Allergy to diazepam. Br Med J 1977; 1:575–6.
Paradis NA, Martin GB, Rosenberg J, et al. The effect of standard- and high-dose epinephrine on coronary perfusion pressure during prolonged cardiopulmonary resuscitation. JAMA 1991; 9:1139–22.
Park W, Balinget P, Kenmore P, Macnamara TE. Changes in arterial oxygen tension during total hip replacement. Anesthesiology 1973; 39:642–6.
Parker CW. Drug allergy. N Engl J Med 1975; 292:511–4; 732–6; 957–60.
Parker CW. Leukotrienes: their metabolism, structure, and role in allergic responses. In: Samuelsson B, Paoletti R, eds. Leukotrienes and other Lipoxygenase Products. New York, Raven Press, 1982: 115–26.
Parker WA, Martin ME, Reid MJ. Cephalosporins and the penicillin-allergic patient. N Engl J Med 1987; 319:520.
Patkar SA, Diamant B. Mechanism of histamine release from rat peritoneal mast cells. Klin Wochenschr 1982; 60:948–53.
Patrick RA, Johnson RE. Complement inhibitors. In: Annual Reports in Medicinal Chemistry, vol 15. London, Academic Press, 1980:193–201.
Patterson R, Anderson J. Allergic reactions to drugs and biologic agents. JAMA 1982; 248:2637–45.
Patterson R. Early recognition of allergic reactions to new drugs. J Allergy Clin Immunol 1984; 74:641–2.
Patterson R, DeSwarte RD, Greenberger PA, Grammer LC. Drug allergy and protocols for management of drug allergies. N Engl Reg Allergy Proceedings 1986; 4:325–42.

Pavek K, Wegmann A, Nordström L, Schwander D. Cardiovascular and respiratory mechanisms in anaphylactic and anaphylactoid shock reactions. Klin Wochenschr 1982; 60:941–7.
Payan DG. Neuropeptides and inflammation: the role of substance P. Ann Rev Med 1989; 40:341–52.
Payne R. The development and persistence of leukoagglutinins in parous women. Blood 1962; 19:411–24.
Pearce FL. Functional heterogeneity of mast cells from different species and tissues. Klin Wochenschr 1982; 60:954–7.
Pearce FL. Calcium and mast cell activation. Br J Clin Pharmacol 1985; 20:267S–274S.
Pearce FL, Ali H, Barrett KE, et al. Functional characteristics of mucosal and connective tissue mast cells of man, the rat and other animals. Int Arch Allergy Appl Immunol 1985; 77:274–6.
Pelc LR, Christensen CW, Gross GJ, Wartlier DC. Direct cardiac actions of the H_2 receptor agonists, impromidine and dimaprit. Eur J Pharmacol 1985; 107:379–84.
Peller JS, Bardana EJ Jr. Anaphylactoid reaction to corticosteroid: case report and review of the literature. Ann Allergy 1985; 54:302–5.
Petz LD. Immunologic reactions of humans to cephalosporins. Post-grad Med J 1971; 47:64–9.
Petz L. Immunologic cross-reactivity between penicillins and cephalosporins: a review. J Infect Dis 1978; 137:S74–S79.
Pevny I, Danhauser I. Anaphylaktischer shock während der narkose mit positivem hauttest auf fentanyl und alloferin. Anaesthesist 1981; 30:400–4.
Philbin DM, Moss J, Akins CW, et al. The use of H_1 and H_2 histamine antagonists with morphine anesthesia: a double-blind study. Anesthesiology 1981; 55:292–6.
Phillips H, Cole P, Lettin A. Cardiovascular effects of implanted acrylic bone cement. Br Med J 1971; 3:460–1.
Pienkowski MM, Kazmier WJ, Adkinson NF Jr. Basophil histamine release remains unaffected by clinical desensitization to penicillin. J Allergy Clin Immunol 1988; 82:171–8.
Pilato MA, Fleming NW, Katz NM, et al. Treatment of non-cardiogenic pulmonary edema following cardiopulmonary bypass with veno-venous extracorporeal membrane oxygenation. Anesthesiology 1988; 69:609–14.
Pineda AA, Taswell HF, Brzica SM Jr. Delayed hemolytic transfusion reaction: an immunologic hazard of blood transfusion. Transfusion 1978; 18:1–7.
Piper PJ. Release of active substances during anaphylaxis. Agents Actions 1976; 6:547–50.
Pitt BR. Metabolic functions of the lung and systemic vasoregulation. Fed Proc 1984; 43:2574–7.
Pixley RA, Schapira M, Colman RW. Effect of heparin on the inactivation rate of human activated factor XII by antithrombin III. Blood 1985; 86:198–203.
Plaut M. Histamine, H1 and H2 antihistamines, and immediate hypersensitivity reactions. J Allergy Clin Immunol 1979; 63:371–5.
Pollock I, Murdoch RD. Pharmacokinetics of infused histamine in normal, atopic, and urticarial subjects. J Allergy Clin Immunol 1989; 83:A218.
Popovsky MA, Abel MD, Moore SB. Transfusion-related acute lung injury associated with passive transfer of antileukocyte antibodies. Am Rev Respir Dis 1983; 128:185–9.
Popovsky MA, Moore SB. Diagnostic and pathogenetic considerations in transfusion-related acute lung injury. Transfusion 1985; 25:573–7.
Poppers PJ. Anaesthetic implications of hereditary angioneurotic oedema. Can J Anaesth 1987; 34:76–8.
Porter J, Jick H. Drug-induced anaphylaxis, convulsions, deafness, and extrapyramidal symptoms. Lancet 1977; 1:587.

Portier MM, Richet C. De l'action anaphylactique de certains venins. C R Soc Biol 1902; 54:170–2.
Powell JR, Brody JM. Participation of H_1 and H_2 histamine receptors in physiological vasodilator responses. Am J Physiol 1976; 231:1002–9.
Pretty HM, Fudenberg HH, Perkins HA, Gerbode F. Anti-gamma globulin antibodies after open heart surgery. Blood 1968; 32:205–16.
Prograis LJ, Brickman CM, Frank MM. C1-inhibitor. In: Murano G, ed. Protease Inhibitors of Human Plasma: Biochemistry and Pathophysiology. New York, PJD Publications, 1986: 303–50.
Pryse-Phillips WEM, Chandra RK, Rose B. Anaphylactoid reaction to methylprednisolone pulsed therapy for multiple sclerosis. Neurology 1984; 34:1119–20.
Radermacker M, Gustin M. An in vivo demonstration of the antianaphylactic effect of terbutaline. Clin Allergy 1981; 11:79–86.
Radford SG, Lockyer JA, Simpson PJ. Immunological aspects of adverse reactions to Althesin. Br J Anaesth 1982; 54:859–64.
Rafferty P, Holgate ST. Histamine and its antagonists in asthma. J Allergy Clin Immunol 1989; 84:144–50.
Raper RF, Fisher MMcD. Profound reversible myocardial depression after anaphylaxis. Lancet 1988; 1:386–8.
Ratnoff OD, Pensky J, Ogston D, Naff GB. The inhibition of plasma kallikrein, plasma permeability factor, and C1r subcomponent of the first component of complement by serum C1 esterase inhibitor. J Exp Med 1969; 129:215–331.
Ratnoff OD, Nossel HL. Wasp sting anaphylaxis. Blood 1983; 61:132–9.
Reed WP, Chick TW, Jutila K, Butler C, Goldblum S. Pulmonary leukostasis in fatal human pneumococcal bacteremia without pneumonia. Am Rev Respir Dis 1984; 130:1184–7.
Reinhardt D, Borchard V. H1 receptor antagonists: comparative pharmacology and clinical use. Klin Wochenschr 1982; 60:983–90.
Rent R, Ertel N, Eisenstein R, Gewurz H. Complement activation by interaction of polyanions and polycations: 1. Heparin-protamine induced consumption of complement. J Immunol 1975; 114:120–4.
Revak SD, Cochrane CG, Johnston AR, Hugli TH. Structural changes accompanying enzymatic activation of Hageman factor. J Clin Invest 1974; 54:619–27.
Revak SD, Cochrane CG. The relationship of structure and function in human Hageman factor: the association of enzymatic binding activities with separate regions of the molecule. J Clin Invest 1976; 57:852–60.
Revak SD, Cochrane CG, Griffin JH. The binding and cleavage characteristics of human Hageman factor during contact activation: a comparison of normal plasma with plasmas deficient in Factor XI, prekallikrein, or high molecular weight kininogen. J Clin Invest 1977; 59:1167–75.
Revenäs B. Anaphylactic shock in the monkey: early circulatory response in aggregate anaphylaxis. Uppsala, Doctoral thesis, 1979.
Revenäs B, Smedegård G, Arfors K. Anaphylactic shock in the monkey: respiratory mechanics, acidbox status, and blood gases. Acta Anaesthesiol Scand 1979; 23:278–84.
Revenäs B, Smedegård G. Aggregate anaphylaxis in the monkey: attenuation of the pulmonary response by pretreatment with indomethacin. Circ Shock 1981; 8:21–9.
Rhoden KJ, Meldrum LA, Barnes PJ. Inhibition of cholinergic neurotransmission in human airways by beta2-adrenoceptors. J Appl Physiol 1988; 65:700–5.
Rich CE, Drage CN. Severe complications of intravenous phytadione therapy: two cases with one fatality. Postgrad Med 1982; 72:303–6.
Rieder MJ, Uetrecht J, Shear NG, Cannon M, Miller M, Spielberg SP. Diagnosis of sulfonamide hypersensitivity reactions in vitro "rechallenge" with hydroxylamine metabolites. Ann Intern Med 1989; 110:286–9.

Rinaldo JE, Rogers RM. Adult respiratory distress syndrome: changing concepts of lung injury and repair. N Engl J Med 1982; 306:900–9.
Ring J, Seifert J, Messmer K, Brendel W. Anaphylactoid reactions due to hydroxyethel starch infusion. Eur Surg Res 1976; 8:389–99.
Ring J, Messmer K. Incidence and severity of anaphylactoid reactions to colloid volume substitutes. Lancet 1977; 1:466–9.
Ring J, Arroyave CM, Fritzler MJ, Tan EM. In vitro histamine and serotonin release by radiographic contrast media in man. J Allergy Clin Immunol 1978; 61:145.
Ring J, Stephan W, Brendel W. Anaphylactoid reactions to infusions of plasma protein and human serum albumin. Clin Allergy 1979; 9:89–97.
Ring J. In vitro studies involving histamine and lysosomal enzyme release from human peripheral leukocytes with different human serum albumin (HSA) preparations. Int Arch Allergy Appl Immunol 1984; 74:71–5.
Robertson EN, Booij LH, Fragen RJ, Crul JF. Intradermal histamine release by 3 muscle relaxants. Acta Anaesthesiol Scand 1983; 27:203–5.
Robinson JA, Klodnycky ML, Loeb HS, Racic MR, Gunnar RM. Endotoxin, prekallikrein, complement and systemic vascular resistance. Sequential measurements in man. Am J Med 1975; 59:61–7.
Roitt I, Brostoff J, Male D, eds. Immunology. St. Louis, CV Mosby, 1989.
Roizen MF, Rodgers GM, Valone FH, et al. Anaphylactoid reactions to vascular graft material presenting with vasodilation and subsequent disseminated intravascular coagulation. Anesthesiology 1989; 71:331–8.
Rosenblatt H, Lawlor G. Anaphylaxis. In: Lawlor G, Fisher T, eds. Manual of allergy and immunology. Boston, Little, Brown, 1981: 215–22.
Rosenthal ME, Dervinis A, Kassarich J. Bronchodilator activity of the prostaglandins, E_1 and E_2. J Pharmacol Exp Ther 1971; 178:541–8.
Rosow CE, Moss J, Philbin DM, Savarese JJ. Histamine release during morphine and fentanyl anesthesia. Anesthesiology 1982; 56:93–6.
Rosow CE, Philbin DM, Keegan CR, Moss J. Hemodynamics and histamine release during induction with sufentanil or fentanyl. Anesthesiology 1984; 60:489–91.
Ross JM, Murali MR, Delara TC, Cheron RG. Anaphylaxis and immunologic insulin resistance in a diabetic woman with ketoacidosis. Diabetes Care 1984; 7:276–9.
Ross JM. Allergy to insulin. Pediatr Clin North Am 1984; 31:675–87.
Royston D, Wilkes RG. True anaphylaxis to suxamethonium chloride: a case report. Br J Anaesth 1978; 50:611–5.
Royston D, Taylor KM, Bidstrup BP, Sapsfort RN. Effect of aprotinin on need for blood transfusion after repeat open-heart surgery. Lancet 1987; 2:1289–91.
Royston D. Aprotinin in open heart surgery: background and results in patients having aortocoronary bypass grafts. Perfusion 1990; 5(S):63–72.
Ruddy S, Gigli I, Austen KF. The complement system of man. N Engl J Med 1972; 287:489–95; 592–6; 642–6.
Rush B, Lee NLY. Clinical presentation of nonhaemolytic transfusion reactions. Anaesth Intensive Care 1980; 8:125–31.
Rydzynski K, Kolago B, Zaslonka J, Kuroczynski W. Distribution of mast cells in human heart auricles and correlation with tissue histamine. Agents Actions 1988; 23:273–5.
Safwat A, Dror A. Pulmonary capillary leak associated with methyl methacrylate during general anesthesia: a case report. Clin Orthop 1982; 168:59–63.
Sage D. Intradermal drug testing following anaphylactoid reactions during anaesthesia. Anaesth Intensive Care 1981; 9:381–6.
Sakuma I, Genovese A, Gross SS, et al. Histamine-induced atrioventricular conduction block is mediated by adenosine. Circulation 1988; 78:II–349.
Salem DN, Findlay SR, Isner JM, Konstam MA, Cohen PF. Comparison of histamine release effects of ionic and non-ionic radiographic contrast media. Am J Med 1986; 80:382–4.

Samuel T, Kolk AHJ, Rümke P. Autoimmunity to sperm antigens in vasectomized men. Clin Exp Immunol 1975; 21:65–74.

Samuel T. Antibodies reacting with salmon and human protamines in sera from infertile men and from vasectomized men and monkeys. Clin Exp Immunol 1977; 30: 181–7.

Samuel T. Differentiation between antibodies to protamines and somatic nuclear antigens by means of a comparative fluorescence study on swollen nuclei of spermatozoa and somatic cells. Clin Exp Immunol 1978; 32:290–8.

Samuel T, Linnet L, Rümke P. Post-vasectomy autoimmunity to protamines in relation to the formation of granulomas and sperm agglutinating antibodies. Clin Exp Immunol 1978; 33:251–69.

Samuelsson B, Hammarström S, Murphy RC, Borgeat P. Leukotrienes and slow reacting substance of anaphylaxis (SRS-A). Allergy 1980; 35:375–81.

Sanchez MB, Paolillo M, Chacon RS, et al. Protamine as a cause of generalized allergic reactions to NPH insulin. Lancet 1982; 1:1243.

Sandoz Inc. Sandimmune.® Drug bulletin, 1984.

Santrach PJ, Parker JL, Jones RT, Yunginger JW. Diagnostic and therapeutic applications of a modified radioallergosorbent test and comparison with the conventional radioallergosorbent test. J Allergy Clin Immunol 1981; 67:97–105.

Saucedo R, Erill S. Morphine-induced skin wheals: a possible model for the study of histamine release. Clin Pharmacol Ther 1985; 38:365–70.

Sauder RA, Hirshman CA. Protamine-induced histamine release in human skin mast cells. Anesthesiology 1990; 73:165–7.

Saxon A, Beall GN, Rohr AS, Adelman DC. Immediate hypersensitivity reactions to beta-lactam antibiotics. Ann Intern Med 1987; 107:204–15.

Schapira M, Scott DF, Colman RW. Protection of human plasma kallikrein from inactivation by C1 inhibitor and other protease inhibitors: the role of high molecular weight kininogen. Biochemistry 1981; 20:2738–43.

Schapira M, Scott CF, James A, et al. High molecular weight kininogen or its light chain protects human plasma kallikrein from inactivation by plasma protease inhibitors. Biochemistry 1982a; 21:567–72.

Schapira M, Scott CF, Colman RW. Contribution of plasma protease inhibitors to the inactivation of kallikrein in plasma. J Clin Invest 1982b: 462–8.

Schatz M, Wasserman S, Patterson R. The eosinophil and the lung. Arch Intern Med 1978; 142:1515–19.

Schatz M. Skin testing and incremental challenge in the evaluation of adverse reactions to local anesthetics. J Allergy Clin Immunol 1984; 74:606–16.

Schellenberg RR, Duff MJ, Foster A, Paddon HB. Histamine releases PGI_2 from human pulmonary artery. Prostagl 1986; 32:201–9.

Schellenberg RR, Ohtaka H, Paddon HB, Bramble SE, Rangno RE. Catecholamine responses to histamine infusion in man. J Allergy Clin Immunol 1991; 87:499–504.

Schleimer RP, MacGlashan DW Jr, Schulman ES, et al. Human mast cells and basophils-structure, function, pharmacology, and biochemistry. Clin Rev Allergy 1983; 1:327–41.

Schleimer RP, Schulman ES, MacGlashan DW Jr, et al. Effects of dexamethasone on mediator release from human lung fragments and purified human lung mast cells. J Clin Invest 1983; 71:1830–5.

Schleimer RP, MacGlashan DW Jr, Peters SP. Inflammatory mediators and mechanisms of release from purified human basophils and mast cells. J Allergy Clin Immunol 1984; 74:473–81.

Schmidt AP, Taswell HF, Gleich GJ. Anaphylactic transfusion reactions associated with anti-IgA antibody. N Engl J Med 1969; 280:188–93.

Schneiderman H, Hammerschmidt DE, McCall AR, Jacob HS. Fatal complement-induced leukostasis after diatrizoate injection. JAMA 1983; 250:2340–2.

Schnitzler S, Renner H, Pfüller W. Histamine release from rat mast cells induced by protamine sulfate and polyethylene imine. Agents Actions 1981; 11:73–4.
Schoeffter P, Godfraine T. Histamine receptors in the smooth muscle of human internal mammary artery and saphenous vein. Pharmacol Toxicol 1989; 64:64–71.
Schreiber AD, Kaplan AP, Austen KF. Inhibition by C1 INH of Hageman factor fragment activation of coagulation, fibrinolysis and kinin generation. J Clin Invest 1973; 52:1402.
Schreiber AD. Clinical immunology of the corticosteroids. Prog Clin Immunol 1977; 3:103–14.
Schreiber AD. Immunohematology. JAMA 1982; 248:1380–5.
Schuler TM, Frosch PJ, Arza D, Wahl R. Allergie vom Soforttyp: anaphylaktische reaktion auf aprotinin. Munch Med Wschr 1987; 129:816–7.
Schulman ES, Newball HH, Demers LM, Fitzpatrick FA, Adkinson NF. Anaphylactic release of thromboxane A_2, prostaglandin D_2, and prostacyclin from human lung parenchyma. Am Rev Respir Dis 1981; 124:402–6.
Schwartz LB. Enzyme mediators of mast cells and basophils. Clin Rev Allergy 1983; 1:397–416.
Schwartz H, Sher TH. Bisulfite sensitivity manifesting as allergy to local dental anesthesia. J Allergy Clin Immunol 1985; 75:525–7.
Schwartz LB, Metcalfe DD, Miller JS, Earl H, Sullivan T. Tryptase levels as an indicator of mast-cell activation in systemic anaphylaxis and mastocytosis. N Engl J Med 1987; 316:1622–6.
Schwartz LB, Yunginger JW, Miller J, Bokhari R, Dull D. Time course of appearance and disappearance of human mast cell tryptase in the circulation after anaphylaxis. J Clin Invest 1989; 83:1551–5.
Schwartz LB. Tryptase, a mediator of human mast cells. J Allergy Clin Immunol 1990; 86:594–8.
Schwarz A, McKenna E, Vaghy PL. Receptors for calcium antagonists. Am J Cardiol 1988; 62:3G–6G.
Scott HW, Parris WCV, Sandidge PC, Oates JA, Roberts LJ. Hazards in operative management of patients with systemic mastocytosis. Ann Surg 1983; 197:507–14.
Scott RPF, Savarese JJ, Basta SJ, et al. Atracurium: clinical strategies for preventing histamine release and attenuating the haemodynamic response. Br J Anaesth 1985; 57:550–3.
Sczeklik J, Dubiel JS, Mieczyslaw M, Puzik Z, Krol R, Horzela T. Effects of prostaglandin E_1 on pulmonary circulation in patients with pulmonary hypertension. Br Heart J 1978; 40:1397–401.
Sellow JE, Mendelson LM, Rosen JP. Anaphylactic reaction in skin test-negative patients. J Allergy Clin Immunol 1980; 65:400.
Serafin WE, Austen FK. Mediators of immediate hypersensitivity reactions. N Engl J Med 1987; 317:30–4.
Shapira N, Schaff HV, Piehler JM, White RD, Sill JC, Pluth JR. Cardiovascular effects of protamine sulfate in man. J Thorac Cardiovasc Surg 1982; 84:505–14.
Shapiro S, Siskin V, Slone D, Lewis GP, Jick H. Drug rash with ampicillin and other penicillins. Lancet 1969; 2:7628.
Sheagren JN. Septic shock and corticosteroids (editorial). N Engl J Med 1981; 305:456–8.
Sheffer AL, Fearon DT, Austen KF, Rosen FS. Tranexamic acid: preoperative prophylactic therapy for patients with hereditary angioneurotic edema. J Allergy Clin Immunol 1977; 60:38–40.
Sheffer AL, Pennoyer DS. Management of adverse drug reactions. J Allergy Clin Immunol 1984; 74:580–8.
Sheffer AL. Unravelling the mystery of idiopathic anaphylaxis. N Engl J Med 1984; 311:1248–9.
Sheffer AL, Tong AKF, Murphy GF, Lewis RA, McFadden ER, Austen KF. Exercise-

induced anaphylaxis: a serious form of physical allergy associated with mast cell degranulation. J Allergy Clin Immunol 1985; 75:479–84.
Sheffer AL. Anaphylaxis. J Allergy Clin Immunol 1985; 75:227–33.
Shehadi WH. Adverse reactions to intravascularly administered contrast media. Am J Roentgenol 1975; 124:145–52.
Shehadi WH, Toniolo G. Adverse reactions to contrast media. Radiology 1980; 136:299–302.
Sher MR, Suchar C, Lockey RF. Anaphylactic shock induced by oral desensitization to trimethoprim/sulfmethoxazole (TMP-SMZ). J Allergy Clin Immunol 1986; 77:133.
Shibata K, Atsumi T, Itorivchi Y, Mashimo K. Immunological cross-reactivities of cephalothin and its related compounds with benzylpenicillin (penicillin G). Nature 1966; 212:419–20.
Siegel J, Rent R, Gewurz H. Interactions of C-reactive protein with the complement system: I. Protamine-induced consumption of complement in acute phase sera. J Exp Med 1974; 140:637–47.
Silver PJ. Biochemical aspects of inhibition of low (km) cyclic adenosine monophosphate phosphodiesterase. Am J Cardiol 1989; 63:2A–8A.
Silverman JH, Van Hook C, Haponik EF. Hemodynamic changes in human anaphylaxis. Am J Med 1984; 77:341–44.
Simon RA, Shatz M, Stevenson DD, et al. Radiographic contrast media infusions: measurements of histamine, complement, and fibrin split products and correlation with clinical parameters. J Allergy Clin Immunol 1979; 63:281–8.
Simon RA, Green L, Stevenson DD. The incidence of sulfite sensitivity in an asthmatic population. J Allergy Clin Immunol 1982; 69:118.
Simon RA. Adverse reactions to drug additives. J Allergy Clin Immunol 1984; 74:623–30.
Simons FER: H_1-receptor antagonists: clinical pharmacology and therapeutics. J Allergy Clin Immunol 1989; 84:845–66.
Sinha AK, Colman RW. Prostaglandin E_1 inhibits platelet aggregation by a pathway independent of adenosine 3′,5′-monophosphate. Science 1978; 200:202–3.
Slade MS, Simmons RL, Yunis E, Greenberg LJ. Immunodepression after major surgery in normal patients. Surgery 1975; 78:363–72.
Slater JE. Rubber anaphylaxis. N Engl J Med 1989; 1126–30.
Smedegärd G, Revenäs B, Arfors K. Anaphylaxis in the monkey: hemodynamics and blood flow distribution. Acta Physiol Scand 1979; 106:191–8.
Smedegärd G, Revenäs B, Saldeen T. Aggregate anaphylaxis in the monkey: haematological and histological findings. Int Arch Allergy Appl Immunol 1980; 61:117–24.
Smedegärd G, Revenäs B, Lundberg C, Arfors K. Anaphylactic shock in monkeys passively sensitized with human reaginic serum: I. Hemodynamic and cardiac performance. Acta Physiol Scand 1981; 111:239–47.
Smedegärd G, Hedqvist P, Dahlén SE, Revenäs B, Hammarström Samuelsson B. Leukotriene C_4 affects pulmonary and cardiovascular dynamics in monkey. Nature 1982; 295:327–9.
Smith PL, Kagey-Sobotka A, Bleecker ER, et al. Physiologic manifestations of human anaphylaxis. J Clin Invest 1980; 66:1072–80.
Smith Laboratories. Chymodiactin® post marking surveillance report, 1984.
Sofer S, Bar-Ziv J, Scharf SM. Pulmonary edema following relief of upper airway obstruction. Chest 1984; 86:401–3.
Sogn DD. Penicillin allergy. J Allergy Clin Immunol 1984; 74:589–93.
Sogn DD. Prevention of allergic reactions to penicillin. J Allergy Clin Immunol 1987; 78:1051–2.
Solanki D, McCurdy PR. Delayed hemolytic transfusion reactions. JAMA 1978; 239:729–31.

Sold M, Rothhammer A. Life-threatening anaphylactoid reaction following etomidate. Anaesthetist 1985; 34:208–10.
Spaner D, Dolovich J, Tarlo S, Sussman G, Butto K. Hypersensitivity to natural latex. J Allergy Clin Immunol 1989; 83:1135–7.
Spruill FG, Minette LJ, Sturner WQ. Two surgical deaths associated with cephalothin. JAMA 1974; 229:440–1.
Squire JR. Tissue reactions to protein sensitization. Br Med J 1952; 1:1–7.
Stark BJ, Sullivan TJ. Biphasic and protracted anaphylaxis. J Allergy Clin Immunol 1986; 78:76–83.
Steen PA, Tinker JH, Pluth JR. Efficacy of dopamine, dobutamine, and epinephrine during emergence from cardiopulmonary bypass. Circulation 1978; 57:378–84.
Stellato C, de Paulis A, Cirillo R, Mastronardi P, Mazzarella B, Marone G. Heterogeneity of human mast cells and basophils in response to muscle relaxants. Anesthesiology 1991; 74:1078–86.
Stenlake JB, Waigh RD, Urwin J, et al. Atracurium conception and inception. Br J Anaesth 1983; 55:3S–5S.
Stenson WF, Parker CW. Metabolites of arachidonic acid. Clin Rev Allergy 1983; 1:369–84.
Sterback GL. Dermatologic problems. In: Rosen P, Baker FJ, Braen GR, et al., eds. Emergency Medicine: Concepts and Clinical Practice. St. Louis, CV Mosby, 1983: 1297.
Stevenson DD. Diagnosis, prevention, and treatment of adverse reactions to aspirin (ASA) and nonsteroidal anti-inflammatory drugs. J Allergy Clin Immunol 1984; 74:617–22.
Stevenson GW, Hall SC, Rudnick S, Seleny FL, Stevenson HC. The effect of anesthetic agents on the human immune response. Anesthesiology 1990; 72:542–52.
Stewart WJ, McSweeney SM, Kellett MA, et al. Increased risk of severe protamine reactions in NPH insulin-dependent diabetics undergoing cardiac catheterization. Circulation 1984; 70:788–92.
Stiles GL, Caron MG, Lefkowitz RJ. β-Adrenergic receptors: biochemical mechanisms of physiological regulation. Physiol Rev 1984; 64: 661–743.
Stoelting RK, Miller RD. Pharmacology of the autonomic nervous system. In: Miller RD, ed. Anesthesia. New York, Churchill Livingstone, 1981; 539–60.
Stoelting RK. Allergic reactions during anesthesia. Anesth Analg 1983; 62:341–56.
Stoelting RK, Henry DP, Verburg KM, McCammon RL, King RD, Brown JW. Haemodynamic changes and circulating histamine concentrations following protamine administration to patients and dogs. Can Anaesth Soc J 1984; 31:534–40.
Sullivan TJ. Cardiac disorders in penicillin induced anaphylaxis: association with intravenous therapy. JAMA 1982; 248:2161–2.
Sullivan TJ, Yecies LD, Shatz GS, Parker CW, Wedner HJ. Desensitization of patients allergic to penicillin using orally administered beta-lactam antibiotics. J Allergy Clin Immunol 1982; 69:275–82.
Sullivan TJ. Allergic reactions to antimicrobial agents: a review of reactions to drugs not in the beta lactam antibiotic class. J Allergy Clin Immunol 1984; 74:594–9.
Sullivan TJ. Facilitated haptenation of human proteins by penicillin (abstract). J Allergy Clin Immunol 1989; 83:255.
Sullivan TJ. Cross-reactions among furosemide, hydrochlorthiazide, and sulfonamides. JAMA 1991; 265:120–1.
Svensjoe A, Romempke K. Dose related antipermeability effects of terbutalene and its inhibition by a selective beta$_2$ receptor blocking agent. Agents Actions 1985; 16:1–2.
Swank DW, Moore SB. Roles of the neutrophil and other mediators in adult respiratory distress syndrome. Mayo Clin Proc 1989; 64:1118–32.
Szczeklik A. Adverse reactions to aspirin and nonsteroidal anti-inflammatory drugs. Ann Allergy 1987; 59:113–8.

Tan F, Jackman H, Skidgel RA, Szigmond EK, Erdös EG. Protamine inhibits plasma carboxypeptidase N, the inactivator of anaphylatoxins and kinins. Anesthesiology 1989; 70:267–75.

Tannenbaum H, Ruddy S, Schur PH. Acute anaphylaxis associated with serum complement depletion. J Allergy Clin Immunol 1975; 56:226–34.

Tanz RD, Kettlekamp N, Hirshman CA. The effect of calcium on cardiac anaphylaxis in guinea pig Lagendorff heart preparations. Agents Actions 1985; 16:415–28.

Tauber AI, Kabner N, Stechschulte PJ, Austen KF. Immunologic release of histamine and slow reacting substances of anaphylaxis from human lung vs effects of prostaglandins on release of histamine. J Immunol 1973; 111:27–32.

Teissner B, Brandslund I, Grunnet N, Hansen LK, Thellesen J, Svehag SE. Acute complement activation during an anaphylactoid reaction to blood transfusion and the disappearance rate of C3c and C3d from the circulation. J Clin Lab Immunol 1983; 12:63–7.

Terr AI. Anaphylaxis. Clin Rev Allergy 1985; 3–23.

Thaler M, Shamiss A, Orgad S, et al. The role of blood from HLA-homozygous donors in fatal transfusion-associated graft-versus-host disease after open-heart surgery. N Engl J Med 1989; 321:25–8.

Tharp MD, Suvonrungsi RT, Sullivan TH. IgE-mediated release of histamine from human cutaneous mast cells. J Immunol 1982; 130:1896–901.

Tharp MD, Thirlby R, Sullivan TJ. Gastrin induces histamine release from human cutaneous mast cells. J Allergy Clin Immunol 1984; 74:159–65.

Tharp MD, Kagey-Sobotka A, Fox CC, Marone G, Lichtenstein LM, Sullivan TJ. Functional heterogeneity of human mast cells from different anatomic sites: in vitro responses to morphine sulfate. J Allergy Clin Immunol 1987; 79:646–53.

Thornton JA, Lorenz W. Histamine and antihistamine in anaesthesia and surgery. Anaesthesia 1983; 38:373–9.

Thulstrip M. The influence of leukocyte and thrombocyte incompatibility of non-haemolytic transfusion reactions. Vox Sang 1971; 21:233–50.

Toda N. Responses to prostaglandins H_2 and I_2 of isolated dog cerebral and peripheral arteries. Am J Physiol 1980; 238(Heart Circ Physiol 7):H111–H117.

Toda N. Isolated human coronary arteries in response to vasoconstrictor substances. Am J Physiol 1983; 245:H937–H941.

Toda N. Mechanism of histamine actions in human coronary arteries. Circ Res 1987; 61:280–6.

Toda N. Heterogeneous responses to histamine in blood vessels. In: Vanhoutte P, ed. Vasodilatation: Vascular Smooth Muscle, Peptides, Autonomic Nerves, and Endothelium. New York, Raven Press, 1988:469–74.

Tomasi TB. Human immunoglobulin A. N Engl J Med 1968; 279:1327–30.

Tomicheck RC, Rosow CG, Philben DM, Moss J, Teplick RS, Schneider RC. Diazepam-fentanyl interaction—hemodynamic and hormonal effects in coronary artery surgery. Anesth Anal 1983; 62:881–4.

Toniolo C. Secondary structure prediction of fish protamines. Biochim Biophys Acta 1980; 626:420–7.

Toogood JH. Risk of anaphylaxis in patients receiving beta-blocker drugs. J Allergy Clin Immunol 1988; 81:1–5.

Travis DW, Todres ID, Shannon DC. Pulmonary edema associated with croup and epiglottitis. Pediatrics 1977; 59:695–8.

Turjanmaa K, Reunala T, Tuimala R, Karkkainen T. Allergy to latex gloves: Unusual complication during delivery. Br Med J 1988; 297:1029.

Vallota EH, Muller-Ebehard HJ. Formation of C3a and C5a anaphylatoxins in human serum after inhibition of the anaphylatoxin inactivator. J Exp Med 1973; 137:1109–23.

van Oeveren W, Jansen NJG, Bidstrup BP, et al. Effects of aprotinin on hemostatic mechanisms during cardiopulmonary bypass. Ann Thorac Surg 1987; 44:640–5.

Vashuk VV. Shock reaction following the repeated use of Trasylol. Clin Med 1971; 49:128–30.
Venkateswara Rao K, Anderson RC, O'Brien TJ. Successful renal transplantation in a patient with anaphylactic reaction to solu-medrol (methylprednisolone sodium succinate). Am J Med 1982; 72:161–3.
Verburg KM, Bowsher RR, Israel KS, Black HR, Henry DP. Histamine release by vancomycin in humans. Fed Proc 1985; 44:1247.
Vercellotti GM, Hammerschmidt DE, Jacob HS, Craddock PR. Activation of plasma complement by perfluorocarbon artificial blood, mechanism and prevention of adverse pulmonary reaction. Clin Res 1981; 29:572A.
Vercellotti GM, Hammerschmidt DE, Craddock PR, Jacob HS. Activation of plasma complement by perfluorocarbon artificial blood: probable mechanism of adverse pulmonary reactions in treated patients and rationale for corticosteroid prophylaxis. Blood 1982; 59:1299–304.
Verstraete M. Clinical application of inhibitors of fibrinolysis. Drugs 1985; 29:236–61.
Vervloet D, Nizankowska M, Arnaud A, Senft M, Alazi M, Charpin J. Adverse reactions to suxamethonium and other muscle relaxants under general anesthesia. J Allergy Clin Immunol 1983; 71:552–8.
Vervloet D, Arnaud A, Senft N, et al. Anaphylactic reactions to suxamethonium prevention of mediatory release by choline. J Allergy Clin Immunol 1985a; 76:225–31.
Vervloet D, Arnaud A, Senft M, et al. Anaphylactic reactions to suxamethonium prevention of mediator release by choline. J Allergy Clin Immunol 1985b; 76:222–5.
Vervloet D, Arnaud A, Senft M, et al. Leukocyte histamine release to suxamethonium in patients with adverse reactions to muscle relaxants. J Allergy Clin Immunol 1985c; 75:338–42.
Vigorito C, Russo P, Picotti GB, Chiariello M, Poto S, Marone G. Cardiovascular effects of histamine infusion in man. J Cardiovasc Pharmacol 1983; 5:531–7.
Vigorito C, Poto S, Picotti GB, Triggiani M, Marone G. Effects of activation of the H_1 receptor on coronary hemodynamics in man. Circulation 1986; 73:1175–82.
Vigorito C, Giordano A, De Caprio L, et al. Effects of histamine on coronary hemodynamics in man: role of H_1 and H_2 receptors. J Am Coll Cardiol 1987; 10:1207–13.
von der Graaf F, Koedam JA, Bouma BN. Inactivation of kallikrein in human plasma. J Clin Invest 1983; 71:149–58.
Vontz FK, Puestow EC, Cahill DJ Jr. Anaphylactic shock following protamine administration. Am Surg 1982; 48:549–51.
Vyas GN, Perkins HA, Yang YM. Healthy blood donors with selective absence of immunoglobulin A: prevention of anaphylactic transfusion reactions caused by antibodies to IgA. J Lab Clin Med 1975; 85:838–42.
Wakkers-Garritsen BG, Houwerziji J, Nater JP, Wakkers PJM. IgE mediated adverse reactivity to a radiocontrast medium. Ann Allergy 1976; 36:122–6.
Wall RT, Frank M, Hahn M. A review of 25 patients with hereditary angioedema requiring surgery. Anesthesiology 1989; 71:309–11.
Ward HN, Lipscomb T, Cawley LP. Pulmonary hypersensitivity reaction after blood transfusion. Arch Intern Med 1968; 122:362–6.
Ward HN. Pulmonary infiltrates associated with leukoagglutinin transfusion reactions. Ann Intern Med 1970; 73:669–94.
Warner MA, Weber JG, Warner ME. Etiologies and incidence of acute pulmonary edema in the immediate perioperative period. Anesth Analg 1990; 70:S421.
Warner JA, MacGlashan DW, Peters SP, Kagey-Sobotka A, Lichtenstein LM. The pharmacologic modulation of mediator release from human basophils. J Allergy Clin Immunol 1988; 82:432–8.
Wasserman SI, Goetzl EJ, Austen KF. Preformed eosinophil chemotactic factor of anaphylaxis (ECF-A). J Immunol 1974; 112:351–8.
Wasserman SI. Mediators of immediate hypersensitivity. J Allergy Clin Immunol 1983; 72:101–6.

Wasserman SI. Anaphylaxis. In: Middleton E, Reed CR, Ellis EF, eds. Allergy Principles and Practice. St. Louis, CV Mosby, 1983: 689–99.
Wasserman SI. Mast cell biology. J Allergy Clin Immunol 1990; 86:590–3.
Watkins J, Clark A, Appleyard TN, Padfield M. Immune mediated reactions to althesin (alphaxalone). Br J Anaesth 1976; 55:231.
Watkins J, Clarke RSJ. Report of a symposium: adverse responses to intravenous agents. Br J Anaesth 1978; 50:1159–64.
Watkins J. Anaphylactoid reactions to I.V. substances. Br J Anaesth 1979; 51:51–60.
Watkins J, Clarke RSJ, Fee JPH. The relationship between reported atopy or allergy and immunoglobulins: a preliminary study. Anaesthesia 1981; 36:582–5.
Watkins J, Salo M. Hypersensitivity response to drugs and plasma substitutes used in anesthesia and surgery. In: Watkins J, Salo M eds. Trauma, Stress and Immunity in Anaesthesia and Surgery. London, Butterworth & Co. Ltd., 1982:254–91.
Watkins J, Thornton JA. Immunological and nonimmunological mechanisms involved in adverse reactions to drugs. Klin Wochenschr 1982; 60:958–64.
Watkins J. Etomidate: an immunologically safe anesthetic agent. Anaesthesia 1983; 38 (suppl):34–8.
Watson RA, Ansbacher R, Barry M, Deshon GE, Ogee RE. Allergic reaction to protamine: a late complication of elective vasectomy? Urology 1983; 22:493–5.
Weatherbee TC, Esterbrooks DJ, Katz DA, Aronow WS, Kenik JG, Mohiuddin SM. Serum sickness following selective intracoronary streptokinase. Curr Ther Res 1984; 35:433–8.
Webb-Johnson DC, Andrews JL Jr. Bronchodilator therapy. N Engl J Med 1977; 297:476–82.
Webster BH. Clinical presentation of haemolytic transfusion reactions. Anaesth Intensive Care 1980; 8:115–19.
Weiler JM, Freiman P, Shareath MD, et al. Serious adverse reactions to protamine sulfate: are alternatives needed? J Allergy Clin Immunol 1985; 75:297–303.
Weiler JM, Gellhaus MA, Carter JG, et al. A prospective study of the risk of an immediate adverse reaction to protamine sulfate during cardiopulmonary bypass surgery. J Allergy Clin Immunol 1990; 85:713–9.
Weishaar RE, Burrows SD, Kobylarz DC, Quade MM, Evans DB. Multiple molecular forms of cyclic nucleotide phosphodiesterase in cardiac and smooth muscle and in platelets: isolation, characterization, and effects of various reference phosphodiesterase inhibitors and cardiotonic agents. Biochem Pharmacol 1986; 35:787–800.
Weiss JW, Drazen JM, Coles N, et al. Bronchoconstrictor effects of leukotriene C in humans. Science 1982; 216:196–8.
Weiss JW, Drazen JM, McFadden R Jr, et al. Airway constriction in normal humans produced by inhalation of leukotriene D. JAMA 1983; 249:2814–23.
Weiss ME, Adkinson NF Jr. Immediate hypersensitivity reactions to penicillin and related antibiotics. Clin Allergy 1988; 18:515–40.
Weiss ME, Levy JH. Allergic and transfusion reactions. In: Speiss BD, Vender JS, eds. Acute Postoperative Care. Philadelphia, WB Saunders, in press.
Weiss ME, Nyhan D, Peng Z, et al. Association of protamine IgE and IgG antibodies with life-threatening reactions to intravenous protamine. N Engl J Med 1989; 320:886–92.
Weiss WA, Gilman JS, Catenacci AJ, Osterberg AE. Heparin neutralization with polybrene administered intravenously. JAMA 1958; 166:603–7.
Weissman G, Smolen JE, Korchak HM. Release of inflammatory mediators from stimulated neutrophils. N Engl J Med 1980; 303:27–34.
Weller PF. Eosinophilia. J Allergy Clin Immunol 1984; 73:1–10.
Whalen JP. Hypersensitivity to cimetidine. J Clin Pharmacol 1985; 25:610.
Whaley K. Complement in Health and Disease. Boston, MTP Press, 1987.

White MV. The role of histamine in allergic diseases. J Allergy Clin Immunol 1990; 86:599–605.
White RD. Cardiovascular pharmacology, part 1. In: McIntyre KM, Lewis AJ, eds. Textbook of Advanced Cardiac Life Support. Dallas, American Heart Association, 1981: VIII-4.
Wide L, Juhlin L. Detection of penicillin allergy of the immediate type by radioimmunoassay of reagins (IgE) to penicillin conjugates. Clin Allergy 1971; 1:171–7.
Wide L. Clinical significance of measurements of reaginic (IgE) antibody by RAST. Clin Allergy 1973; 3:583–95.
Wiggins CA, Dykewicz MS, Patterson R. Idiopathic anaphylaxis: classification, evaluation, and treatment of 123 patients. J Allergy Clin Immunol 1988; 82:849–56.
Wiggins RC, Cochrane CG, Griffin JH. Rabbit blood coagulation factor XI: mechanism of activation by rabbit Hageman factor. Thromb Res 1979; 15:487.
Wiggins RC, Cochrane CC. Kinins and kinin-forming system. In: Dale MM, Foreman J, eds. Textbook of Immunopharmacology. London, Blackwell Scientific Publications, 1984:158–69.
Winslow CM, Austen KF. Enzymatic regulation of mast cell activation and secretion by adenylate cyclase and cyclic AMP-dependent protein kinases. Fed Proc 1982; 41:22–9.
Withington DE, Leung KBP, Bromley L, Scadding GK, Pearce FL. Basophil histamine release: a study in allergy to suxamethonium. Anaesthesia 1987; 42:850–4.
Wolff AA, Levi R. Histamine and cardiac arrhythmias. Circ Res 1986; 58:1–16.
Woodward JK. Pharmacology of antihistamines. J Allergy Clin Immunol 1990; 86:606–12.
Yanagihara Y, Shida T. Immunological studies on patients who recieved aprotinin therapy. Jpn J Allergol 1985; 34:899–904.
Youngman PR, Taylor KM, Wilson JD. Anaphylactoid reactions to neuromuscular blocking agents: a commonly undiagnosed condition? Lancet 1983; 2:597–9.
Zapol WM, Falker J, eds. Acute Respiratory Failure. New York, Marcel Dekker, 1985.
Zeiss CR, Grammer LC, Levitz D. Comparison of the radioallergosorbent test and a quantitative solid-phase radioimmunoassay for the detection of ragweed-specific immunoglobulin E antibody in patients undergoing immunotherapy. J Allergy Clin Immunol 1981; 67:105–10.
Zucker-Pinchoff B, Ramanathan S. Anaphylactic reaction to epidural fentanyl. Anesthesiology 1989; 71:599–601.
Zweiman B. Mast cells in human disease. Clin Rev Allergy 1983; 1:417–26.

Index

Abdomen, examination of, after anaphylactic reactions, 177
Abdominal pain, in anaphylaxis, 19
ABO blood groups, antibodies against, 8
Acetylcholine, 67
Acid-base status, 169. *See also* Metabolic acidosis
Acid hydrolases, 43
Acquired immunodeficiency syndrome, 11
Activated partial thromboplastin times, in anaphylaxis, 30
Adenylate cyclase, 146
β_2-Adrenergic agents
   for bronchospasm, 171–172
   metered-dose inhalational therapy with, 171–172
     adaptor for administering, 172f
   in treatment of anaphylaxis, 134
α_1-Adrenergic agonists, 143
β_1-Adrenergic agonists, 143
β_2-Adrenergic agonists, 146
   antipermeability effects of, 160
β-Adrenergic blocking agents, and vasodilation after epinephrine administration, 168
α-Adrenergic receptor stimulation, by catecholamines, 143–144
β-Adrenergic receptor stimulation, by catecholamines, 146
Adult respiratory distress syndrome, 55, 180–182. *See also* Respiratory distress

Adverse drug reaction(s), 121. *See also* Allergic drug reaction(s)
   causes of, 121
   frequency of, in patients with atopy, 124
   incidence of, 121
   predictable, 121–122
     characteristics of, 122t
     classification of, 122f
     versus unpredictable, 121
   unpredictable, 122–124
     classification of, 123f
AIDS. *See* Acquired immunodeficiency syndrome
Air embolism, 141
Air trapping, prevention of, 171
Airway
   evaluation, in anaphylactic reactions, 169–170
   inflammation, in anaphylaxis, mediators of, 26t
   management, in initial therapy of anaphylaxis, 162–163
   manipulation, in patients with hereditary angioedema, 61–62
   obstruction, in anaphylaxis, 18, 18t, 26–27
   mechanisms of, 25f
Albumin (human serum), anaphylactic/anaphylactoid reactions to, 85t, 107
Albuterol, 171–172
Alcuronium, anaphylactic/anaphylactoid reactions to, 90, 90t, 92

Alfentanil
  administration of, and histamine release, 74
  dilution used for skin testing, 128t
Allergen
  identification
    in anaphylactic reactions, 126
    skin testing for, 126–129
  suspected
    intravenous challenges with, antibody levels after, 129
    stopping administration of, 162
Allergic drug reaction(s), 4, 83–84, 122–124. *See also* Adverse drug reaction(s)
  diagnosis of, 121
  diagnostic criteria for, 123
  prevalence of, 121
  risk of, and previous reactions to that drug, 125
Allergic patient(s)
  management of, 124–126
  preoperative considerations with, 121–134
Allergic reaction(s), 8
  definition of, 3
  to drugs. *See* Allergic drug reaction(s)
  type I, 13
Allergic rhinitis, 8
Alpha interferon, 11
Alphaxalone/alphadolone, 84, 86
Althesin. *See* Alphaxalone/alphadolone
Alveolar edema, in anaphylaxis, 29
Alypin. *See* Amiydricaine
Amides
  allergic reactions to, 88
  anaphylactic/anaphylactoid reactions to, 85t
  indications for, 88–89
ε-Aminocaproic acid, 154
Aminoglycosides, anaphylactic/anaphylactoid reactions to, 85t
Aminophylline, 190
  antiinflammatory action of, 150
  effects on respiratory function, 149–150
  indications for, 145t, 172–173
  mechanism of action, 149–150
  pharmacologic effects of, 145t, 149

  in treatment of pulmonary hypertension and right heart failure, 159
Amiydricaine, classification of, 89t
Amrinone, 202
  cardiovascular effects of, 150
  hemodynamic effects of, 150, 151f
  indications for, 145t
  mechanism of action, 149
  pharmacologic effects of, 145t
  in treatment of pulmonary hypertension and right heart failure, 159, 173
Anamnestic responses, 3
Anamnestic responses, to transfused red blood cells, 99
Anaphylactic mediators. *See* Mediators
Anaphylactic reaction(s), 8. *See also* Anaphylaxis
  agents most likely to cause, 84, 85t
  allergen identification in, 126
  cause of, determining, 126–132
  fatal, 93
  mediators of. *See* Mediators
  pathophysiologic changes producing, 52f
  patients with prior history of, management of, 125–126, 206
  perioperative, incidence of, 83
  pretreatment for, 133–134, 195
  prevention of, 205–206
  protracted, management of, 161
  treatment protocol for, 161
Anaphylactic shock
  cardiac output during, 22–23
  irreversible, 183
  mortality rate with, 161
  persistent hypotension after, 180
  resuscitation after, 181
Anaphylactoid reaction(s)
  agents most likely to cause, 84, 85t
  agents producing, 51
  during anesthesia, incidence of allergic history in patients with, 124, 124t
  definition of, 51
  pathogenesis of, 53f
  pathophysiologic changes producing, 52f
  pathways for, 51

Calcium *(continued)*
  pretreatment for, 133–134
  prevention of, 205–206
  treatment protocol for, 161
Anaphylatoxin(s), 10, 13, 115
  complement, 54–55
    biologic effects of, 55t
    histamine release caused by, 77–79
Anaphylaxis, 9t, 42–43. *See also* Anaphylactic reaction(s)
  activation of coagulation system during, 30, 51, 56, 57f
  chemotactic factors in, 13, 26t, 42–43
  clinical observations of patients after, 175
  definition of, 3
  dextran-induced, 29, 85t, 107
  diagnosis of, 135
  differential diagnosis of, 135–141, 136t
  dog model for, 13
  effector cells of, 14
  first report of, 3
  immediate cause of death in, 28
  immunoglobulin E-mediated, 13, 15f
  immunoglobulin G-mediated, 13
  initial cell activation in, 13–14
  initial therapy for, 162t, 162–166
  initiation of, 13–17
  intraoperative, 19–21, 20t
  management of, 161–174
  mechanisms of, 3
  mediators of. *See* Mediators
  mortality rate from, 83–84
  onset of reaction, 17, 17f
  pathologic findings in, 28–30
  pathophysiology of, 3, 21–28
  in patients with preexisting asthma, 27
  perioperative, epidemiologic studies of, 21
  pretreatment for, 133–134, 195, 206
  prompt recognition of, 206
  recurrence of, 170, 175
  respiratory involvement during, 42
    mediators of, 26t
    pathologic features of, 26t
  risk of, in patients with allergic history, 124

  secondary treatment for, 162t, 167–170
  signs and symptoms of, 3, 18t, 18–19, 206
  therapeutic approaches to, 144f
Anesthesia
  complement activation during, 55
    agents producing, 55, 56t
  effects of, on immune response, 11
Anesthetic agent(s)
  administration of, precipitous hypotension after, 135
  anaphylactic/anaphylactoid reactions to, 84–93, 85t
  cross-reactions between, 126
  discontinuation of, during anaphylaxis, 163
  patient with history of allergic reaction to, approach to, 125–126, 206
Anesthetic management, in patients with hereditary angioedema, 61–62
Angina, histamine-induced, 40–41
Angioedema
  acquired, 61
  in anaphylaxis, 19, 27–28
  with angiotensin converting enzyme inhibitors, 49
  definition of, 27
  hereditary
    cardinal symptoms of, 60
    contact activation and, 60–61
    diagnosis of, 138
    management of surgical patient with, 61–62
  transfusion-associated, 102
Angioneurotic edema. *See* Angioedema, hereditary
Angiotensin-converting enzyme. *See* Kininase II
Angiotensin-converting enzyme inhibitors, 49
Antibiotic(s)
  anaphylactic/anaphylactoid reactions to, 84, 85t, 93–97
  histamine release caused by, 64t, 65, 65f
  intraoperative administration of, 206

Antibody(ies), 5–8. *See also* Immunoglobulin(s)
  definition of, 4–5
  levels of, after intravenous challenges of suspected allergen, 129
  serum, 6
  structures of, 5, 5f
  synthesis of, 5–6
Anticholinergic drug(s)
  mechanism of action, 152
  for severe bronchospasm, 172
  in treatment of anaphylaxis, 152
Antigen(s)
  complete, 4, 4t
  definition of, 4
  immunologic response to, factors influencing, 15
  molecules that function as, 4t
  polyvalent, 13
  properties of, 4–5
Antigen-antibody interaction, 10
  immunologic activation during, 53
Antigen-immunoglobulin E interactions, cutaneous mast cells as immunologic window to evaluate, 28
Antihistamine(s)
  as adjuvant therapy, 167
  anaphylactic/anaphylactoid reactions to, 85t, 97
  indications for, 145t
  parenteral formulations of, 148t
  pharmacologic effects of, 145t
  pretreatment with, 148, 206
  receptor effects of, 145t
  site of action, 148
  in treatment of anaphylaxis, 143, 148–149
Antileukocyte antibodies, 101
α_2-Antiplasmin, 58t
Antithrombin III, 57, 58t
α_1-Antitrypsin, 57, 58t
Aprotinin, 58–60, 154
  activity of, 97
  anaphylactic/anaphylactoid reactions to, 85t, 97–98
Arachidonic acid
  in anaphylaxis, 48–49
  metabolism, 14, 17
  and nonsteroidal antiinflammatory drugs, 112
  metabolites, 43–46
Arterial pressure. *See also* Hypotension; Mean arterial pressure
  in anaphylaxis, 23
  effects of histamine infusion on, 36t, 36
    diastolic, 36t, 36
    systolic, 36t, 36
Arylsulfatase, 42
Asphyxiation, in anaphylaxis, 28
Aspirin, patient with history of allergic reaction to, approach to, 125–126
Asthma, 26–27
  versus anaphylaxis, 136
  extrinsic, 8, 9t
  and nonsteroidal antiinflammatory drugs, 125
  pathologic features of, 26–27
  prostaglandin $F_2\alpha$ in, 46
  pulmonary dysfunction in, 42
Atarax. *See* Hydroxyzine
Atenolol, and hemodynamic response to epinephrine administration, 168, 176
Atracurium, 66
  administration of, 205
  anaphylactic/anaphylactoid reactions to, 85t, 90, 90t
  dilution used for skin testing, 128t
  hemodynamic response to, 67, 70f
  histamine release caused by, 63, 64t, 68–69, 73, 80
  mast cell degranulation by, 80
  molecular structure responsible for, 70
  wheal and flare responses to, 68–72, 71f–72f
Atrioventricular nodal conduction, histamine's actions on, 36–37
Atropine
  anaphylactic/anaphylactoid reactions to, 85t, 98
  dilution used for skin testing, 128t
  pharmacologic effects of, 152
Aztreonam, 96

Barbiturate(s)
  allergy to, skin testing in evaluation of, 126
  anaphylactic/anaphylactoid reactions to, 85t, 86
    in patients with history of allergy or atopy, 124
    histamine release caused by, 64t, 65–66
Basophil(s)
  activation of, factors influencing, 15
  granular constituents of, 31, 32t
  granule size of, 14
  location of, 14
  membrane receptors for immunoglobulin E, 14
  normal physiologic role of, 14
  in pathogenesis of immediate hypersensitivity reactions, 14–17
Bee-sting reactions, 8
Benadryl. See Diphenhydramine
Benzocaine, classification of, 89t
Benzodiazepines, anaphylactic/anaphylactoid reactions to, 84, 85t, 86
Benzylisoquinoline-derived muscle relaxants
  adverse hemodynamic reactions to, 67
  allergic reactions to, 83
  histamine release caused by, 63, 64t, 67–72
  histamine-releasing potency of, 67–68
  mast cell degranulation by, 80
Beta-lactam antibiotics, new classes of, anaphylactic/anaphylactoid reactions to, 96
Bisulfite, 88, 109
Bleeding, in hemolytic transfusion reactions, 98
Blood glucose, measured during epinephrine infusions, 181
Blood group antigens, 8, 10
Blood pressure. See also Arterial pressure; Hypotension; Mean arterial pressure; Systemic vascular resistance
  monitoring, automated, in recovery room and intensive care unit, 179
Blood products, 205
  anaphylactic/anaphylactoid reactions to, 84, 85t, 98. See also Transfusion reactions
  leukocyte-poor, 101
Blood/surface interaction
  contact activation by, in generation of intrinsic coagulation cascade, kallikrein and plasmin, 58, 59f
  inflammatory response after, effects of drugs used to inhibit, 58, 59f
Blood urea nitrogen, evaluated after persistent hypotension, 178
Bone cement. See Methylmethacrylate
Bradykinin
  in anaphylaxis, 26t, 48
  biologic properties of, 47f, 48, 115
  effect on vascular responses, 47f
  in gram-negative bacteremia, 60
  vasodilation produced by, 23t
Bronchial hyperresponsiveness, inflammatory cell-induced, 146
Bronchoconstriction
  leukotrienes in, 44–45
  platelet-activating factor in, 48
  prostaglandin-induced, 45–46
Bronchospasm, 83, 136
  in anaphylaxis, 21, 22t, 22, 26–27
    mechanisms of, 25f
    mediators of, 26t
  persistent, 196
  refractory, 167–168
    treatment of, 170–171, 171t
  and right ventricular failure, 170, 170f
  severe, treatment of, 171–173
  transfusion-associated, 102
Bupivicaine
  classification of, 89t
  dilution used for skin testing, 128t
Butacaine, classification of, 89t
Butyn. See Butacaine

Calcium, 144, 146, 153–154, 197
  administration of, increased pulmonary vasoconstriction seen with, 203
  in anaphylaxis, 48–49
  effects of, on mast cell and basophil secretory activity, 16–17

in vascular relaxation and vasodilation, 47f
Calcium channel (entry) blockers, 158, 203
  mechanism of action, 153
  in pretreatment for anaphylactic reactions, 153
  in treatment of anaphylaxis, 144f
Calcium channels, functional heterogeneity of, 153
Calcium chloride, 153–154
Calcium-dependent phospholipase A_2, 17
Calcium ionophores, histamine release caused by, 64t
Capillary permeability
  histamine-induced, 33, 41
  increased, pharmacologic approaches to, 160
Carbapenems, 96
Carbocaine. See Mepivacaine
Carboxypeptidase N, 49, 115
Cardiac dysfunction. See also Right heart failure
  acute, in anaphylaxis, 23–24
Cardiac index
  in anaphylaxis, 24f
  effects of histamine infusion on, 36t, 36
Cardiac output
  during anaphylactic/anaphylactoid reactions, 20t, 23
  decreased, during anaphylactic shock, 22–23
  effects of histamine infusion on, 36t, 36
  monitoring, 180
Cardiogenic shock, 139
  signs and symptoms of, 137
Cardiopulmonary bypass
  contact activation and, 58–60
  in treatment of refractory hypoxemia, 173
  in treatment of right ventricular failure, 174
Cardiovascular collapse
  in anaphylaxis, 21–25
    in intubated patients, 20t
    clinical manifestations of, 31

with intraoperative anaphylaxis, 19–21
with mastocytosis, 138
Cardiovascular system
  in anaphylaxis, 31
    pathologic findings in, 29
    signs and symptoms in, 18t, 19
  examination of, after anaphylaxis, 176
Catecholamine(s)
  effects on α_1-, β_1-, and β_2-adrenergic receptors, 143–144, 145t, 146
  infusions of, indications for, 167–168
  pharmacologic effects of, 145t
  for pulmonary hypertension and right ventricular failure, 173
  receptor effects of, 145t
  in treatment of anaphylactic reactions, 143–148
  indications for, 145t, 167–168
Cefazolin, suspected anaphylaxis to, 187f, 187–188
Cell-mediated immunity, 9t, 10
  abnormalities in, 10–11
Central venous cannula, 179
Central venous pressure, during anaphylactic/anaphylactoid reactions, 20t
Cephalosporins
  anaphylactic/anaphylactoid reactions to, 85t, 95–96
  and penicillins, cross-reactivity between, 95–96
Cephalothin, dilution used for skin testing, 128t
C1 esterase, deficiency of, 60–61
C1 esterase inhibitor, 53, 54f, 57, 58t, 60
  biologic half-life of, 62
  deficiency of, 61
  replacement therapy with, 61–62
cGMP phosphodiesterase, 149
Chemotactic factors. See also Eosinophilic chemotactic factor of anaphylaxis; Neutrophilic chemotactic factor
  in anaphylaxis, 13, 26t, 42–43
  in immediate hypersensitivity reactions, 42

Chest, examination of, after anaphylaxis, 176–177
Chest discomfort, in anaphylaxis, 18, 18t
Chest radiograph, following resuscitation after anaphylaxis, 177
Chlorpheniramine, 148t
  indications for, 145t
  pharmacologic effects of, 145t
  receptor effects of, 145t
Chlorprocaine, classification of, 89t
Chlor-Trimeton. *See* Chlorpheniramine
Chondroitin 4 and 6 sulfates, in basophils, 43
Chromogen, definition of, 131
Chymase, in mast cells, 43
Chymodiactin, 206
  immunoglobulin E concentration, and chymopapain injections, 132
ChymoFAST, 106
Chymopapain
  allergy to
    preoperative evaluation for, 205–206
    skin testing in evaluation of, 126
  anaphylactic/anaphylactoid reactions to, 84, 85t, 106
    despite pretreatment of, 194f, 195–196
  immunoglobulin E antibody to
    enzyme-linked immunosorbent assay for, 131
    radioallergosorbent test for, 131
Cimetidine, 148t, 167
  anaphylactic/anaphylactoid reactions to, 97
  indications for, 145t
  pharmacologic effects of, 145t
  receptor effects of, 145t
C1 inhibitor. *See* C1 esterase inhibitor
Clotting parameters, after anaphylaxis, 178
Coagulation. *See also* Disseminated intravascular coagulation
  activation of, 30, 51, 56, 57f
  interactions with classical complement cascade, 56
Codeine, 92
  histamine release caused by, 63, 64t, 74f, 74–77

Colloid solutions
  anaphylactic/anaphylactoid reactions to, 85t, 106–107
  intravascular volume expansion with, 163
Complement
  activation of, 6, 10, 51–54, 54f, 56, 57f
    during anesthesia, 55
    agents producing, 55, 56t
    drugs that inhibit, 154, 156t
    by endotoxin, 55
    immunoglobulin G in, 6, 7t
    immunoglobulin M in, 7t
    and pathologic effects, 54–55
    by protamine-heparin interactions, 115
  alternative pathway, 53–54, 54f
  anaphylatoxins, 54–55
    biologic effects of, 55t
  classical pathway, 53, 54f
  coagulation interactions with, 56
  interactions with fibrinolytic pathway, 56
  effects of, reversal of, 154, 156t
  histamine release caused by, 64t
  levels of, followed during anaphylactoid reactions, 130
Complement system, 51–55
Complete blood count, 177
Complete heart block, during histamine infusions, 37
Consciousness, loss of, in anaphylaxis, 18t, 19, 22t
Contact activation, 56–62
  by blood/surface interaction, in generation of intrinsic coagulation cascade, kallikrein and plasmin, 58, 59f
  and cardiopulmonary bypass, 58–60
  clinical significance of, 58–62
  by factor XII, 56, 57f
  and hereditary angioedema, 60–61
  plasma inhibitors of, 57, 58t
  plasma system, 51
  regulation of, 57
  and sepsis, 60
Contact dermatitis, 9t
  with penicillin, 94

Coronary arteries, effects of histamine on, 38f, 38–40
Coronary blood flow, effects of histamine on, 40–41
Coronary spasm, histamine's role in, 40–41
Coronary vascular changes, histamine-induced, 40–41
Coronary vasoconstriction, H_1-mediated, 39
Cor pulmonale, in anaphylaxis, 27
Corticosteroid(s), 67, 154
  as adjuncts to therapy in anaphylactic reactions, 152
  anaphylactic/anaphylactoid reactions to, 85t, 108
  effects of, on allergic reactions, 152
  indications for, 168, 172
  mechanism of action, 152
  pharmacologic effects of, 145t
  pretreatment with, 134, 188, 206
  in treatment of anaphylaxis, 143, 150–152
Coughing, in anaphylaxis, 22t
Creatinine, evaluated after persistent hypotension, 178
Cremophor EL. *See* Polyoxyethylated castor oil
Cremophor-solubilized drugs, anaphylactic/anaphylactoid reactions to, 84, 85t, 86–87
Cricothyrotomy, 163
CVP. *See* Central venous pressure
Cyanosis, 19
  in anaphylaxis, 22t
  in intubated patients, 20t
Cyclic adenosine monophosphate, 146, 149, 164
  increasing, in vascular smooth muscle, in therapy of acute pulmonary vasoconstriction, 158
Cyclic adenosine monophosphate-specific phosphodiesterase, 149
  inhibitors of, 150
Cyclic nucleotide(s)
  formation in pulmonary vasculature, stimulation of, 159, 159f
  metabolism, in anaphylaxis, 48–49
  in vascular relaxation and vasodilation, 47f
Cyclic nucleotide phosphodiesterase(s), 149
Cyclomethycaine, classification of, 89t
Cyclooxygenase, metabolism, 14, 17, 44–46
Cyclooxygenase inhibitors, 154, 155f, 156
Cyclosporin, anaphylactic/anaphylactoid reactions to, 85t, 108
Cytotoxic antibodies, 10
Cytotoxic reactions, 9t, 10
Cytotoxic-suppressor cells, in acquired immunodeficiency syndrome, 11

Dacron, adverse reactions to, 120
DAP. *See* Diastolic aortic pressure
Deaths
  due to adverse drug reactions, frequency of, 121
  with anaphylactic shock, 161
  in anaphylaxis, 83–84
    immediate cause of, 28
  after radiocontrast media administration, 118
  with transfusion-related acute lung injury, 104
Delayed hypersensitivity reaction(s), 9t, 10
Dexamethasone, 190–191
  in pretreatment for anaphylaxis, 134
Dextrans, anaphylactic/anaphylactoid reactions to, 29, 85t, 107
Diacylglycerol, 144
Diacylglycerol lipase, 44
Diarrhea, in anaphylaxis, 19
Diastolic aortic pressure, during anaphylactic/anaphylactoid reactions, 20t
Diazepam, anaphylactic/anaphylactoid reactions to, 86
Dibucaine, classification of, 89t
Dicycloine, classification of, 89t
Dihydropyridine analogues, mechanism of action, 153
Dimaprit, 37
Dimethylthiourea, 155f, 156

Diphenhydramine, 148t, 167
  indications for, 145t
  pharmacologic effects of, 145t, 148
  receptor effects of, 145t, 148
Diprivan. See Propofol
Dipyridamole, mechanism of action, 149
Disseminated intravascular coagulation
  after anaphylaxis, 178
  in hemolytic transfusion reactions, 98–99
  with vascular graft reaction, 120
Diuresis, following resuscitation after anaphylaxis, 177
Dizziness, in anaphylaxis, 18t, 19
Dobutamine, for pulmonary hypertension and right ventricular failure, 173
Doxacurium, 66
  administration of, 67
  anaphylactic/anaphylactoid reactions to, 85t
  histamine release caused by, 63, 64t, 67
Droperidol
  anaphylactic/anaphylactoid reactions to, 85t, 108
  dilution used for skin testing, 128t
Drug(s)
  allergic reactions to. See Allergic drug reaction(s)
  histamine-releasing potency and cutaneous vascular reactions to, evaluating and comparing, 63–64
  idiosyncratic reactions to, 122
  immunologic response to, 122–124
  intolerance, 122
  secondary effects of, 122
  in therapy of anaphylactic reactions, 143, 144f
Drug additives/preservatives, anaphylactic/anaphylactoid reactions to, 85t, 108
Drug allergy. See Allergic drug reaction(s)
Drug interactions, 122
Dyclone. See Dicycloine
Dynorphin, wheal and flare responses to, 77

Dyspnea
  in anaphylaxis, 18, 18t
  in hemolytic transfusion reactions, 98
Dysrhythmias
  in anaphylaxis, 18t, 19, 23, 138
  in intubated patients, 20t
  in shock, 138

ECF-A. See Eosinophilic chemotactic factor of anaphylaxis
Echocardiographic changes, in anaphylaxis, 24f
Edema
  in anaphylaxis, 22t
  histamine-induced, 33
  laryngeal. See Laryngeal edema
  mucosal. See Mucosal edema
  perioral, in anaphylaxis, 18t, 19, 27
    in intubated patients, 20t
  periorbital, in anaphylaxis, 18t, 19, 27
    in intubated patients, 20t
  pharyngeal, in anaphylaxis, 27
  upper respiratory tract. See also Pulmonary edema
    in anaphylaxis, 28
Ejection fraction, in anaphylaxis, 23, 24f
Electrocardiography
  after resuscitation, 177–178
  in anaphylaxis, 19, 23
  monitoring with, after anaphylactic reactions, 178
Emphysema, acute, in anaphylaxis, 29
β-Endorphin, wheal and flare responses to, 77
Endothelial cells
  H_1 receptors, 41
  release of platelet-activating factor from, 48
Endothelial leaks, histamine-induced, 33
Endothelium, 37
  histamine metabolism in, 34
  histamine's actions on, 37, 38f, 41
Endothelium-derived relaxing factor(s), 22, 37, 159
  action of, on vascular responses, 47f
  in coronary vasomotor action of histamine, 39
  release of, 37, 38f, 49

Endotoxin, activation of complement by, 55
Endotracheal intubation. *See also* Intubated patient(s)
  in initial therapy of anaphylaxis, 163
End-tidal CO_2 monitoring, 171–172, 178–179
Enflurane, 163
Enkephalin, wheal and flare responses to, 77
Enoximone, 202
  cardiovascular effects of, 150
  hemodynamic effects of, 150
  indications for, 145t
  mechanism of action, 149
  pharmacologic effects of, 145t
  in treatment of right ventricular failure, 173
Enzyme-linked immunoabsorbent assay
  for antigen-specific antibodies, 131–132
  for immunoglobulin E antibodies to chymopapain, 106
Enzyme mediators, 43
Eosinophil, in allergic response, 42
Eosinophilic chemotactic factor of anaphylaxis, 42
  biologic actions of, 32t
  manifestations of, 32t
Ephedrine
  pretreatment with, for potential anaphylactic reactions, 206
  radiocontrast media pretreatment modifications using, 133–134
Epinephrine, 188, 193–196
  administration of, in acute anaphylaxis, 164–166
  dosage of, 146–147
  for hypotension, dosage and administration of, 164–165, 166f–167f
  indications for, 145t, 146
  intramuscular or subcutaneous administration of, 166
  intratracheal administration of, 166
  intravenous
    cardiopulmonary resuscitative doses of, 165–166, 167f
    for persistent hypotension after initial resuscitation, 167–168
  mechanism of action, 144, 145t, 146
  pharmacologic effects of, 145t, 146
  plasma, effects of histamine infusion on, 36t, 36
  for pulmonary hypertension and right ventricular failure, 173
  receptor effects of, 145t, 146
  site of action, 145t, 146
  in treatment of anaphylaxis, 144f
Epontol. *See* Propanidid
Etomidate, anaphylactic/anaphylactoid reactions to, 85t, 87
Extremities, examination of, after anaphylactic reactions, 177

Factor V, in anaphylaxis, 30
Factor VIII, in anaphylaxis, 30
Factor XI, 56
  activation of, 57
Factor XIa, inactivation of, 57
Factor XII, 56, 60
  activation of, 56
  in anaphylaxis, 30
  contact activation initiated by, 56, 57f
Factor XIIa, 56–57
α-Factor XIIa. *See* Factor XIIa
β-Factor XIIa. *See* Factor XIIf
Factor XIIf, 56–57
Famotidine, 148t
  indications for, 145t
  pharmacologic effects of, 145t
  receptor effects of, 145t
Fatal reactions. *See* Deaths
Fentanyl
  administration of, and histamine release, 72f–73f, 74
  anaphylactic/anaphylactoid reactions to, 85t, 93
  dilution used for skin testing, 128t
Fever, transfusion-associated, 102
Fibrinogen, in anaphylaxis, 30
Fibrinolytic pathway(s)
  activation of, 51, 56, 57f
  interactions with classical complement cascade, 56
Fish, allergy to, and theoretical risk for protamine reactions, 114
Fletcher factor. *See* Prekallikrein

Flunitrazepam, anaphylactic/anaphylactoid reactions to, 86
Flushing
  in anaphylaxis, 18t, 19, 21, 22t
  in intubated patients, 20t
  in hemolytic transfusion reactions, 98
  with nonimmunologic histamine release, 63
  and plasma histamine level, 35t, 35
Foley catheter, indications for, after resuscitation, 180
Foreignness, of molecule, and antibody formation, 4–5
Functional residual capacity, in anaphylaxis, 27
Furosemide, anaphylactic/anaphylactoid reactions to, 85t, 109
FUT-175. *See* Nafamstat mesilate

Gallamine, anaphylactic/anaphylactoid reactions to, 85t, 90, 90t, 92
Gamma globulin, antibodies against, 104
Gamma interferon, 11
Gastrin, histamine release caused by, 64t, 77–79
Gastrointestinal system, in anaphylaxis, 29
  signs and symptoms in, 18t, 19
General anesthesia, anaphylaxis during
  incidence of, 106
  recognition of, 18t
Glomerulonephritis, 9t
Glycopeptide antibiotics, histamine release caused by, 63, 64t
Glycopyrrolate
  pharmacologic effects of, 152
  for severe bronchospasm, 172
Goodpasture syndrome, 10
Graft rejection, 10
Gram-negative sepsis, 55, 60
Granulocyte colony-stimulating factors, 11
Granulocyte-monocyte colony-stimulating factor, 11
Granulocyte-specific antigens, 98, 99t

Hageman factor. *See* Factor XII
Halothane, 163
Haptens, 4, 4t, 10
Headache, and plasma histamine level, 35t, 35
Heart rate
  during anaphylactic/anaphylactoid reactions, 20t, 24f
  effects of histamine infusion on, 36t, 36
  and plasma histamine level, 35t, 35
Helium-oxygen mixture (Heliox), administration of, 182–183
Hemodynamic instability, after anaphylaxis, measurements useful in managing, 179–180
Hemodynamic manifestations and symptoms, histamine levels and, 35t, 35–36
Hemodynamic monitoring
  after resuscitation, 178–180
  in anaphylactic/anaphylactoid reactions, 19–21, 20t, 23, 24f
Hemoglobinuria, in hemolytic transfusion reactions, 98
Hemolytic anemia, 9t, 10
  with penicillin, 94
Hemostatic changes. *See also* Coagulation
  in anaphylaxis, 30
Heparin, 57
  biologic actions of, 32t
  complement-inhibiting effects of, 154
  in human lung or cutaneous mast cells, 43
  manifestations of, 32t
  neutralization, possible substitutes for protamine in, 126
  release of, 13
  to reverse acute cardiovascular dysfunction after protamine reactions, 174
Heparinase, 126
Heparin-binding filters, 126
Hereditary angioedema. *See* Angioedema, hereditary
Hetastarch. *See* Hydroxyethyl starch
Hexadimethrine, 125
HFa. *See* Factor XIIa
HFf. *See* Factor XIIf

Histaminase, 42
Histamine, 148
  in basophils, 33
  biochemistry of, 31–33
  biologic actions of, 32t, 33, 34t
    on vascular smooth muscle, 37
  cardiovascular effects of, 34t, 35–41
  cutaneous effects of, 27–28
  effects of
    on cardiac contractility, 37
    on conduction in heart, 36–37
    on contractile state of endothelium, 41
    on coronary arteries, 38f, 38–40
    on coronary blood flow, 40–41
    on endothelium, 37, 38f, 41
    on regional vascular beds, 37–38, 38f–39f
    on vascular permeability, 41
    on veins, 41
  effects on arterial pressure, 36t, 36
  hemodynamic effects of, in humans, 35t, 35–36
  H_1 receptor effects of, 26t, 33–35, 34t
    action of, on vascular responses, 47f
  H_2 receptor effects of, 33–35, 34t
  inotropic effects of, 23, 25, 37
  manifestations of, 32t
  in mast cell granules, 33
  metabolism, 34–35
    in endothelium, 34
  negative dromotropic effects of, 37
  physiologic dose-response curve, alteration of, 134
  plasma half-life of, 34
  plasma levels of
    radioimmunoassay of, 35
    and symptoms, 35t, 35
  positive chronotropic effects of, 36–37
  positive inotropic effects of, 37
  pulmonary effects of, 41–42
  radioenzymatic assays of, 35
  receptors, 33–34, 34t, 37. See also H_1 receptors; H_2 receptors; H_3 receptors
  release of, 13, 16, 64f
    allergen-mediated, pretreatment for, 134
    caused by antibiotics, 64t, 65, 65f
    caused by atracurium, 63, 64t, 68–69, 73, 80
    flushing with, 35t, 35, 63, 72f–73f, 74
    nonimmunologic, 51, 63–80, 185
      clinical significance of, 79–80
    role of, in anaphylaxis, 26t
  tissue and cellular distribution of, 31–33
  vasoactive effects of, 23t, 27, 33–35, 35t, 38–41
  vasodilation produced by, 23t, 33, 38
  wheal and flare responses to, 68, 70–72, 71f–72f
Histamine N-methyltransferase, 35
History
  in diagnosis of drug allergy, 125
  pertinent to patient following anaphylactic reaction, 176
HIV. See Human immunodeficiency virus
Hives. See Urticaria
HMWK. See Kininogen, high-molecular weight
Holocaine. See Phenacaine
Horse sera, allergic reactions to, 5
H_1 receptor antagonist(s), 148t
  pretreatment with, 134, 206
H_2 receptor antagonist(s), 148t
  pretreatment with, 134, 206
H_1 receptors, 26t, 33–35, 37, 38f, 39, 41
  distribution of, 34t
H_2 receptors, 33–34, 37
  distribution of, 34t
H_3 receptors, 33–34, 37
Human immunodeficiency virus, 11
Hydrocortisone, 152, 168
  pharmacologic effects of, 145t
Hydroxyethyl starch
  anaphylactic/anaphylactoid reactions to, 85t, 107
  intravascular volume expansion with, 163
Hydroxyzine, 148t
Hymenoptera anaphylaxis, experimentally induced, 19, 30
Hypercapnia, during anaphylactic reactions, 162

Hyperglycemia, 181
Hyperosmotic agents, histamine release caused by, 64t, 110
Hypersensitivity reactions, classification of, 8
Hypnotics, administration of, precipitous hypotension after, 135
Hypotension, 83
  after anaphylaxis, 195–196
  in anaphylaxis, 18t, 19, 22–23
    in intubated patients, 20t
  definition of, 135
  epinephrine for, dosage and administration of, 164–165, 166f–167f
  in hemolytic transfusion reactions, 98
  induced by d-tubocurarine, 39f
  intravenous drugs that produce, 137t
  persistent, 167–168, 177
    after anaphylactic shock, 180
    blood urea nitrogen evaluated after, 178
    creatinine evaluated after, 178
    renal function tests evaluated after, 178
  and plasma histamine level, 35t, 35
  precipitous
    after administration of anesthetic agents, 135
    after hypnotic administration, 135
    after sedative administration, 135
    with inadvertent discontinuation of vasoconstrictor infusions, 137
    with overdosage of vasoactive drug infusion, 137
  with protamine, 115, 117f, 168, 169f
  in septic shock, 140
  with tension pneumothorax, 140–141
  transfusion-associated, 102
  with vancomycin administration, 96–97
  with venous air embolism, 141
Hypoxemia, 137, 178, 180
  during anaphylactic reactions, 162

Iloprost, 46
Imipenem, 96
Immediate hypersensitivity reaction(s), 3, 5, 8, 9t
  agents producing, 51
  with anesthetic drugs, 84
  chemotactic factors in, 42
  definition of, 3
  pathogenesis of
    basophils in, 14–17
    mast cells in, 14–17
  pathophysiologic mechanisms of, 130
  pathways for, 51
  types I–IV, 6, 8–11, 15t
Immune complex reactions, 9t, 10
Immune system, effects of anesthetic agents on, 11
Immunogenicity, definition of, 4
Immunoglobulin(s)
  antibody function of, 5
  classes of, 6
  disulfide linkages, 5
  Fab fragments, 5, 5f
  Fc fragments, 5, 5f
  Fc region (constant region) of, and biologic behavior, 6
  heavy chains, 5
  intravenous, anaphylactic/anaphylactoid reactions to, 104
  light chains, 5
  synthesis of, 5–6
  in transfusion reactions, 104–106
Immunoglobulin A
  antibodies against, 104–105
  biologic characteristics of, 7t
  deficiency of, 8, 104–105
  function of, 7t, 8
  molecular weight of, 7t
  serum concentration of, 7t
  structure of, 8
  synthesis of, 8
Immunoglobulin D
  biologic characteristics of, 7t
  function of, 6, 7t
  molecular weight of, 7t
  serum concentration of, 7t
Immunoglobulin E
  in anaphylactic reactions to protamine, 193
  in anaphylaxis, 13, 15f
  in anaphylaxis to muscle relaxant, 90
  anti-immunoglobulin A, 105

anti-insulin, radioallergosorbent test
for, 131
anti-muscle relaxant, radioallergosorbent test for, 131
anti-penicillin, radioallergosorbent test
for, 131
anti-protamine
enzyme-linked immunosorbent assay
for, 131
radioallergosorbent test for, 131
anti-thiopental, 86
radioallergosorbent test for, 131
basophil membrane receptors for, 14
biologic characteristics of, 7t
epsilon chain, 6
Fc region of, 6
function of, 6, 7t, 8, 9t
half-life of, 106
levels of, after intravenous challenges
of suspected allergen, 129
mast cell binding, 6, 7t
mast cell membrane receptors for,
14
molecular weight of, 7t
morphine binding, structural features
of, 93
in penicillin allergy, skin testing in
evaluation of, 126
properties of, 6
in reactions to local anesthetics, 88
in sensitivity to parabens, 88–89
serum concentration of, 7t
transfusion of, in blood products,
105–106
Immunoglobulin G
in anaphylaxis, 13
antibodies against, 104
anti-immunoglobulin A, 105
anti-penicillin, 123
anti-protamine, 115–117, 193
biologic characteristics of, 7t
in complement activation, 6, 7t
in complement binding, 105
Fab regions of, 6
Fc regions of, 6
function of, 7t, 9t, 10
heavy chains, 6
light chains, 6

molecular weight of, 7t
serum concentration of, 7t
structure of, 5, 5f, 6
subclasses of, 6
Immunoglobulin M
antibodies against, 105
anti-penicillin, 123
biologic characteristics of, 7t
in complement activation, 7t
function of, 7t, 9t, 10
molecular weight of, 7t
serum concentration of, 7t
structure of, 6
Immunologic reaction(s)
characteristics of, 3–4
classification of, 8–11
gel and classification of, 8–11, 9t
pathophysiology of, 8
specificity of, 4
spectrum of, 8
type I, 8, 9t
type II, 9t, 10
type III, 9t, 10
type IV, 9t, 10–11
Impromidine, 37
Indomethacin, 156
Induction agent(s), anaphylactic/anaphylactoid reactions to, 84–87, 85t
incidence of, 83
Insulin
allergy to, skin testing in evaluation
of, 126
anaphylactic/anaphylactoid reactions
to, 85t, 109
immunogenicity, 110
immunoglobulin E antibody to, radioallergosorbent test for, 131
NPH, allergic reactions to, 113,
118
Integumentary system, signs and symptoms of anaphylaxis in, 18t, 19
Intensive care unit
management in, after anaphylactic reaction, 175–183
observation in, for patients resuscitated after anaphylactic reaction,
170
Interleukins, 11

254 | INDEX

Intraalveolar hemorrhage, in anaphylaxis, 28
Intraaortic balloon pump, with acute right ventricular failure, 174
Intraarterial cannula, indications for, after resuscitation, 180
Intradermal testing. See Skin testing
Intravascular volume expansion
  after anaphylaxis, 179
  in initial therapy of anaphylaxis, 163–164
Intubated patient(s). See also Endotracheal intubation
  anaphylactic reactions in, signs and symptoms of, 19, 20t
Ipratropium
  pharmacologic effects of, 152
  for severe bronchospasm, 172
Isobucaine, classification of, 89t
Isoflurane, 163
Isohemagglutinins, 8
Isoproterenol, 191–192, 199
  antipermeability effects of, 160
  indications for, 145t, 147, 168, 169f
  mechanism of action, 145t, 147
  pharmacologic effects of, 145t, 147
  for pulmonary hypertension and right ventricular failure, 173
  receptor effects of, 145t, 147
  site of action, 145t, 147
Isradipine, 158
  mechanism of action, 153
Itching, in anaphylaxis, 18t, 19

Jarisch-Herxheimer reactions, 138
J chain, 8

Kallikrein
  biologic actions of, 48, 56
  in gram-negative bacteremia, 60
  inactivator of, 57
    units of, 97
  vasodilation produced by, 23t
Kaposi's sarcoma, 11
Ketamine reactions, 84–87
Ketorolac
  anaphylactic/anaphylactoid reactions to, 112
  treatment of protamine-induced pulmonary hypertension following cardiopulmonary bypass, 156, 157f
Kincaine. See Isobucaine
Kinin(s)
  activation of, 56, 57f
  in anaphylaxis, 48
  biologic properties of, 48
  inactivation of, 49
  metabolism of, 49
  physiologic effects of, 48–49
  synthesis of, 43
  vasodilation produced by, 23t, 48
Kininase I, 49
Kininase II, 49
Kininogen
  high-molecular weight, 48, 56
    in anaphylaxis, 30
  low-molecular weight, 48

L-6705696, thromboxane A_2 receptor blockade with, 156
Laboratory evaluation, after anaphylactic reaction, 177
Laryngeal edema, 163, 169
  in anaphylaxis, 18, 18t, 28–29
  epinephrine for, 166
  management of, 182
  residual, 182
Laryngospasm, 163
Late-phase reactions, 146, 170, 175
Latex (rubber)
  allergy to, preoperative evaluation for, 205
  anaphylactic/anaphylactoid reactions to, 84, 85t, 110
  medical products that may contain, 111t
Left ventricular diastolic dysfunction, and pulmonary edema, 139
Left ventricular dP/dT max, and plasma histamine level, 35t, 35, 36t, 36
Left ventricular dysfunction, in anaphylaxis, 22
Left ventricular end-diastolic cross-sectional area, in anaphylaxis, 24f

Index | 255

Left ventricular end-diastolic pressure, effects of histamine infusion on, 36t, 36
Left ventricular end-diastolic volumes, precipitous decreases in, during anaphylaxis, 163
Left ventricular end-systolic cross-sectional area, in anaphylaxis, 24f
Left ventricular failure, 180
Left ventricular volume, in anaphylaxis, 23, 24f, 163
Leukoagglutinin(s), 101–103, 182, 200–203
Leukoagglutinin reaction(s), 180
  agents producing, 103
  incidence of, 103
  suspected, 197–203
  treatment of, 103–104
Leukocyte antigens, 99t
Leukocyte histamine release, in vitro, to explore pathophysiologic mechanisms of immediate hypersensitivity reactions, 130
Leukotriene(s), 44–45, 148
  action of, on vascular responses, 47f
  pulmonary effects of, 42
  role of, in anaphylaxis, 26t
  synthesis of, 44
  vasodilation produced by, 23t
Leukotriene antagonists, in treatment of anaphylaxis, 144f
Leukotriene B_4
  chemotactic and chemokinetic properties of, 44
  effects of, 44
  role of, in anaphylaxis, 26t
Leukotriene C_4
  biologic actions of, 32t, 44–45
  cardiovascular effects of, 45
  manifestations of, 32t
  negative inotropic effects of, 45
  release of, 64f
  role of, in anaphylaxis, 26t
  source of, 44
  vasoconstriction caused by, 45
Leukotriene D_4
  biologic actions of, 32t, 45
  coronary vasoconstriction caused by, 45
  manifestations of, 32t
  role of, in anaphylaxis, 26t
Leukotriene E_4
  biologic actions of, 32t
  manifestations of, 32t
  role of, in anaphylaxis, 26t
Levarterenol. See Norepinephrine
Levophed. See Norepinephrine
Lidocaine
  classification of, 89t
  dilution used for skin testing, 128t
  evaluation of allergic reactions to, 88–89
Lipoxygenase, metabolism, 14, 17, 44
Local anesthetic(s)
  adverse drug reactions to, 88
  allergic reactions to, 87–88
    clinical manifestations of, 88
    evaluation of patient with history of, 88–89
  anaphylactic/anaphylactoid reactions to, 85t, 87–89
  classification of, 89t
  cross-reactivity to, 88–89
  direct challenge test, 88, 89t
  immunoglobulin E-mediated reactions to, 88
  provocative dose testing, 88, 89t
  toxic effects of, 88
  vasovagal reactions with, 88
Lopressor. See Metoprolol
Lung(s)
  granulocyte aggregation in, 102–103, 103f
  hyperinflation of, in anaphylaxis, 28
Lung Hageman activator, 43
Lung injury, acute, 182
  transfusion-related, 100t, 101–104, 102t, 197–203
    hemodynamic changes during, 196f, 197
    morbidity of, 103–104, 105t
    mortality of, 104
    right heart failure (right ventricular failure) after, 202–203
    pulmonary edema secondary to, 164
Lymphoid cells, 10

Lymphokines, 10
Lymphoproliferative syndromes, 11
Lymphotoxin, 11

α_2-Macroglobulin, 57, 58t
Management, of anaphylaxis, 161–174
Mannitol
  anaphylactic/anaphylactoid reactions to, 85t
  histamine release caused by, 110
MAP. *See* Mean arterial pressure
Marcaine. *See* Bupivicaine
Mast cell(s)
  activation of, 17
    factors influencing, 15
  biosynthetic products of, 14
  chymase in, 43
  degranulation of, nonimmunologic, 70, 80
  effects of muscle relaxants on, 66–73
  functional characteristics of, 14
  granular constituents of, 31, 32t
  granules, 14, 16f
    histamine in, 33
    size of, 14
  half-life of, 14
  heparin in, 43
  heterogeneity of, 14
  immunoglobulin E binding, 6, 7t, 14
  in initial host defense, 14
  location of, 14
  membrane receptors for immunoglobulin E, 14
  nonimmunologic responses to drugs and neuropeptides, 63
  normal physiologic role of, 14
  opiate effects on, 77
  in pathogenesis of immediate hypersensitivity reactions, 14–17
  protamine effects on, 115
  secretory activity, effects of calcium on, 16–17
  skin
    as immunologic window to evaluate antigen-immunoglobulin E interactions, 28
    mediator release from, 64f
    substance P effects on, 77–78, 78f
  tryptase in, 43

Mastocytosis
  anesthetic management of patients with, 138
  cutaneous, 138
  systemic, 138
MAST suit. *See* Military antishock trousers
Mean arterial pressure
  during anaphylactic/anaphylactoid reactions, 20t, 24f
  effects of histamine infusion on, 36t, 36
Mean pulmonary arterial pressure
  during anaphylactic/anaphylactoid reactions, 20t, 21, 21f
  effects of histamine infusion on, 36t, 36
Mechanical ventilation
  after anaphylactic reaction, 182
  with positive end-expiratory pressure, 190–192, 200, 203
Mediators, 148–149, 161. *See also* specific mediator
  of airway inflammation in anaphylaxis, 26t
  of anaphylaxis/anaphylactic reactions, 13–14, 31–49
    clinical manifestations of, 31, 32t
    lipid-derived, 43
    physiologic effects of, 31
    protein-derived, 43
    stored, 31–43
    synthesized, 43–49
  of bronchospasm in anaphylaxis, 26t
  enzyme, 43
  during immunoglobulin E-mediated anaphylaxis to protamine, 193
  of mucosal edema in anaphylaxis, 26t
  release
    effects of calcium channel blockers on, 153
    from skin mast cells, 64f
  vasoactive, 22, 23t, 34
Medic-Alert bracelet, 125
Medical history, 205
Medications, that may contribute to shock, 176
Membrane phospholipids, turnover of, 144

Mental status, after resuscitation, 176
Meperidine
    administration of, 205
    allergic reactions to, 83
    anaphylactic/anaphylactoid reactions to, 85t, 92–93, 188–192, 189t
    dilution used for skin testing, 128t
    histamine release caused by, 63, 64t, 74f, 74–77
    wheal and flare responses to, 74, 75f
Mepivacaine
    classification of, 89t
    dilution used for skin testing, 128t
Meprylcaine, classification of, 89t
Metabisulfite, 88, 109
Metabolic acidosis, 181
Metabolic status, after resuscitation following anaphylactic shock, 181
Metabulethamine, classification of, 89t
Methohexital, 84
    anaphylactic/anaphylactoid reactions to, 86
    dilution used for skin testing, 128t
    histamine release caused by, 66f
Methylmethacrylate
    anaphylactic/anaphylactoid reactions to, 85t
    cardiopulmonary complications with, 111–112
Methylprednisolone, 152, 168
    anaphylactic/anaphylactoid reactions to, 108
    pharmacologic effects of, 145t
    in pretreatment for anaphylaxis, 134
Metocurine, 66–67
    administration of, 205
    anaphylactic/anaphylactoid reactions to, 85t
    dilution used for skin testing, 128t
    histamine release caused by, 63, 64t, 68–69
    wheal and flare responses to, 68–69, 71f
Metoprolol, and hemodynamic response to epinephrine administration, 168, 176
Metycaine. *See* Pipercocaine
Midazolam, dilution used for skin testing, 128t

Military antishock trousers, 164
Milrinone, 202
    cardiovascular effects of, 150
    hemodynamic effects of, 150
    indications for, 145t
    mechanism of action, 149
    pharmacologic effects of, 145t
    in treatment of right ventricular failure, 173
Mirror molecules, 4t
Mivacurium, 66
    administration of, 67, 205
    anaphylactic/anaphylactoid reactions to, 85t
    histamine release caused by, 63, 64t, 67
Monobactams, 96
Morphiceptin, wheal and flare responses to, 77
Morphine, 92
    administration of, 205
    adverse hemodynamic effects of, antagonism of, 75–77
    allergic reactions to, 83
    anaphylactic/anaphylactoid reactions to, 85t
    cardiovascular responses to, 79
    dilution used for skin testing, 128t
    effects of, on calculated systemic vascular resistance, 79, 79f
    hemodynamic effects of, 75–80
    histamine release caused by, 63, 64t, 72f, 74f, 74–77, 79–80
    hypotensive response associated with, 79–80
    wheal and flare responses to, 68, 70–72, 71f–72f, 74, 75f
Morphine-immunoglobulin E binding, structural features of, 93
MPAP. *See* Mean pulmonary arterial pressure
Mucosal edema, in anaphylaxis, mediators of, 26t
Muscle relaxant(s). *See also* Benzylisoquinoline-derived muscle relaxants
    allergy to
        approach to patient with history of, 125–126

Muscle relaxant(s) *(continued)*
  skin testing in evaluation of, 126
  anaphylactic/anaphylactoid reactions to, 84, 85t, 90–92
  incidence of, 83
  cross-reactivity to, 90
  histamine release caused by, 66–73
  immunoglobulin E antibody to, radioallergosorbent test for, 131
  immunoglobulin E-mediated anaphylaxis to, 90
  steroidal, wheal and flare responses to, 73
  structure of, 67t
  wheal and flare responses to, 66, 67f, 67–68, 71f, 73
Myocardial function, in anaphylaxis, 23
Myocardial ischemia
  after resuscitation, 178
  in anaphylaxis, 22, 25, 29
Myocardial ischemia/infarction, pulmonary edema caused by, 139
Myocardial lesions, in anaphylaxis, 29
Myosin light-chain kinase, 144

Nafamstat mesilate, 154
Natural killer cell factor, 11
Nausea, in anaphylaxis, 19
NCA. *See* Neutrophilic chemotactic factor
Neostigmine, dilution used for skin testing, 128t
Nesacaine. *See* Chlorprocaine
Neuropeptides, histamine release caused by, 77–79
Neutral proteases
  biologic actions of, 32t
  manifestations of, 32t
Neutrophilic chemotactic factor, 42
  biologic actions of, 32t
  manifestations of, 32t
Nicardipine, 158
  mechanism of action, 153
Nifedipine, 158
  mechanism of action, 153
  pharmacologic effects of, 153
Nitroglycerine, indications for, 173
Nonsteroidal antiinflammatory drugs, 154
  adverse drug reactions to, 112
  allergic reaction to, approach to patient with history of, 125–126
  anaphylactic/anaphylactoid reactions to, 85t, 112–113
  in treatment of anaphylaxis, 144f
Norepinephrine, 193–196, 199
  dosage of, 147
  indications for, 145t, 147–148, 168, 174, 176
  left atrial administration of, 158, 173–174, 199, 202
  mechanism of action, 144, 145t
  pharmacologic effects of, 145t, 147
  plasma, effects of histamine infusion on, 36t, 36
  receptor effects of, 145t, 147
  site of action, 145t
Novocaine. *See* Procaine
NPH. *See* Insulin, NPH
NSAIDs. *See* Nonsteroidal antiinflammatory drugs
Nupercaine. *See* Dibucaine

Oliguria, after resuscitation following anaphylactic shock, 181
Opioid(s), 135
  adverse hemodynamic effects of, 80
  antagonism of, 75–77
  anaphylactic/anaphylactoid reactions to, 84, 85t, 92–93
  histamine release caused by, 63, 64t, 74f, 74–77
  vascular effects of, 80
  wheal and flare responses to, 74–75
  antagonism of, 74–75, 76f
Opioid receptor, 77
Opioid receptor agonists, intradermal skin tests with, 77
Opportunistic infections, 11
Oxaine. *See* Oxethazine
Oxethazine, classification of, 89t
Oxygenation, in initial therapy of anaphylaxis, 162–163

Pacing, atrial or ventricular, 179
Packed red blood cells, 205
PAF. *See* Platelet-activating factor
Pain, back and flank, in hemolytic transfusion reactions, 98

Pancuronium, 67
  anaphylactic/anaphylactoid reactions to, 85t, 90, 90t
  dilution used for skin testing, 128t
  wheal and flare responses to, 68, 71f
Papaveretum, anaphylactic/anaphylactoid reactions to, 93
Papaverine, 69–70
  mechanism of action, 149
  wheal and flare responses to, 68, 71f
Para-aminobenzoic ester agents, anaphylactic/anaphylactoid reactions to, 85t
Parabens
  hypersensitivity reactions to, 108–109
  immunoglobulin E-mediated sensitivity to, 88–89
Partial thromboplastin time, after anaphylaxis, 178
Passive transfer of cutaneous reactivity, 129
Peak airway pressure, increased, in anaphylaxis, in intubated patients, 20t
Penicillin
  administration of, and allergic reactions, 94
  allergy to, 8, 93–94
    immunoglobulin E-mediated, skin testing in evaluation of, 126
    and route of administration, 94
  anaphylactic/anaphylactoid reactions to, 28, 84, 85t, 93–95, 123–124
    fatality from, 93
    pathogenesis of, 94
    types of, 94
  antibodies against, 123, 126, 131
  and cephalosporins, cross-reactivity between, 95–96
  contact dermatitis with, 94
  desensitization, 95
  dosage of, and allergic reactions, 94
  hemolytic anemia with, 94
  immune responses to, 123–124
  immunoglobulin E antibody to, radioallergosorbent test for, 131
  immunoglobulin G antibody to, 123
  route of administration of, and allergic reactions, 94
  serum sickness with, 94
  skin tests, 95, 126
  use of, in atopic patients, 124
  vasculitis after, 10
Pentobarbital, histamine release caused by, 66f
Pepsid. See Famotidine
Peptides, histamine release caused by, 63, 64t, 77–79
Pericardial tamponade
  diagnosis of, 139
  signs and symptoms of, 139
  therapy for, 139
Peroxidase, 43
Pharmacologic therapy, for anaphylaxis, 143–160
Phenacaine, classification of, 89t
Phenergan. See Promethazine
Phentolamine, 199
Phosphodiesterase(s), 47f
  fraction I, 149
  fraction III, 149
  inhibitors of, 150
  substrate specificity of, 149
  tissue distribution of, 149
Phosphodiesterase inhibitors, 150t
  antipermeability effects of, 160
  cyclic adenosine monophosphate-specific (fraction III), 173
  indications for, 145t
  mechanism of action, 149
  pharmacologic effects of, 145t
  physiologic effects of, 149
  in treatment of anaphylaxis, 143, 149
  in treatment of pulmonary hypertension, 159
  in treatment of right ventricular failure, 173
Phospholipase A_2, 44, 47
Phospholipase C, 44, 144
Physical examination, after resuscitation, 176–177
Physiologic responses, during anaphylactic or anaphylactoid reactions, 185–203
Phytonadione. See Vitamin K
Pipercocaine, classification of, 89t
Piroximone, mechanism of action, 149

Plasma contact activation system, 51.
See also Contact activation
Plasma protein fractions, anaphylactic/
anaphylactoid reactions to, 85t,
107
Plasma thromboplastin antecedent. See
Factor XI
Plasmin, 56
complement activation by, 56
inactivation of, 57
inhibitors of, 154
Platelet-activating factor
biologic actions of, 32t
manifestations of, 32t
negative inotropic effects of, 48
physiologic effects of, 47–48
release of, 45
role of, in anaphylaxis, 26t
synthesis of, 43, 46–47
vasodilation produced by, 23t
Platelet antigens, 99t
Platelet count, after anaphylaxis, 178
Platelet Factor 4, to reverse protamine,
126
Pneumocystis carinii, 11
Poison ivy, allergy to, 10
Polybasic compounds, histamine release
caused by, 64t
Polybrene. See Hexadimethrine
Polyoxyethylated castor oil, intravenous,
anaphylactoid reactions to, 120
Pontocaine. See Tetracaine
Positive pressure ventilation
indications for, 183
in initial therapy of anaphylaxis, 163
Potassium, serum, after massive volume
resuscitation, 177
Potassium supplementations, 177
Prausnitz-K&uuml§ner testing, 91–92.
See also Passive transfer of cuta-
neous reactivity
Prekallikrein, 56, 60
activator of, biologic actions of, 48
in anaphylaxis, 30, 48
biologic actions of, 48
Preoperative considerations, with allergic
patients, 121–134
Preoperative evaluation
for chymopapain allergy, 205–206

for latex (rubber) allergy, 205
Pretreatment
for allergen-mediated histamine release, 134
for anaphylactic/anaphylactoid reactions, 133–134, 195, 206
with antihistamines, 148, 206
with calcium entry blockers, 153
with corticosteroids, 188, 206
with dexamethasone, 134
with ephedrine, 133–134, 206
with H_1 receptor antagonists, 134,
206
with H_2 receptor antagonists, 134,
206
with methylprednisolone, 134
with steroids in combination with antihistamines, 134
Prilocaine, dilution used for skin testing,
128t
Procaine
classification of, 89t
dilution used for skin testing, 128t
Promethazine, 148t
pharmacologic effects of, 148
receptor effects of, 148
Promoxine, classification of, 89t
Propanidid, 84, 86
Propofol
anaphylactic/anaphylactoid reactions
to, 85t, 87
dilution used for skin testing, 128t
Prostacyclin (prostaglandin I_2)
biologic action of, 46
effects on vascular responses, 46, 47f
release of, 37, 38f
source of, 46
synthesis of, 45–46
vasodilation produced by, 23t
Prostaglandin(s), 148
biologic actions of, 45
pulmonary effects of, 42
receptors of, on vascular smooth muscle, 47f
release of, 49
synthesis of, 45
vasodilation produced by, 45–46
Prostaglandin A_2, vasodilation produced
by, 23t

Prostaglandin D_2
  biologic actions of, 32t, 45–46
  manifestations of, 32t
  release of, 45, 64f
  source of, 45
  vasodilation produced by, 23t
Prostaglandin E_1
  administration of, 158
  antiinflammatory effects of, 157–158, 202
  antipermeability effects of, 160
  in combination with left atrial norepinephrine infusion, 158, 174, 199
  effects of, 158t
  for pulmonary hypertension and right heart failure, 159
    after cardiopulmonary bypass, 157
  for refractory pulmonary artery hypertension, and noncardiogenic pulmonary edema after protamine, 158
  right atrial infusion of, 174, 199, 202
  vasodilation produced by, 23t
Prostaglandin E_2
  biologic action of, 46
  role of, in anaphylaxis, 26t
  source of, 46
  vasodilation produced by, 23t
Prostaglandin $F_2\alpha$
  biologic action of, 46
  effects of, on vasculature, 46
  release of, 45
  role of, in anaphylaxis, 26t
Prostaglandin I_2. See Prostacyclin
Prostin VR. See Prostaglandin E_1
Protamine
  adverse reactions to, 113
  allergy to, management of patient with, 125–126
  anaphylactic/anaphylactoid reactions to, 55, 84, 85t, 116f, 117, 192–195
    incidence of, 83
    mechanisms of, 114–115
    patients at risk for, 113–114
    pulmonary hypertension with left atrial and systemic hypotension during, 168, 169f
  desensitization, 126
  dilution used for skin testing, 128t
  effects of, on mast cells, 115
  hemodynamic effects of, 113, 115
  histamine release caused by, 77
  hypotension with, 115, 117f, 168, 169f
  immunoglobulin E antibody to
    enzyme-linked immunosorbent assay for, 131
    radioallergosorbent test for, 131
  immunoglobulin E-mediated anaphylactic reaction to, 193
  immunoglobulin G antibody to, 115–117, 193
  intraaortic injection of, 118
  pulmonary hypertension with, 115, 117, 117f
  test dose of, 132
Protamine-zinc insulin, allergic reactions to, 113, 118
Protein kinase A, 146
Protein kinase C, 144
Prothrombin time(s)
  after anaphylaxis, 178
  in anaphylaxis, 30
Pruritus
  in anaphylaxis, 27
  transfusion-associated, 102
Pulmonary artery catheter, 179
Pulmonary artery pressure, monitoring, 180
Pulmonary capillary wedge pressure
  after anaphylaxis, 179
  in anaphylaxis, 23, 24f, 163
Pulmonary circulation, air in, 141
Pulmonary congestion, in anaphylaxis, 28
Pulmonary edema, 190–191, 197, 200
  after relief of upper airway obstruction, 139
  in anaphylaxis, 18, 18t, 28
    in intubated patients, 20t
  caused by myocardial ischemia/infarction, 139
  noncardiogenic, 103, 139, 182, 202
    causes of, 139, 140t
    treatment of, 164, 168
  perioperative, causes of, 139
  reperfusion, 139

Pulmonary edema *(continued)*
  secondary to transfusion-related acute lung injury, with right heart failure, 164
Pulmonary embolism
  versus anaphylaxis, 140
  risk factors for, 140
  signs and symptoms of, 140
Pulmonary hypertension, 180. *See also* Right heart failure, and pulmonary hypertension
  in anaphylaxis, 18t, 19
  in intubated patients, 20t
  protamine-induced, 115, 117, 117f, 168, 169f
    treatment of, 156, 157f
  and right ventricular failure, therapeutic interventions for, 159, 170–171, 173–174
  treatment of, 157–159, 173
Pulmonary leukostasis, 102–103, 103f
Pulmonary microemboli, in anaphylaxis, 29
Pulmonary vascular resistance
  in anaphylaxis, 22–23, 27
  calculation of, 180
  effects of histamine infusion on, 36t, 36
  increased, 180
    in anaphylaxis, 29
Pulmonary vascular resistance index, in anaphylaxis, 24f
Pulmonary vasculature
  cyclic nucleotide formation in, stimulation of, 159, 159f
  effects of histamine on, 41–42
Pulmonary vasoconstriction
  with calcium administration, 203
  pharmacologic approaches to, 158–159
  reversal of, 154, 155f, 159f
  treatment of, 156, 157f, 158
Pulse, not palpable, in anaphylaxis, 22t
Pulse oximetry, after anaphylactic reactions, 178
Pulse pressure, and plasma histamine level, 35t, 35

Quaternary ammonium compounds
  cross-reactivity to, 90–91
  sensitization to, 91

Radioallergosorbent test, antigen-specific immunoglobulin E antibody measurement using, 130–131
Radiocontrast dye (media), anaphylactic/ anaphylactoid reactions to, 85t, 118–119
  pretreatment of adult patients with history of, 133–134
Ranitidine, 148t, 167
  anaphylactic/anaphylactoid reactions to, 97
  indications for, 145t
  pharmacologic effects of, 145t
  receptor effects of, 145t
RAST. *See* Radioallergosorbent test
Reaginic antibody, 6
Recovery room, management in, after anaphylactic reaction, 175–183
Red cell antigens, 98, 99t
Red man syndrome, after vancomycin use, 97
Regional anesthesia, recognition of anaphylaxis during, 18t
Regional vasculature, effects of histamine on, 37–38, 38f–39f
Releasibility, definition of, 16
Renal failure, in hemolytic transfusion reactions, 98
Renal function, after resuscitation following anaphylactic shock, 181
Reperfusion, pulmonary edema in, 139
Respiratory distress. *See also* Adult respiratory distress syndrome
  in anaphylaxis, 18t, 19
  transfusion-associated, 102
Respiratory failure, 190–191
Respiratory system
  in anaphylaxis
    pathologic findings in, 28–29
    signs and symptoms of, 18t, 18
  management, after anaphylaxis, 181–183
Restlessness, in hemolytic transfusion reactions, 98
Rh disease, 9t, 10
Right heart failure (right ventricular failure)
  after transfusion-related acute lung injury, 202–203

in anaphylaxis, 22, 29
   treatment of, 171t
and bronchospasm, 170, 170f
intraaortic balloon pumping with, 174
and pulmonary hypertension, treatment of, 159, 170–171, 173–174
and refractory pulmonary hypertension, after cardiopulmonary bypass, PGE_1 for, 157
treatment of, 156, 157f
Rigor, in hemolytic transfusion reactions, 98
Rocuronium, 67

Sandimmune. See Cyclosporin
SAP. See Systolic arterial pressure
Sedatives, administration of, precipitous hypotension after, 135
Seizures, after anaphylaxis, 176
Sepsis, contact activation and, 60
Septic shock
   versus anaphylactic shock, 140
   signs and symptoms of, 140
Sequelae, management of, 175–183
Serum electrolytes, after massive volume resuscitation, 177
Serum sickness, 9t, 10, 55
   with penicillin, 94
Shock, 135. See also Anaphylactic shock; Cardiogenic shock; Septic shock
   dysrhythmias in, 138
   in hemolytic transfusion reactions, 98
   irreversible, 183
   medications that may contribute to, 176
   refractory, 176
Side effects, definition of, 121
Skin testing
   for allergen identification, 126–129
   anaphylaxis caused by, 127
   for diagnosis in patients with history of anaphylaxis during anesthesia, 126
   for drug allergy, 125
   drug dilutions used for, 128t
   for evaluation of chymopapain anaphylaxis, 106

false-negative results of, 127
false-positive results of, 127
Fisher protocol for, 127–129
interpretation of, 129
for penicillin allergy, 95, 126
for streptokinase allergy, 119, 126
Slow-reacting substance of anaphylaxis, 44
Smooth muscle, histamine's actions on, 37, 38f
Sodium benzoate, cross-reactivity, with parabens, 109
Sodium bicarbonate, 199
   indications for, 169
Sodium cephalothin sodium, anaphylaxis with, 84
Somatostatin, histamine release caused by, 64t
Sperm antibodies, and risk for protamine reactions, 114
Streptokinase
   allergic reactions to
      incidence of, 119
      signs and symptoms of, 119
   skin testing in evaluation of, 126
   anaphylactic/anaphylactoid reactions to, 85t
   thrombolytic therapy, skin testing before, 119
Stridor
   postextubation, 139, 182–183
   reintubation of patient with, 183
Stroke index
   in anaphylaxis, 24f
   effects of histamine infusion on, 36t, 36
Stroke volume, during anaphylactic/anaphylactoid reactions, 20t, 23
Subjective complaint, in anaphylaxis, 22t
Substance P
   effects of
      on cutaneous mast cells, 77–78, 78f
      on vascular responses, 47f
   histamine release caused by, 64t, 77–79
   vasodilation produced by, 23t
Succinylcholine, 67, 70
   anaphylactic/anaphylactoid reactions to, 85t, 90, 90t, 92

Succinylcholine *(continued)*
  dilution used for skin testing, 128t
  molecular structure of, 91
  wheal and flare responses to, 68, 71f
Sufentanil
  administration of, and histamine release, 73f, 74
  adverse hemodynamic effects of, antagonism of, 75–77
  dilution used for skin testing, 128t
  wheal and flare responses to, 74, 75f
Sulfiting agents, 109
Sulfonamides, anaphylactic/anaphylactoid reactions to, 85t, 96
Surfacaine. *See* Cyclomethycaine
Surgery, trauma of, and postoperative immunodepression, 11
SVR. *See* Systemic vascular resistance
Systemic lupus erythematosus, drug-induced, 10
Systemic vascular resistance
  during anaphylactic/anaphylactoid reactions, 18t, 19, 20t, 23
  in intubated patients, 20t
  effects of histamine infusion on, 36t, 36
Systemic vascular resistance index, in anaphylaxis, 24f
Systolic arterial pressure, during anaphylactic/anaphylactoid reactions, 20t

Tachycardia, in anaphylaxis, 18t, 19, 21
  in intubated patients, 20t
Tagamet. *See* Cimetidine
T cells, activated, 10
Tenormin. *See* Atenolol
Tension pneumothorax, 140–141
Terbutaline, 171–172, 188
  antianaphylactic effects of, 134
  antipermeability effects of, 160
Test dose, clinical use of, 132–133
Tetracaine, classification of, 89t
Theophylline, 149–150
Thiamylal, histamine release caused by, 64t, 65–66, 66f, 86
Thiazide diuretics, anaphylactic/anaphylactoid reactions to, 109
Thiobarbiturate(s)
  allergic reactions to, 83
  approach to patient with history of, 125–126
  histamine release caused by, 63, 64t
Thiopental, 84
  anaphylactic/anaphylactoid reactions to, 86
  dilution used for skin testing, 128t
  histamine release caused by, 64t, 65–66, 66f, 80, 86
  immunoglobulin E antibody to, 86
  radioallergosorbent test for, 131
  test dose of, 133
Thrombin inhibitor, in anaphylaxis, 30
Thromboxane, synthesis of, 45
Thromboxane A_2
  in anaphylaxis, 22, 26t
  biologic action of, 46
  effects of, on vascular responses, 47f
  release of, 45
  source of, 46
  vasoconstriction produced by, 46
Thromboxane A_2 receptor antagonists, 156
Thromboxane synthetase inhibitors, 154–156, 155f
Thymus-derived lymphocytes, 10
Tissue plasminogen activator, 119
Toradol. *See* Ketorolac
Tranexamic acid, 154
Transfusion reactions, 9t, 10, 55, 100t
  acute lung injury in, 100t, 101–104, 102t, 164, 196f, 197–203
  allergic, 101–104
  alloimmunization, 100t
  anaphylactic, 100t, 101
  classification of, 98
  febrile nonhemolytic, 100t, 101
  graft versus host disease, 100t
  hemolytic, 98–99
    acute, 100t
    definition of, 98
    delayed, 99, 100f
    therapy for, 99
  immunoglobulin-associated, 104–106
  nonhemolytic, 101–104
    classification of, 101
  to packed red blood cells, 206t
  pulmonary edema in, 139

urticarial, 100t, 101
  to whole blood, 206t
Transfusion-related acute lung injury, 100t, 101–104, 102t, 197–203
Transplantation antigens, 98, 99t
Trayslol. *See* Aprotinin
Trimethoprim-sulfamethoxazole, anaphylactic/anaphylactoid reactions to, 96
Triple response of Lewis, 28
Tronothane. *See* Promoxine
Tryptase
  as marker for anaphylaxis, 132
  in mast cells, 43
  radioimmunoassay of, 132
  in serum or plasma, 43
Tuberculin immunity, 9t
Tuberculin skin testing, 10
d-Tubocurarine, 66
  administration of, 67, 205
  adverse hemodynamic reactions to, 67
  and plasma histamine levels, 67, 69f
  anaphylactic/anaphylactoid reactions to, 85t, 90, 90t, 92
  dilution used for skin testing, 128t
  histamine release caused by, 63, 64t, 67–69
  contribution of prostacyclin to, 39f
  hypotension induced by, 39f
  wheal and flare responses to, 68–69, 71f
Tumor necrosis factor, 11

Upper airway edema, 139
Urine output, after resuscitation following anaphylactic shock, 181
Urokinase 38-485, 156
Urticaria, 83
  in anaphylaxis, 18t, 19, 22t, 27–28
  in intubated patients, 20t
  definition of, 27
  transfusion-associated, 102
Urticaria pigmentosa, 138

Vancomycin
  administration of, 97, 185, 205
    hemodynamic parameters after, 65f
    histamine levels after, 65f
  allergic reactions to, 83
  anaphylactic/anaphylactoid reactions to, 85t, 96, 185–187, 186f
  dilution used for skin testing, 128t
  histamine release caused by, 63, 64t, 65f, 65, 97
  hypotension with, 96–97
Vascular endothelium. *See* Endothelium
Vascular graft material
  adverse reactions to, 120
  anaphylactic/anaphylactoid reactions to, 85t, 120
Vascular permeability
  effects of histamine on, 41
  effects of kinins on, 48–49
  effects of prostaglandins on, 46
  increases in, pharmacologic approaches to, 160
Vascular relaxation, histamine-induced, 38
Vascular smooth muscle, histamine's actions on, 37, 38f
Vasculitis, 10
Vasectomy, and risk for protamine reactions, 114
Vasoactive drug infusions, overdosage of, precipitous hypotension with, 137
Vasoactive intestinal peptide, histamine release caused by, 64t, 77–79
Vasoactive mediators, 22, 23t, 34
Vasoconstriction. *See also* Pulmonary vasoconstriction
  H_1-mediated, 37
Vasoconstrictor infusions, inadvertent discontinuation of, precipitous hypotension with, 137
Vasodilation
  cyclic nucleotides in, 47f
  drugs causing, 135
  epinephrine-induced, and β-adrenergic blocking agents, 168
  histamine-induced, 23t, 33, 38
  in intraoperative cardiovascular collapse, 22
  intravenous drugs that produce, 137t
  leukotriene-induced, 23t, 45
  mechanisms of, 22
  mediators that produce, 22, 23t, 48

Vasodilation *(continued)*
  with nonimmunologic histamine release, 63
  opioid-mediated, 75–77
  prostaglandin-induced, 23t, 45–46
Vasorelaxation
  H_1-mediated, 37, 38f
  H_2-mediated, 37, 38f
Vasovagal reactions, 141
  with local anesthetics, 88
Vecuronium, 67
  anaphylactic/anaphylactoid reactions to, 85t
  dilution used for skin testing, 128t
  hemodynamic response to, 67, 70f
  histamine release caused by, 73
  wheal and flare responses to, 68, 71f
Veins, effects of histamine on, 41
Venous air embolism, 141
Venovenous extracorporeal membrane oxygenation, in treatment of refractory hypoxemia, 173
Ventilation-perfusion mismatching, 178
Ventilatory mode, for patients with severe bronchospasm and air trapping, 171
Ventricular assist devices, after cardiopulmonary bypass surgery, 174
Ventricular dysfunction
  in anaphylaxis, 25
  pulmonary edema caused by, 139
Verapamil
  mechanism of action, 153
  pharmacologic effects of, 153
Vistaril. *See* Hydroxyzine
Vitamin K, anaphylactic/anaphylactoid reactions to, 85t, 120
Volume overloading, 139
Vomiting, in anaphylaxis, 19

Wheal and flare reaction, 9t, 27–28, 47
  in anaphylaxis, 19
  to atracurium, 68–72, 71f–72f
  to dynorphin, 77
  to β-endorphin, 77
  to enkephalin, 77
  to histamine, 68, 70–72, 71f–72f
  to meperidine, 74, 75f
  to metocurine, 68–69, 71f
  to morphiceptin, 77
  to morphine, 68, 70–72, 71f–72f, 74, 75f
  to muscle relaxant(s), 66, 67f, 67–68, 71f, 73
  with nonimmunologic histamine release, 63
  to opioids, 74–75
    antagonism of, 74–75, 76f
  to pancuronium, 68, 71f
  to papaverine, 68, 71f
  to steroidal muscle relaxants, 73
  to succinylcholine, 68, 71f
  to sufentanil, 74, 75f
  to *d*-tubocurarine, 68–69, 71f
  to vecuronium, 68, 71f
Wheezing, 136, 190–191
  in anaphylaxis, in intubated patients, 20t
  intraoperative causes of, 136, 136t
  postextubation, 182–183
Whole blood, reaction to, 205, 206t

Xantac. *See* Ranitidine
Xylocaine. *See* Lidocaine

Zaprinast, mechanism of action, 149